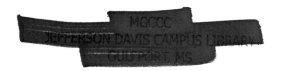

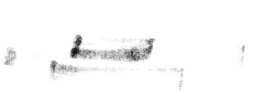

MEDICAL ILLNESS AND POSITIVE LIFE CHANGE

MEDICAL ILLNESS AND POSITIVE LIFE CHANGE

Can Crisis Lead to Personal Transformation?

Edited by
Crystal L. Park
Suzanne C. Lechner
Michael H. Antoni
Annette L. Stanton

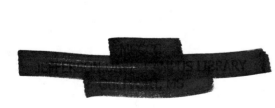

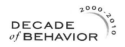

DECADE
of BEHAVIOR
2000·2010

American Psychological Association
Washington, DC

Published by
American Psychological Association
750 First Street, NE
Washington, DC 20002
www.apa.org

To order
APA Order Department
P.O. Box 92984
Washington, DC 20090-2984
Tel: (800) 374-2721
Direct: (202) 336-5510
Fax: (202) 336-5502
TDD/TTY: (202) 336-6123
Online: www.apa.org/books/
E-mail: order@apa.org

In the U.K., Europe, Africa, and the Middle East, copies may be ordered from
American Psychological Association
3 Henrietta Street
Covent Garden, London
WC2E 8LU England

Typeset in New Century Schoolbook by Circle Graphics, Inc., Columbia, MD

Printer: Data Reproductions, Auburn Hills, MI
Cover Designer: Watermark Design Office, Alexandria, VA
Technical/Production Editor: Devon Bourexis

The opinions and statements published are the responsibility of the authors, and such opinions and statements do not necessarily represent the policies of the American Psychological Association.

Library of Congress Cataloging-in-Publication Data

Medical illness and positive life change : can crisis lead to personal transformation? / edited by Crystal L. Park ... [et al.]. — 1st ed.
    p. ; cm. — (Decade of behavior)
 Includes bibliographical references and index.
 ISBN-13: 978-1-4338-0396-3
 ISBN-10: 1-4338-0396-8
1. Sick—Psychology. 2. Life change events. 3. Clinical health psychology. 4. Self-actualization (Psychology) I. Park, Crystal L. II. American Psychological Association. III. Series.
 [DNLM: 1. Life Change Events. 2. Adaptation, Psychological. 3. Personality Development. BF 637.L53 M489 2009]

 R726.7.M43 2009
 616.001'9—dc22

                                                                           2008014268

British Library Cataloguing-in-Publication Data
A CIP record is available from the British Library.

Printed in the United States of America
First Edition

APA Science Volumes

APA Decade of Behavior Volumes

Contents

Contributors

Glenn Affleck, PhD, University of Connecticut Health Center, Farmington
Carolyn M. Aldwin, PhD, Oregon State University, Corvallis
Sara B. Algoe, PhD, University of North Carolina, Chapel Hill
Michael H. Antoni, PhD, University of Miami, Miami, FL
Julienne E. Bower, PhD, University of California, Los Angeles
Lawrence G. Calhoun, PhD, University of North Carolina, Charlotte
Charles S. Carver, PhD, University of Miami, Coral Gables, FL
Arden Corter, MSc, University of Auckland, Auckland, New Zealand
Elissa Epel, PhD, University of California, San Francisco
Vicki S. Helgeson, PhD, Carnegie Mellon University, Pittsburgh, PA
Linda Kelly, PhD, University of California, Davis
William D. Kernan, EdD, William Paterson University, Wayne, NJ
Suzanne C. Lechner, PhD, University of Miami, Miami, FL
Stephen J. Lepore, PhD, Temple University, Philadelphia, PA
Michael R. Levenson, PhD, Oregon State University, Corvallis
Lindsey Lopez, BA, Carnegie Mellon University, Pittsburgh, PA
Constance Mennella, BA, Carnegie Mellon University, Pittsburgh, PA
Judith Tedlie Moskowitz, PhD, MPH, University of California,
    San Francisco
Crystal L. Park, PhD, University of Connecticut, Storrs
Keith J. Petrie, PhD, University of Auckland, Auckland, New Zealand
Annette L. Stanton, PhD, University of California, Los Angeles
Richard G. Tedeschi, PhD, University of North Carolina, Charlotte
Howard Tennen, PhD, University of Connecticut Health Center,
    Farmington
Kathryn E. Weaver, PhD, MPH, National Cancer Institute, Bethesda, MD

Foreword

In early 1988, the American Psychological Association (APA) Science Directorate began its sponsorship of what would become an exceptionally successful activity in support of psychological science—the APA Scientific Conferences program. This program has showcased some of the most important topics in psychological science and has provided a forum for collaboration among many leading figures in the field.

The program has inspired a series of books that have presented cutting-edge work in all areas of psychology. At the turn of the millennium, the series was renamed the Decade of Behavior Series to help advance the goals of this important initiative. The Decade of Behavior is a major interdisciplinary campaign designed to promote the contributions of the behavioral and social sciences to our most important societal challenges in the decade leading up to 2010. Although a key goal has been to inform the public about these scientific contributions, other activities have been designed to encourage and further collaboration among scientists. Hence, the series that was the "APA Science Series" has continued as the "Decade of Behavior Series." This represents one element in APA's efforts to promote the Decade of Behavior initiative as one of its endorsing organizations. For additional information about the Decade of Behavior, please visit http://www.decadeofbehavior.org.

Over the course of the past years, the Science Conference and Decade of Behavior Series has allowed psychological scientists to share and explore cutting-edge findings in psychology. The APA Science Directorate looks forward to continuing this successful program and to sponsoring other conferences and books in the years ahead. This series has been so successful that we have chosen to extend it to include books that, although they do not arise from conferences, report with the same high quality of scholarship on the latest research.

We are pleased that this important contribution to the literature was supported in part by the Decade of Behavior program. Congratulations to the editors and contributors of this volume on their sterling effort.

Steven J. Breckler, PhD
Executive Director for Science

Virginia E. Holt
*Assistant Executive Director
for Science*

Preface

The idea for this book arose in a hotel lobby bar during a scientific conference in 2004. We (Crystal and Suzanne) were lamenting that recent research reports on the phenomena of stress-related growth and benefit finding were often confusing and contradictory. Crystal commented that it would be nice if everyone working in these areas were to be in the same room for an in-depth discussion. We felt that the study of growth had reached a point at which it was imperative to review and integrate the progress that had been made over the past 2 decades and to chart a course for future directions. Later, Annette and Mike concurred about the need for such an event and joined us in its planning.

The chapters in this book are based on presentations at the first Positive Life Changes in the Context of Medical Illness conference held in 2005, sponsored by the Science Directorate of the American Psychological Association (APA). We enlisted respected researchers to present their thoughts about growth. Throughout the days and evenings of the conference, we had lively discussions about aspects of growth, particularly in the context of medical illness. We are extremely grateful to our colleagues who shared their wisdom, time, and effort in preparing thoughtful and thought-provoking presentations. Many of those presentations were the basis for the chapters in this book.

Several successful collaborations began that weekend in Storrs, Connecticut. For many, it represented a meeting of the minds and generated fuel for future theory-building and research. Research questions for several studies were conceived, and several of those studies are now under way.

All of us would like to express our appreciation to our fine colleagues and students who attended the conference and contributed their perspectives and knowledge to the event. Graduate students and research assistants Julie Fenster, Betina Yanez, Mary Alice Mills, and Donald Edmondson assisted us with planning, organizing, and hosting the meeting, and we would not have succeeded without their help. We are grateful to APA; the University of Connecticut Center for Health, Intervention, and Prevention; and the University of Connecticut Department of Psychology for their financial and logistical assistance in bringing this work to a larger audience. We thank Jessica Tocco for her assistance with manuscript preparation and Susan Reynolds, our acquisitions editor in the APA Books Department, for helping us bring this book to fruition. Finally, we are indebted to the hundreds of individuals who were willing to share their lives with us as they experienced profound health challenges; we hope this book does their experience justice, posing vital questions that will move the field forward.

MEDICAL ILLNESS AND POSITIVE LIFE CHANGE

Introduction

Suzanne C. Lechner, Crystal L. Park,
Annette L. Stanton, and Michael H. Antoni

How do people adapt to physical health problems and medical illnesses? What psychological processes are involved in adaptation? What should psychologists make of people's reports that their lives are enriched by their experience with illness? How do perceptions of such benefits occur? How can positive and negative changes co-occur following illness?

These questions reflect the growing consensus that even highly taxing life events can have positive consequences. Traditionally, the field of clinical health psychology has focused on the negative sequelae that follow the diagnosis of chronic or life-threatening illnesses. However, anecdotal, qualitative, and quantitative reports suggest that many individuals also experience positive life changes as a result of serious illness. Sometimes called *stress-related growth, benefit finding,* or *posttraumatic growth,* this construct refers to the positive life changes that people make in their struggle to cope with negative life events (Antoni et al., 2001; Lechner, Carver, Antoni, Weaver, & Phillips, 2006; Park, Cohen, & Murch, 1996; Sears, Stanton, & Danoff-Burg, 2003; Tedeschi & Calhoun, 1996). Such changes can include improved relationships with family and friends, a clearer sense of one's own strengths and resilience, and changed priorities about what is important in life. Although the idea that people experience positive life changes is not new, it has only recently generated widespread empirical attention (see Tedeschi, Park, & Calhoun, 1998). Presentations on growth and benefit finding appear with increasing frequency at scientific conferences, including those of the American Psychological Association (APA) and the Society of Behavioral Medicine. A special section of the *Journal of Consulting and Clinical Psychology* devoted to research on positive life change was published in 2006 (Park & Helgeson, 2006). At this point, we saw a sufficient development of theory, measurement, methods, and findings, as well as articulation of critical questions, to collate and integrate the state of the science into an edited volume focusing specifically on positive life change as it relates to clinical health psychology and behavioral medicine. One of the primary areas in which the relationship between benefit finding and growth has been examined is in the context of serious physical illness, although there has been little attempt to integrate findings from various diseases and conditions. This book focuses on the phenomenon of positive life change in the context of physical illness and health psychology.

The purpose of this volume is to combine and integrate the thinking of scientists working in the area of positive life changes, based on a recent APA-funded conference in which they presented theoretical perspectives, empirical data, and emerging questions. Clinicians and researchers alike are interested in the role of positive life changes in psychological adjustment, physical health, and adherence to treatments, as well as the potential for psychosocial interventions to catalyze positive life change (Bower & Segerstrom, 2004; Chesney, Chambers, Taylor, Johnson, & Folkman, 2003; Lepore, Helgeson, Eton, & Schulz, 2003; Petrie, Cameron, Ellis, Buick, & Weinman, 2002). By bringing together a prominent group of researchers who use diverse methodologies and theories in their studies of positive life change, the conference served to strengthen the knowledge base in this area. Theoretical bases for the chapters range from existential psychology to cognitive–behavioral approaches. The empirical basis for each chapter includes research designs ranging from cross-sectional and longitudinal approaches to randomized, controlled intervention trials. Targeted populations primarily include persons confronting acute and chronic medical illnesses; associated research with healthy individuals dealing with traumatic events is discussed where relevant.

A Note on Terminology

Perusing the chapters in this volume, astute readers will note the variety of terminology used by different chapter authors. As noted by Park in chapter 1, the perception of positive change following stressful experiences is known by many names but generally refers to the same phenomenon. The chapter authors, like other researchers in the field, have not yet arrived at a consensus on terminology. Thus, throughout the book, they use the following terms interchangeably to refer to positive life change: *stress-related growth, posttraumatic growth,* just plain *growth,* or *benefit finding.* As the field matures, researchers will no doubt have to decide on a precise terminology that can be used consistently.

Overview of the Book

This book comprises 12 chapters and is organized into 5 major parts.

Part I: Conceptual and Methodological Issues

In chapter 1, Park presents the theoretical perspectives on positive life change that guide investigations of this topic. This chapter serves as an introduction to the book by discussing the predominant current theory of how positive life change may occur (i.e., meaning making), as well as other potential meanings of positive life changes (e.g., defense, illusion, temporal comparison) and the empirical support that has accrued for each of these. In chapter 2, Tennen and Affleck present unique perspectives on the conceptual, methodological, statistical, and political challenges related to assessing reported positive life change.

This thought-provoking chapter raises several pertinent questions about the nature of positive life change, the development of growth, and the meaning of such change to individuals. Shifting the focus to empirical investigations and statistical strategies for examining positive life change, in chapter 3, Carver, Lechner, and Antoni provide an example statistical strategy for assessing reported positive life changes among individuals with breast cancer. This chapter exemplifies the need to use a sophisticated methodology and nonlinear models of positive life changes.

Part II: Developmental Issues

In chapter 4, Helgeson, Lopez, and Mennella focus on reported positive life changes among children and adolescents with chronic illness, focusing on diabetes as an example. Aldwin, Levenson, and Kelly address life span developmental perspectives on perceived positive life change following illness in chapter 5. They discuss whether perceived positive life change differs in quantity or type by age and whether there are qualitative differences in developmental processes at different phases of the life cycle that may lead to those differences.

Part III: Factors That Influence Positive Life Change

In chapter 6, Lechner and Weaver highlight some of the lessons that have been learned about perceived positive life change in individuals with cancer and HIV. Focusing on the content as well as predictors and consequences of perceived positive life change, the chapter reveals the similarities and differences in positive life change among individuals with cancer and HIV and the ways in which contextual factors may play a role in its development. In chapter 7, Petrie and Corter examine the role of illness perceptions on a person's subsequent perceptions of positive life change, focusing in particular on breast cancer, acoustic neuroma, and heart disease. In chapter 8, Lepore and Kernan address the importance of the social context of illness, including social roles, the availability and quality of social support, and social conflict, all of which can potentially hamper or facilitate positive life change. They give special attention to social influences on meaning making, drawing on data from several longitudinal studies with survivors of traumatic experiences, including cancer and bereavement, to illustrate their key points.

Part IV: Effects of Positive Life Change

In chapter 9, Bower, Epel, and Moskowitz examine the biological correlates of perceived positive life change in health psychology populations. They evaluate psychological and physiological mechanisms through which perceived positive life changes may influence health. On the basis of research drawn from persons dealing with cancer and HIV infection, the chapter focuses on appraisal and coping processes, positive affect, social support, and expectancies/goal engagement as plausible mediators of this relationship. In chapter 10, Algoe and Stanton address the question of whether benefit finding is good for individuals with chronic disease. This chapter reviews the literature showing that individuals report a range of benefits arising from their experience with chronic disease. The chapter authors examine the literature linking reports of benefit finding to outcomes in the domains of psychological and physical health among persons with chronic disease and discuss implications of the findings for theory development and future research.

Part V: Clinical Applications

In chapter 11, Antoni, Carver, and Lechner present the outcomes of an intervention trial that had the notable effect of enhancing benefit finding among women with breast cancer. The chapter focuses specifically on the biobehavioral processes that are involved in this intervention effect. Finally, in chapter 12, Tedeschi and Calhoun propose a model for clinical practice in which the clinician assumes the role of *expert companion,* struggling alongside the patient in the process of making sense of the illness. This chapter stresses the importance of having humility and empathy for patients with medical illnesses and suggests the possibility for clinicians to experience positive life change alongside their patients.

Overall Objective

We expect that this book will be of interest to clinical health psychologists and professionals from a variety of other specialties (e.g., mental health counselors, physicians, social workers, nurses) who work with a broad range of clientele, including trauma survivors, families, and those dealing with life crises. In addition, this book is relevant to the work of researchers in behavioral and psychosomatic medicine, and in clinical and health psychology. Behavioral and social scientists involved in the study and graduate level teaching of individual differences in health-promoting behaviors and disease risk behaviors, adjustment to specific illnesses, and the role of comorbid mental health processes in medical patients may also find this book appealing. If the ideas in this book contribute productively to the next generation of critical inquiry and application of the positive life change construct, we will have accomplished our goal.

References

Antoni, M. H., Lehman, J. M., Kilbourn, K. M., Boyers, A. E., Culver, J. L., Alferi, S. M., et al. (2001). Cognitive–behavioral stress management intervention decreases the prevalence of depression and enhances benefit finding among women under treatment for early-stage breast cancer. *Health Psychology, 20,* 20–32.

Bower, J. E., & Segerstrom, S. C. (2004). Stress management, finding benefit, and immune function: Positive mechanisms for intervention effects on physiology. *Journal of Psychosomatic Research, 56,* 9–11.

Chesney, M., Chambers, D., Taylor, J., Johnson, L., & Folkman, S. (2003). Coping effectiveness training for men living with HIV: Results from a randomized clinical trial testing a group-based intervention. *Psychosomatic Medicine, 65,* 1038–1046.

Lechner, S. C., Carver, C. S., Antoni, M. H., Weaver, K., & Phillips, K. (2006). Curvilinear associations between benefit finding and adjustment to breast cancer. *Journal of Consulting and Clinical Psychology, 74,* 828–840.

Lepore, S. J., Helgeson, V. S., Eton, D. T., & Schulz, R. (2003). Improving quality of life in men with prostate cancer: A randomized controlled trial of group education interventions. *Health Psychology, 22,* 443–452.

Park, C. L., Cohen, L. H., & Murch, R. L. (1996). Assessment and prediction of stress-related growth. *Journal of Personality, 64,* 71–105.

Park, C. L., & Helgeson, V. S. (2006). Growth following highly stressful events: Current status and future directions. *Journal of Consulting and Clinical Psychology, 74,* 791–796.

Petrie, K. J., Cameron, L. D., Ellis, C. J., Buick, D. L., & Weinman, J. (2002). Changing illness perceptions after myocardial infarction: An early intervention randomized controlled trial. *Psychosomatic Medicine, 64,* 580–586.

Sears, S. R., Stanton, A. L., & Danoff-Burg, S. (2003). The Yellow Brick Road and the Emerald City: Benefit finding, positive reappraisal coping and posttraumatic growth in women with early-stage breast cancer. *Health Psychology, 22,* 487–497.

Tedeschi, R. G., & Calhoun, L. G. (1996). The Posttraumatic Growth Inventory: Measuring the positive legacy of trauma. *Journal of Traumatic Stress, 9,* 455–471.

Tedeschi, R. G., Park, C. L., & Calhoun, L. G. (Eds.). (1998). *Posttraumatic growth: Positive changes in the aftermath of crisis.* Mahwah, NJ: Erlbaum.

Part I

Conceptual and Methodological Issues

1

Overview of
Theoretical Perspectives

Crystal L. Park

Although the literature on stress and crisis is replete with studies of the damage people sustain following stressful encounters, researchers and clinicians are increasingly interested in the potentially beneficial aspects of life crises. This affirmative focus parallels in some ways the increased interest in *positive psychology* in general. Proposed as an alternative to traditional psychology, which many feel has overemphasized the negative aspects of human experience (Seligman & Csikszentmihalyi, 2000), positive psychology emphasizes human strengths and resilience, providing a counterbalance to the focus on pathology and dysfunction.

However, just as positive psychology has deep historical roots within many areas of psychology (see Fernández-Ballesteros, 2003), the perspective that positive outcomes can result from crisis is better viewed as a renewed emphasis on old ideas rather than as a newly discovered phenomenon. Over the millennia, many religious and philosophical systems have promoted the notion that through suffering can come transformation (Aldwin, 2007). Even within psychology, these ideas have a long history. In the 1960s, Caplan (1964) proposed that although ineffective coping with a crisis may lead to significant psychiatric problems, crises also present opportunities, through constructive resolution, for greater personality integration and the development of coping abilities. Similarly, the surge in interest in resilience that developed in the 1980s and continues today, focuses on how people—primarily children—can develop normally, or perhaps even thrive, in the context of terrible family and social circumstances, including poverty, neglect, and abuse (see Lepore & Revenson, 2006). Two studies published in 1980 heralded the systematic study of perceived positive changes in individuals experiencing highly stressful encounters. One study, described in Yalom's (1980) classic *Existential Psychotherapy,* detailed the positive life changes reported by terminal cancer patients. The other study reported the unexpected finding of little psychopathology and, instead, much reported positive change in a sample of prisoners of war returning from Vietnam (Sledge, Boydstun, & Rabe, 1980).

In the 1990s, research assessing positive life changes burgeoned (see Calhoun & Tedeschi, 2006; Linley & Joseph, 2004; Park & Helgeson, 2006, for reviews). In fact, this phenomenon, which is known by a number of names (e.g., stress-related growth, adversarial growth, posttraumatic growth, benefit finding),[1] has been the subject of over 100 empirical studies in just the past 10 years. High levels of self-reported growth have been documented in samples of people dealing with events as disparate as relationship dissolution, bereavement, sexual assault, and even terrorist attacks (Calhoun & Tedeschi, 2006). Many types of stressful, traumatic, and transitional events have been examined as the impetus for the growth that people report experiencing, and researchers have increasingly turned to adverse health conditions as an ideal crucible in which to study the phenomenon. In this volume, researchers review research literature on growth reported by individuals with a range of illnesses, including cancer, HIV, diabetes, SARS, cardiovascular disorders, and many other medical conditions.

To provide an overview of growth in the context of medical illness, I first describe the meanings of the phenomenon of growth. I then briefly review the prominent theories regarding how growth occurs, as well as evidence for these theories. Next, I describe the application of this area of research to the arena of health, illness, and disease. I then discuss three important issues currently at the forefront of this field, particularly as applied to medical illness: measurement, implications for individuals' well-being, and clinical and therapeutic applications. Finally, I discuss directions for future research.

The Meaning of Stress-Related Growth

Delving into the area of growth requires, first, venturing into the difficult issue of definition: What do researchers mean when they refer to *growth* or use other terms such as *stress-related growth, posttraumatic growth, benefit finding,* and so forth? The definition can be approached in two ways, conceptual and operational.

Regarding conceptual definition, there is fairly good consensus among researchers that these terms generally refer to actual or veridical changes that people have made in relation to their experience with an identified stressful or traumatic event. One notable exception to this is the work on benefit finding by Tennen and Affleck (e.g., see Tennen & Affleck, 2002; see also chap. 2, this volume), who are careful to refer to the construct that they measure as *perceptions* and to distinguish the construct of perceptions of change from that of veridical change. These positive changes typically occur in the domains of relationships, self-concept, life philosophy, and coping skills.

A number of measures have been developed to generate an operational definition of growth. Typically, these measures have been designed to capture, as closely as possible, the commonly accepted conceptual definition while allowing for the practical conduct of research. This means that researchers usually assess growth through self-report instruments or, less frequently, through coding of open-ended questions or interviews (Park & Lechner, 2006). Virtually all research on this topic, therefore, has been based

---

[1]This chapter uses the term *perceived growth* or *reported growth* because, as is described later, many reports of growth may not comprise veridical growth. Further, the word *trauma* is not used because most of the research described in this volume does not constitute stressors of the magnitude of trauma as conventionally defined.

on self-perceptions of change, which may or may not correspond to veridical change (see chap. 2, this volume).

This disconnection between conceptual and operational definitions calls into question the validity of the instruments used to measure growth and the meaning of the resulting scores. In fact, little research has attended to the issue of demonstrating instrument validity (i.e., the correspondence of scores on a measure and actual real-life change), partly because assessing actual change is so difficult (cf. Frazier & Kaler, 2006). Several studies have shown modest correlations between self- and informant-reports (e.g., see Park, Cohen, & Murch, 1996; Weiss, 2002), although these studies are likely to have been at least somewhat contaminated by shared method variance (i.e., relationship due simply to assessment by common techniques such as questionnaires) as well as by discussion between informants and participants. Another approach to establishing validity involves demonstrating that growth as reported on a questionnaire is similar to that reported in a writing sample (e.g., see Weinrib, Rothrock, Johnsen, & Lutgendorf, 2006), but again, this approach is based solely on self-reported change as opposed to any objective measure of change.

Thus, we are left to contemplate the meaning of scores on growth inventories. What do growth scores on self-report instruments signify? Clearly, without strong evidence of validity, these reports do not necessarily indicate growth, but rather people's perceptions of their growth. Because such reports involve individuals' own perceptions, there are several different perspectives regarding their meaning. One is that the perception of growth, regardless of any veridical change, is an important phenomenon in its own right. For example, a breast cancer survivor might feel that she has a deeper spirituality or an increased appreciation of life, or that she is more capable of handling future stressors because of what she learned through her struggle with cancer. This approach, the benefit-finding perspective, explicitly focuses on the perception of positive outcomes regardless of any actual change.

Clearly, there is some utility in taking reports of growth at face value. However, many researchers and clinicians have an explicit interest in the occurrence of veridical or true (i.e., reflected in external reality) positive change that can result after crisis (e.g., see Tedeschi & Calhoun, 2004). For example, if it were documented that this survivor has indeed learned to handle stress more effectively—a kind of stress-inoculation effect—then it would be important to understand how this increased skill came about. Such information could lead to broadly applied interventions for improving individuals' coping abilities following illness and the expected subsequent improvements in mental and physical health. However, if the self-perceived improvements in coping skills were illusory and the survivor continued to deal with stressors in the same way as she always did, the possibilities for developing interventions to improve public health would be substantially diminished.

On the basis of intensive discussions of these issues, a group of scientists met in 2005 as part of the American Psychological Association's Science Directorate conference on Positive Life Changes in the Context of Medical Illness. Attempting to gain some clarity on issues of definition and operation, the group came to the consensus that self-reports of growth may reflect at least three different phenomena, which are listed in Table 1.1. It should be noted that although these

Table 1.1. Constructs That May Be Reflected in Self-Report Measures of Growth Following Stressful Experiences

Label	Description	Mechanism	Commonality of occurrence	Duration
Posttraumatic growth	Radical and veridical positive transformation in areas such as relationships, spirituality, and appreciation of life.	Arises following traumatic or seismic events and the resulting rebuilding of shattered assumptions and radically restructured lives.	Rare (Tedeschi & Calhoun, 2004). Thus, much of what has been labeled "posttraumatic growth" instead likely reflects either stress-related or perceived but nonveridical growth.	Posited to be permanent (transformative).
Stress-related growth	Veridical positive change in one or more life domains. Less dramatic or radical than posttraumatic growth.	Arises through attempts to make meaning by re-appraising the stressor or one's global beliefs and goals.	Likely very common. Reflected in most research on positive life change.	Relatively permanent, but people may regress toward old habits.
Perceived but nonveridical growth	Reports of growth that do not reflect objective or veridical reality.	Results from inaccuracy in perceptions (e.g., coping efforts, illusions, wishful thinking, cognitive bias).	Fairly common.	May be relatively temporary, possibly while people are in the midst of struggle.

Note. The term *benefit finding* does not refer to any specific construct listed here; instead, benefit finding refers to perceptions of growth and thus may be veridical or nonveridical and arise through any of the mechanisms listed.

constructs are conceptually distinct, it is likely that there are links among them (e.g., positive reappraisal coping may lead to subsequent veridical growth). Both posttraumatic growth and stress-related growth are conceptualized as actual changes that a person experiences, whereas the third meaning of self-reported growth, the inaccurate reporting of growth, is considered an effort to cope. This type of self-reported growth is not conceptualized as reflecting veridical objective change, but only self-perception. Such distinctions are critical in understanding the nature and meaning of reports of growth and in making sense of the literature.

Although the difference shown in Table 1.1 between real growth (shown in the categories "posttraumatic growth" and "stress-related growth") and illusory growth (shown in the category "perceived but nonveridical growth") is important, most researchers in the field do not make this distinction in their terminology. For example, researchers in the field often use the terms *posttraumatic growth* and *stress-related growth* when assessing whether someone *perceives* positive life change in the wake of trauma or stress, but those perceptions may reflect real or illusory change. Indeed, most researchers assume that real change has occurred if there is perceived change, but it is important to keep in mind that this is only an assumption (Tennen & Affleck, 2002), and likely often wrong (see chap. 2, this volume).

Most research measures, including self-report measures, assess only reports of perceptions of positive life change. Thus, the reader must be aware that the majority of research drawn on for this book deals with only perceived positive life change. Chapter 2 is the only chapter in this volume that carefully distinguishes between real and illusory change.

As was mentioned in this book's introduction, the chapter authors of this book, like other researchers in the field, have not yet arrived at a consensus on terminology. Thus, throughout the book, they use the following terms interchangeably to refer to positive life change: *stress-related growth, posttraumatic growth, growth,* or *benefit finding.* As the field matures, researchers will no doubt have to decide on a precise terminology that can be used consistently. The consensus on terminology should reflect an eventual consensus on the conceptualization of the phenomenon of positive life changes. The distinctions among the constructs are useful when considering reported growth following stressful encounters, and will be considered further in the following overview of theories of how growth may occur.

Theories: How Does Growth Occur?

Researchers have proposed a number of conceptualizations of the processes through which growth occurs (see Linley & Joseph, 2004; O'Leary, Alday, & Ickovics, 1998; Tedeschi & Calhoun, 2004, for reviews). In spite of variations in terminologies and details, most of these conceptualizations comprise some variant of a common set of processes, albeit with different emphases. This model will be discussed in some detail, and then alternate theories that have been proposed to account for reports of growth will be briefly discussed.

The General Meaning-Making Model

The general meaning-making model underlying most theories of veridical growth is presented in Figure 1.1.

As Figure 1.1 shows, events appraised as "stressors" by the individuals experiencing them are the starting point of all theories of growth. This distinguishes positive stress-related changes from positive changes that might arise through other processes, such as normative development (cf. chap. 5, this volume). All theories of growth also include, as an implicit but critical element, individuals' *global meaning* prior to the event or trauma (i.e., their status on each domain of potential positive change, such as their religious or spiritual life, the extent to which their behavior is aligned with their values and goals, their relationships with others, their ability to cope with stress, and their perspectives on life). Theories of growth typically propose that when people in their pre-event state encounter highly stressful events, they appraise these events as violating their life schemas or meaning system (e.g., their global beliefs or goals), which creates distress (Park & Folkman, 1997; Tedeschi & Calhoun, 2004). For example, highly stressful or traumatic events may violate an individual's beliefs in the fairness or justice of the world, or one's own sense of control or invulnerability (Janoff-Bulman, 2004). Even events that are not highly inconsistent with one's beliefs, such as an expected disappointment or an on-time death, may still bring a sense of violation of what one had wanted (i.e., one's goals; Klinger, 1998).

Discrepancies between appraised meanings of a situation and one's global beliefs and goals create a strong sense of discomfort or even outright emotional pain; thus, individuals are highly motivated to reduce the sense of discrepancy between their meaning system and their understanding or appraisal of the stressful situation. Often, they can perform behaviors to actually change the situation, typically labeled *problem-focused* or *active coping* (Aldwin, 2007). However, even when problems pass, the fact that such a problem could occur

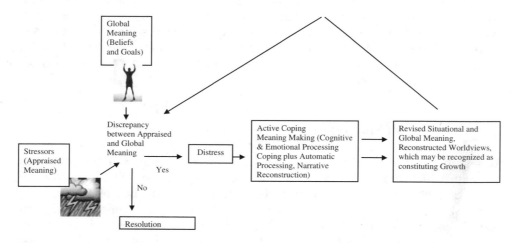

Figure 1.1. The basic hypothesized model of growth.

and may occur again can violate one's beliefs of invulnerability or personal control. In these cases, individuals often engage in more cognitive and emotional efforts to bring their global meaning into alignment with their understanding of the stressful situation. This process is called *meaning making* (Park, 2005).

Meaning making often involves deliberate coping efforts, although it can also take place beneath conscious awareness. These effortful processes involve trying to change one's global meaning or views of the situation, typically through activities such as processing one's emotions internally or with others, searching for a more complete or benign understanding of why the event occurred, thinking through the implications of the event for one's life, discerning ways in which positives can come from the situation, comparing oneself with others who are worse off, and putting the event into a broader context (Park & Folkman, 1997). Automatic meaning making has been conceptualized as an iterative process in which intrusive cognitions and images alternate with efforts to avoid the intrusions or reminders of the painful situation (Horowitz, 1986). These intrusions are thought to reflect the unconscious mind's attempts to integrate the painful material.

These various meaning-making efforts have been posited to result in either *assimilation* (i.e., changing one's view of the stressor so that it is consistent with one's global meaning) or *accommodation* (i.e., changing one's global meaning to incorporate the stressor; Joseph & Linley, 2005). It should be noted that just because meaning-making processes may result in a reevaluation of the stressor as positive (i.e., I have grown from it) does not mean that they actually have! In attempting to distinguish between veridical growth and biased perceptions, Joseph and Linley (2005) noted that perceptions of growth can result from either assimilation (i.e., changing one's view of the situation) or accommodation (i.e., changing global beliefs and goals) but proposed that actual growth only occurs through accommodation.

Virtually all of the commonly discussed theories conceptualize growth as an outcome of this process of meaning making. Drawing on the work of Janoff-Bulman (1989, 1992), Tedeschi and Calhoun (2004) described posttraumatic growth as the rebuilding and reorganization of global beliefs and goals following "seismic events" that threaten or destroy individuals' "schematic structures that have guided understanding, decision-making, and meaningfulness" (p. 5). Tedeschi and Calhoun explained the process as follows:

> Cognitive rebuilding that takes into account the changed reality of one's life after trauma produces schemas that incorporate the trauma and possible events in the future, and that are more resistant to being shattered. These results are experienced as growth. (p. 5)

For example, Janoff-Bulman (2004) described how the existential reevaluations in which individuals engage following highly stressful events can lead to increased appreciation for life or a renewed commitment to one's spiritual values and beliefs.

One unresolved issue in the area of growth following stressful events is the extent to which global beliefs and goals need to be shattered or violated to facilitate growth. As noted in Table 1.1, shattered global beliefs or worldviews has been proposed to be the impetus for posttraumatic growth; more commonly, however, people do not experience such dramatic alterations in their global meaning. Rather, most of the changes reported are less dramatic than total transformation. They may experience some violation and struggle to integrate the new facts and implications of their crisis with their existing global beliefs and goals, but it does not appear that individuals' overarching global meaning must be extensively violated in order for them to make positive changes in their lives following crises.

Alternative Theories of Veridical Growth

In her recent reconceptualization, Janoff-Bulman (2004) speculated that different types of growth following traumatic events may arise through different pathways, only some of which are necessarily mediated by changes in global beliefs. For example, she noted that learning more about one's coping strengths or abilities may not require major cognitive shifts. Rather, simply reflecting back on one's coping efforts or success could change one's estimation of the ability to cope with stressful experiences, without the violation and rebuilding of global meaning.

Janoff-Bulman (2004) also suggested another pathway through which meaning making may result in modified global beliefs that are more realistic, such as less globally positive expectations (e.g., decreased sense of invulnerability or control). Such modified or tempered global meanings may lead to an increased ability to tolerate future stressful circumstances, but, she argued, these changes occur at a level beneath awareness. Therefore, individuals would be unable to accurately report this type of growth on the types of direct self-report inventories of growth currently in use. Instead, more innovative ways of studying global meaning, coping, and outcomes across time and situations is necessary to capture this type of positive change.

Narrative construction and reconstruction may also be part of the meaning-making process (Neimeyer, 2004; Tedeschi & Calhoun, 2004). Through the stories they tell themselves and others, people add coherence and significance to the events in their lives. As part of this storytelling, people receive feedback and are offered validation as well as alternative ways of viewing stressful situations from others in their social networks (see chap. 8, this volume). In addition, this narrative reconstruction introduces another pathway through which growth may occur: People may deliberately implement changes in their life structures as a way to cope (e.g., "I am bound and determined that something good will come from this, and therefore, I am going to quit drinking and tell others about the dangers of drinking and driving"; McMillen, 1999). Thus, transformation in the narrative may actually lead to subsequent veridical change.

Theories of Growth as Nonveridical

In addition to the general theory of meaning making and related views that consider reports of growth as veridical, several other theories have been employed to explain the phenomenon of self-reported growth following stressors; these theories focus on the phenomenon of perceptions of growth but generally do not consider them to be veridical (Tennen & Affleck, 2002). Instead, these theories view reports of growth as a function or byproduct of either hot (i.e., motivated) or cold (i.e., dispassionate) cognitive processes. Among the hot processes, Taylor's (1983, 1989) cognitive adaptation theory is probably the best known. According to *cognitive adaptation theory,* a natural and healthy response to stressful circumstances that threaten one's sense of control or self-esteem involves selectively evaluating a situation and focusing on aspects that allow an individual to maintain his or her positive illusions (Updegraff & Taylor, 2000). Thus, people often perceive that some benefits or growth have come from a stressful situation; these beliefs may be mildly distorted or illusory, but they facilitate adjustment by helping individuals to maintain their positively biased perceptions (Evers et al., 2001; Helgeson & Fritz, 1999).

Temporal comparison, a form of downward comparison (i.e., focusing on others who are perceived as being worse off than one's self), is another well-known theory of adjustment that bears on perceptions of growth following stressful encounters. According to this theory, people are highly motivated to maintain their self-regard, which is generally positive (Taylor & Brown, 1994). When self-regard is threatened, people tend to maintain their positive self-views by constructing a relatively negative past sense of self or a derogatory standing on particular attributes in comparison with their current sense of self (Albert, 1977; Suls & Mullen, 1984).

A *cold cognition perspective* on reports of growth is based on the notion of people's implicit theories of consistency and change (Ross, 1989). According to this theory, when asked to report on life changes following a stressful encounter, people will first note their present status and then use their implicit theory of stability or change to guide a reconstruction of the past. It seems that particularly in the United States, people possess implicit theories of change following stress and trauma that may lead them to overestimate the amount of positive change that has occurred (McFarland & Alvaro, 2000; Wilson & Ross, 2001, 2003; see also chap. 2, this volume). In contrast to theories that posit that the distortions in recollection are motivated to preserve a sense of control or self-esteem, this perspective proposes a dispassionate reconstruction according to one's implicit theory of growth through adversity.

Evidence for Theories of Growth

To date, theoretical developments seem to have far outpaced the evidence regarding the widely accepted general meaning-making theory of growth. Thus, unfortunately, this model remains primarily descriptive, although researchers are now attempting to test specific hypotheses derived from it. Several studies have failed to find evidence for a link between growth and changed global beliefs (e.g., see Carboon, Anderson, Pollard, Szer, & Seymour, 2005; Park & Fenster, 2004), although in these cases global beliefs were not examined prospectively (i.e., before the event occurred). Not all researchers are convinced that violations and rebuilding of global meaning are related to veridical growth. Wortman (2004), for example, chided,

> To my knowledge, there is no real evidence in support of the hypothesis that events that shatter one's basic assumptions are most likely to promote

> growth . . . it is my clear impression that those whose assumptions about the
> world have been most shattered by the event—those who experienced a sud-
> den traumatic loss—are far less likely to experience growth than those in
> other groups. (p. 84)

Studies have found some support for the notion that a certain threshold of perceived threat is necessary for individuals to experience a sense of growth, but it may be that if the threat is too overwhelming or extreme, the likelihood of perceived growth diminishes (e.g., see Lechner, Carver, Antoni, Weaver, & Phillips, 2006; see also chap. 3, this volume). Clearly, more research is needed to understand the extent to which shattering of global beliefs and goals and appraisals of threat impel the process of experiencing growth.

Regarding coping efforts, ample evidence suggests that acknowledging the stressful experience and actively dealing with it are generally associated with higher levels of perceived growth (for reviews, see Linley & Joseph, 2004; Park, 2004; Stanton, Bower, & Low, 2006). In particular, meaning-focused types of coping, which involve positively reappraising or reframing the experience and talking with others about it, are more likely to lead to perceptions of growth (e.g., see Calhoun, Cann, Tedeschi, & McMillan, 2000; Park & Fenster, 2004). In one experimental study of expressive writing, college students were explic- itly instructed to write about their thoughts, feelings, or both thoughts and feelings regarding their most traumatic life event. Those who wrote about thoughts and feelings reported experiencing the most positive changes from this event (Ullrich & Lutgendorf, 2002), suggesting that growth arises from meaning making that involves both cognitive and emotional processing.

In addition to examining deliberate meaning-making coping, researchers have also focused on unintentional or automatic meaning-making processes, typically operationally defined as intrusions and avoidance (e.g., see Roberts, Lepore, & Helgeson, 2005). This type of meaning making is also associated with higher levels of reported growth (e.g., see Calhoun et al., 2000; Park et al., 1996). In spite of the close relations between meaning making and reports of growth, questions have been raised about the adaptiveness of meaning making in terms of psychological or physical adjustment following stressful events (e.g., see Wortman, 2004). Indeed, empirical findings are conflicting: Some have found that meaning making can lead to adaptive adjustment as well as reported growth, whereas others have found meaning making to be related to higher levels of distress and maladjustment (e.g., see Roberts et al., 2005). This lack of consensus is not surprising given that meaning making has sometimes been operationally defined as intrusive thoughts (Park, 2004). More generally, it appears that engaging in meaning making may be an indication of distress, and that eventually, if the meaning-making process produces an acceptable understanding, it may be adaptive (Segerstrom, Stanton, Alden, & Shortridge, 2003). However, at this point, we have a poor understanding of the determi- nants of meaning making that result in perceptions of growth and other indica- tors of adjustment to stressful life events.

Evidence in support of alternative theories that propose that reports of growth may reflect coping or cognitive biases has also been accumulating. A series of studies by McFarland and Alvaro (2000), for example, convincingly documented a consistent downward temporal comparison bias, such that, when asked to remember their attributes prior to a stressful event, people tended to derogate their former selves, which allowed them to make positive assessments of their current status relative to their (recollected) previous status. Results of other studies of growth are consistent with temporal comparison theory (e.g., see Widows, Jacobsen, Booth-Jones, & Fields, 2005). At this point, few researchers have explicitly interpreted their data on growth from the perspective of cognitive adaptation theory or implicit theories of stability and change (cf. Collins, Taylor, & Skokan, 1990).

Growth Within the Context of Medical Illness

As noted earlier, research on stress-related growth in the context of medical illness and health conditions has proliferated, from the early work by Tennen and his colleagues on myocardial infarction and other conditions (Affleck, Tennen, Croog, & Levine, 1987), to the current interest in perceptions of growth in the context of many illnesses. Although cancer is receiving the lion's share of attention (Stanton et al., 2006), growth has been documented in the context of HIV (Bower, Kemeny, Taylor, & Fahey, 1998; Siegel & Schrimshaw, 2000), lupus (Katz, Flasher, Cacciapaglia, & Nelson, 2001), infertility (Mendola, Tennen, Affleck, McCann, & Fitzgerald, 1990), arthritis (Tennen, Affleck, Urrows, Higgins, & Mendola, 1992), psoriasis (Fortune, Richards, Griffiths, & Main, 2005), and many other health problems.

Why is there so much interest in growth in the context of medical illness and health conditions? First, medical illnesses often bring a great deal of uncertainty, fear, suffering, and loss (Falvo, 2005; Holland, 2000). These conditions set the stage for the kind of existential confrontations and global violations of beliefs and goals that are thought to lead to meaning making and, ultimately, to growth, thus leading researchers to look in this direction.

In addition, many people who have encountered serious illnesses have reported growth, both to researchers and in public forums. For example, seven-time Tour de France winner Lance Armstrong wrote the following:

> The truth is that cancer was the best thing that ever happened to me. I don't know why I got the illness, but it did wonders for me, and I wouldn't want to walk away from it. Why would I want to change, even for a day, the most important and shaping event of my life? (Armstrong, 2001, as cited in Sears, Stanton, & Danoff-Burg, 2003)

That serious and even life-threatening illness can lead to positive growth provides drama, fanning public interest and leading to a fair amount of media coverage. These widespread reports of growth in the context of serious illness appear to provide hope to others who find themselves in similar circumstances, and fuel yet further discussion. Such interest may partially be a function of modern U.S. society, a concatenation of Americans' media-driven and health-focused culture as well as their long tradition of optimism and efforts at self-improvement (Held, 2002; McMillen, 2004).

Researchers have other compelling and practical reasons for focusing on health conditions: Many of their most important questions regarding theory, measurement, and implications of growth are relatively easily studied in patient populations who have regular contact with health care systems. Further, growth in this context may have implications for interventions, even at the broad level of public health, where knowledge gained from research in these areas would have substantial impact.

The nature of different types of physical illnesses and health conditions raises different challenges and concerns, which likely influence the levels and types of growth that are reported in their aftermath. Several of these important dimensions, and speculation regarding their implications for experiencing growth, are outlined here:

- *Symptom onset.* Some illnesses may begin with troubling symptoms that are only eventually diagnosed, leading to a gradual recognition that something may be wrong, along with much uncertainty about the problem. Other illnesses begin with a crisis, during which the person may have no time to reflect. For example, an acute myocardial infarction may occur so suddenly that by the time a person realizes what he or she is experiencing, it is already over. Perceiving growth may be more likely in illnesses in which there is more time to process the meanings and implications of the illness before the health challenge is successfully labeled and treated.
- *Presumed etiology.* Some illnesses have no clear etiology, whereas others have known causes or risk factors, some of which are behavioral (e.g., cigarette smoking, sedentary behavior), familial (e.g., genetics), or environmental (e.g., toxins). It may be that a higher sense of self-blame or perception of responsibility for one's illness leads to greater degrees of growth (e.g., improving one's health behaviors), perhaps in an effort to reestablish a sense of control. Struggling to understand why one contracted a disease or health condition may be part of the necessary grappling with violations of global meaning that can lead to meaning making and subsequent growth.
- *Threat to life.* Illnesses vary in the extent to which they force a confrontation with existential issues; such confrontations appear to invoke the kinds of meaning-focused coping that gives rise to reports of growth. In particular, threats of impending mortality may spur individuals to contemplate the meaning of their lives in the context of a shortened life span, leading to perceptions of positive changes (Stanton et al., 2006). Evidence suggests that higher levels of perceived threat to life, but not objective threat, is related to higher levels of reported growth (e.g., see Lechner et al., 2003; Linley & Joseph, 2004; Stanton et al., 2006; see also chap. 3, this volume).
- *Life disruption.* Some illnesses may impact multiple domains of one's life, creating a general sense of crisis; other diseases are more circumscribed, causing less disruption. Illnesses that provoke greater crisis may create more opportunities to grow. For example, the few studies of perceived growth in prostate cancer survivors have found modest

growth relative to survivors of other cancers (e.g., see Thornton & Perez, 2005). These findings have been attributed to the relatively older age and lower sense of crisis and life disruption experienced by prostate cancer survivors.

- *Recovery trajectory.* The course of treatment and recovery varies greatly across illnesses and health conditions. Some illnesses, such as many cancers, involve a long period of treatment, after which individuals remain at elevated risk for recurrence, second primary cancers, and other serious health complications (Demark-Wahnefried, Aziz, Rowland, & Pinto, 2005). Some illnesses may follow a predictable course of gradual or abrupt decline, even toward death (e.g., some cancers, amyotrophic lateral sclerosis), whereas others may have unpredictable exacerbations and remissions (e.g., multiple sclerosis, congestive heart failure). Still other illnesses involve a long period of disability and rehabilitation efforts but may eventually allow individuals to return to their pre-illness lifestyle and level of functioning. These different courses likely have implications for the experience of growth, although little research has yet addressed this aspect of illness and growth.

- *Chronicity.* Although acute stressors have been the focus of much of the research on growth, many health conditions are chronic (e.g., cardiovascular disease, arthritis). Chronic diseases pose a different set of challenges for individuals and may require lifelong attention and radical changes in lifestyle. For example, a diagnosis of diabetes typically involves a daily regimen of medications, glucose monitoring, and strict dietary limits (Koenigsberg, Bartlett, & Cramer, 2004; see also chap. 4, this volume). It may be that growth is more likely for people who have achieved a level of stable postcrisis survivorship, compared with those who live with chronic disease. However, chronic disease might provide individuals with continued opportunities to remind themselves of the positive changes or growth (see chap. 10, this volume). The role of chronicity was demonstrated in a study of women with fibromyalgia; it found that reminding oneself of the positives derived from the illness was related to higher levels of positive mood (Affleck & Tennen, 1996). Chronic pain may or may not provide more challenges to perceptions of growth.

- *Permanence of change.* Some illnesses, such as Bell's palsy, strike suddenly and are severe and mysterious but may allow for complete and rapid recovery. Other illnesses may pass but leave permanent changes, such as mastectomy following cancer. It appears that the less permanent the change, the more possible it is to return to one's pre-illness baseline, which may truncate opportunities to experience growth. However, it is not clear whether people are ever the same after they have had close brushes with death (Martin & Kleiber, 2005). For example, several writers have proposed that cancer survivors do not return to their "normal" lives, but instead experience a "new normal" (e.g., see Magee & Scalzo, 2006). This new normal may involve new knowledge, including an awareness of one's own vulnerability. The extent to which one's life or physical health has permanently changed will lead to greater discrepancy between one's goals and one's experiences (e.g., desire to dance and permanent paralysis). This discrepancy results in an increased need for meaning making, which, theoretically, may lead to more perceived growth. This effect, however, may be complicated, depending on the extent and permanence of the loss or damage that has been sustained and the amount of accommodation needed.

- *Life context.* The context in which the illness occurs (e.g., the individual's age and experience), social support, and available opportunities to process their experience with others (e.g., in support groups) may influence the growth that individuals experience. For example, several studies of cancer survivors have found that age is inversely related to growth (e.g., see Lechner et al., 2003), although these effects may not be due to age per se, but rather may reflect life course or life span developmental issues (see chap. 5, this volume). Social support, particularly opportunities to talk with supportive others, has been related to higher levels of perceived growth (e.g., see Danoff-Burg & Revenson, 2005; see also chap. 8, this volume).

Because illnesses and health conditions differ greatly on these dimensions and therefore present different challenges and concerns, sweeping generalizations about perceptions of growth in the context of illness may be uninformative and inaccurate; instead, it is likely that the pathways to and types of perceived positive changes experienced may differ across illness experiences. Future research is needed to better understand how growth arises in diverse illnesses varying along these different dimensions.

Cutting Edge Issues in the Study of Growth

Research in stress-related growth appears to be maturing. Thus far, researchers have thoroughly documented that growth is commonly reported. They have also suggested measurement strategies, proposed theories, and examined correlates of these positive life changes. Building on this base, researchers have begun implementing more theoretically grounded and empirically sophisticated studies. As discussed earlier, among the most important issues to be examined are defining growth and distinguishing the different meanings of self-reports of growth. Several other issues, and their relevance in the context of health and illness, are outlined here. These include measurement, the meaning of growth in terms of subsequent health or psychological well-being, and implications for interventions in health populations.

Measurement

Attempts to develop psychometrically sound instruments have produced a number of scales specifically designed to assess positive change or growth (see Park & Lechner, 2006, for a review). These scales differ in some respects, but all essentially ask participants to report on whether they have made changes in a number of domains. Scores are considered to indicate the extent of growth. In a critique of these measures, Lechner and I (Park & Lechner, 2006) noted their drawbacks, including limited domains, response biases, and lack of opportunities to report change bidirectionally. Interest in developing better measurement strategies remains, and new measures (e.g., see Joseph, Linley, Shevlin, Goodfellow, & Butler, 2006) and measurement strategies continue to be proposed (e.g., the possibility of allowing individuals to report negative as well as positive changes in domains; Park & Lechner, 2006).

Currently, two different approaches are being advocated in the assessment of growth following stressful experiences. One proposes moving toward increasingly complex measurement schemes, including refinement of items and scoring. At this point, it is not clear whether negative as well as positive change should be assessed and, if so, whether both should be included in a single score (so that they balance each other out), or whether positive life change should be considered a phenomenon distinct from negative change. Tennen and Affleck (see chap. 2, this volume) propose a strategy to assess growth wherein people's scores on a variety of domains that are thought to be likely loci of growth are examined prior to and following a stressful event, producing a true positive change score. The alternate approach proposes that the critical datum regarding perceptions of growth is simply whether any growth is perceived (Nolen-Hoeksema & Davis, 2004). In their study of bereaved family members, Davis, Nolen-Hoeksema, and Larson (1998) found that a dichotomous score of *no growth* versus *at least some growth* predicted adjustment to the death of a family member, arguing that further refinement or assignment of a range of scores leads to an overestimation of positive life changes (Nolen-Hoeksema & Davis, 2004). However, this strategy may not be feasible in many samples, as reports of experiencing at least some positive change may be so high as to eliminate adequate variability. For example, in one study, 83% of breast cancer survivors reported at least one positive life change as a result of their cancer experience (Sears et al., 2003). Comparing three different methods of assessing growth (i.e., any or no growth, number of positive changes reported in response to an open-ended question, and scores on a standard growth inventory), this study indicated that the three methods were only modestly correlated and each had different predictors. The authors concluded that these different ways of assessing growth appear to tap into different, albeit related, constructs (Sears et al., 2003).

Finally, it should be noted that, in spite of researchers' stated interest in veridical change, no current instrument offers a way to assess growth other than through self-report. Alternative assessment strategies, such as the one proposed by Tennen and Affleck (see chap. 2, this volume), may help distinguish individuals who have made actual changes in their lives, at least as reflected in somewhat less obviously biased procedures to assess change, from those who merely report that they have. However, conducting prospective research is a daunting challenge, and, so far, such strategies have failed to document much veridical change (e.g., see Frazier & Kaler, 2006). Other approaches have been proposed, such as examining positive life change observationally rather than through self-report (Park & Lechner, 2006); such approaches await implementation.

Implications of Growth for Individuals' Well-Being

Reasoning that positive life changes should be reflected in improvements in well-being, many researchers have attempted to understand the meaning of reported growth in individuals' lives by examining the extent to which the perceptions of growth are related to aspects of psychological and physical adjustment. This approach has been widely used despite theorists' explicit prediction that growth would not necessarily be related to better well-being, because many of the changes in global meaning may lead individuals to be "sadder but wiser" (e.g., see Tedeschi & Calhoun, 2004). Studies generally find a weak relationship or no relationship between perceived growth and psychological distress. However, positive relationships between perceived growth and positive well-being have been found. This has been demonstrated in samples of people with cancer (see Stanton et al., 2006), arthritis (Evers et al., 2001), multiple sclerosis (Mohr et al., 1999; Pakenham, 2005), and other illnesses (see chap. 10, this volume). Thus, although a growing number of studies have found positive relations between reports of growth and indices of adjustment, the findings are inconsistent, and the possibility of alternative explanations (e.g., unmeasured but important third variables, a nonlinear relationship) remains (Lechner et al., 2006; see also chap. 3, this volume).

In terms of physical health, results of several studies suggest that perceptions of positive changes following illness can lead to subsequent positive health consequences (see chap. 10, this volume). For example, an early study by Affleck and his colleagues (Affleck et al., 1987) found that perceptions of growth following a myocardial infarction were related to a lower likelihood of subsequent myocardial infarction and lower levels of mortality assessed 8 years later. In addition to studies focusing specifically on illness populations, studies of other stressful situations have demonstrated that perceptions of growth were associated with various health benefits. For example, in a study of bereaved family members, Bower, Kemeny, Taylor, and Fahey (2003) found that perceived growth was related to better immune functioning.

Clinical and Therapeutic Applications

This work on growth following stressful experiences, such as serious illness, presents some intriguing questions regarding applications. Should therapists foster perceptions of growth? Can they encourage these perceptions directly? Are there downsides to attempts at facilitating growth? Throughout this volume, the chapter authors address clinical implications for a variety of disorders (e.g., see chaps. 8 and 11). Clinical applications obviously need to be made cautiously; typically, until people are at the point of perceiving, on their own, the positive changes they have made, observations of such positives by others are perceived as insensitive and unwelcome (Tennen & Affleck, 2002).

Future Directions

Research on growth following stressful encounters faces many challenges; fascinating theoretical and empirical questions remain to be answered. We, the volume editors, discuss a number of these overarching questions in the afterword. These questions can be better answered with a new generation of more thoughtful and sophisticated conceptualizations and methodologies, including prospective designs, experimental approaches, observational studies, behavioral assessments, and developmental studies, which may allow us to better distinguish veridical posttraumatic growth and stress-related growth from illusory or nonveridical growth. Playing devil's advocate, Bonanno (2005) challenged researchers, and commented as follows:

> To the best of my knowledge reliable data to support the idea that trauma induces movement toward optimal functioning are not actually available. . . . Virtually all the available research on growth consists of retrospective self-reports. . . . In the absence of more objective and prospective data, one could just as easily argue that reports of growth are simply the result of retrospective reattribution for the pain caused by the recovery process (e.g., "I am better now, so I must have grown"). . . . Convincing evidence of authentic (rather than assumed or imagined) trauma-induced growth and movement toward optimal functioning will require actual pre-event data and objective demonstration that levels of health and well-being had improved after a designated traumatic event. (p. 266)

It behooves researchers to answer such critiques with more convincing data.

Furthering one's knowledge of growth that can arise in the aftermath of highly stressful situations such as illness and suffering holds promise for better understanding the human condition and, perhaps, improving it. As work proceeds in this area, however, a note of caution is in order. It is true that some research participants have gone so far as to say that they are grateful for their health crisis; for example, some participants in Bulman and Wortman's (1977) classic study of paraplegics commented that paralysis was the best thing that had ever happened to them. We must always keep in mind, however, that survivorship implies that one has experienced significant pain or loss. Furthermore, those who report growth in the context of health-related crises often continue to experience negative reverberations, such as long-term side effects, chronic pain, recurrence risks, and other negative sequelae. Surely, many would gladly give up their growth if only they could have their lives return to the way they were before the illness. We must not underestimate or downplay the pain and suffering that serious illness creates, and, as we pursue this intriguing line of research into positive life changes in the context of illness, we must remember to stay close to the experiences of those whom we seek to understand, and to view these positive changes in the context of their suffering and struggle.

References

Affleck, G., & Tennen, H. (1996). Construing benefits from adversity: Adaptational significance and dispositional underpinnings. *Journal of Personality, 64,* 899–922.

Affleck, G., Tennen, H., Croog, S., & Levine, S. (1987). Causal attribution, perceived benefits, and morbidity following a heart attack. *Journal of Consulting and Clinical Psychology, 55,* 29–35.

Albert, S. (1977). Temporal comparison theory. *Psychological Review, 84,* 485–503.

Aldwin, C. M. (2007). *Stress, coping, and development: An integrative approach* (2nd ed.). New York: Guilford Press.

Armstrong, L. (2001). *It's not about the bike: My journey back to life.* New York: Penguin.

Bonanno, G. A. (2005). Clarifying and extending the construct of adult resilience. *American Psychologist, 60,* 265–267.

Bower, J. E., Kemeny, M. E., Taylor, S. E., & Fahey, J. L. (1998). Cognitive processing, discovery of meaning, CD4 decline, and AIDS-related mortality among bereaved HIV-seropositive men. *Journal of Consulting and Clinical Psychology, 66,* 979–986.

Bower, J. E., Kemeny, M. E., Taylor S. E., & Fahey, J. L. (2003). Finding positive meaning and its association with natural killer cell cytotoxicity among participants in a bereavement-related disclosure intervention. *Annals of Behavioral Medicine, 25,* 146–155.

Bulman, R. J., & Wortman, C. B. (1977). Attributions of blame and coping in the "real world": Severe accident victims react to their lot. *Journal of Personality and Social Psychology, 35,* 351–363.

Calhoun, L., Cann, A., Tedeschi, R., & McMillan, J. (2000). A correlational test of the relationship between posttraumatic growth, religion, and cognitive processing. *Journal of Traumatic Stress, 13,* 521–527.

Calhoun, L. G., & Tedeschi, R. G. (2006). *Handbook of posttraumatic growth: Research and practice.* Mahwah, NJ: Erlbaum.

Caplan, G. (1964). *Principles of preventive psychiatry.* New York: Basic Books.

Carboon, I., Anderson, V. A., Pollard, A., Szer, J., & Seymour, J. F. (2005). Posttraumatic growth following a cancer diagnosis: Do world assumptions contribute? *Traumatology, 11,* 269–283.

Collins, R., Taylor, S. E., & Skokan, L. A. (1990). A better world or a shattered vision? Changes in perspectives following victimization. *Social Cognition, 8,* 263–285.

Danoff-Burg, S. A., & Revenson, T. A. (2005). Benefit-finding among patients with rheumatoid arthritis: Positive effects on interpersonal relationships. *Journal of Behavioral Medicine, 28,* 91–103.

Davis, C. G., Nolen-Hoeksema, S., & Larson, J. (1998). Making sense of loss and benefiting from the experience: Two construals of meaning. *Journal of Personality and Social Psychology, 75,* 561–574.

Demark-Wahnefried, W., Aziz, N. M., Rowland, J. H., & Pinto, B. M. (2005). Riding the crest of the teachable moment: Promoting long-term health after the diagnosis of cancer. *Journal of Clinical Oncology, 23,* 5814–5830.

Evers, A. W., Kraaimaat, F. W., van Lankveld, W., Jongen, P. J., Jacobs, J. W., & Bijlsma, J. W. (2001). Beyond unfavorable thinking: The Illness Cognition Questionnaire for chronic diseases. *Journal of Consulting and Clinical Psychology, 69,* 1026–1036.

Falvo, D. R. (2005). *Medical and psychosocial aspects of chronic illness and disability.* Sudbury, MA: Jones & Bartlett.

Fernández-Ballesteros, R. (2003). Light and dark in the psychology of human strengths: The example of psychogerontology. In L. G. Aspinwall & U. M. Staudinger (Eds.), *A psychology of human strengths: Fundamental questions and future directions for a positive psychology* (pp. 131–147). Washington, DC: American Psychological Association.

Fortune, D. G., Richards, H. L., Griffiths, C. E. M., & Main, C. J. (2005). Adversarial growth in patients undergoing treatment for psoriasis: A prospective study of the ability of patients to construe benefits from negative events. *Psychology, Health & Medicine, 10,* 44–56.

Frazier, P. A., & Kaler, M. E. (2006). Assessing the validity of self-reported stress-related growth. *Journal of Consulting and Clinical Psychology, 74,* 859–869.

Held, B. S. (2002). The tyranny of the positive attitude in America: Observation and speculation. *Journal of Clinical Psychology, 58,* 965–991.

Helgeson, V. S., & Fritz, H. L. (1999). Cognitive adaptation as a predictor of new coronary events after percutaneous transluminal coronary angioplasty. *Psychosomatic Medicine, 61,* 488–495.

Holland, J. (2000). Psychosocial distress in the patient with cancer: Standards of care and treatment guidelines. *Oncology Symptom Management, 10,* 19–24.

Horowitz, M. J. (1986). *Stress response syndromes* (2nd ed.). New York: Jason Aronson.

Janoff-Bulman, R. (1989). Assumptive worlds and the stress of traumatic events: Applications of the schema construct. *Social Cognition, 7,* 113–136.

Janoff-Bulman, R. (1992). *Shattered assumptions: Towards a new psychology of trauma.* New York: Free Press.

Janoff-Bulman, R. (2004). Posttraumatic growth: Three models. *Psychological Inquiry, 15,* 30–34.

Joseph, S., & Linley, P. A. (2005). Positive adjustment to threatening events: An organismic valuing theory of growth through adversity. *Review of General Psychology, 9,* 262–280.

Joseph, S., Linley, P. A., Shevlin, M., Goodfellow, B., & Butler, L. D. (2006). Assessing positive and negative changes in the aftermath of adversity: A short form of the Changes in Outlook Questionnaire. *Journal of Loss & Trauma, 11,* 85–99.

Katz, R. C., Flasher, L., Cacciapaglia, H., & Nelson, S. (2001). The psychosocial impact of cancer and lupus: A cross validation study that extends the generality of "benefit-finding" in patients with chronic disease. *Journal of Behavioral Medicine, 24,* 561–571.

Klinger, E. (1998). The search for meaning in evolutionary perspective and its clinical implications. In P. T. P. Wong & P. S. Fry (Eds.), *The human quest for meaning* (pp. 27–50). Mahwah, NJ: Erlbaum.

Koenigsberg, M. R., Bartlett, D., & Cramer, S. (2004). Facilitating treatment adherence with lifestyle changes in diabetes. *American Family Physician, 69,* 309–316.

Lechner, S. C., Carver, C. S., Antoni, M. H., Weaver, K., & Phillips, K. (2006). Curvilinear associations between benefit finding and adjustment to breast cancer. *Journal of Consulting and Clinical Psychology, 74,* 828–840.

Lechner, S. C., Zakowski, S. G., Antoni, M. H., Greenhawt, M., Block, K., & Block, P. (2003). Do sociodemographic and disease-related variables influence benefit-finding in cancer patients? *Psycho-Oncology, 12,* 491–499.

Lepore, S. J., & Revenson, T. A. (2006). Resilience and posttraumatic growth: Recovery, resistance, and reconfiguration. In L. G. Calhoun & R. G. Tedeschi (Eds.), *Handbook of posttraumatic growth: Research and practice* (pp. 24–46). Mahwah, NJ: Erlbaum.

Linley, P. A., & Joseph, S. (2004). Positive change following trauma and adversity: A review. *Journal of Traumatic Stress, 17,* 11–21.

Magee, M., & Scalzo, K. (2006). *Picking up the pieces: Moving forward after surviving cancer.* Vancouver, BC, Canada: Raincoast Books.

Martin, L. L., & Kleiber, D. A. (2005). Letting go of the negative: Psychological growth from a close brush with death. *Traumatology, 11,* 221–232.

McFarland, C., & Alvaro, C. (2000). The impact of motivation on temporal comparisons: Coping with traumatic events by perceiving personal growth. *Journal of Personality and Social Psychology, 79,* 327–343.

McMillen, J. C. (1999). Better for it: How people benefit from adversity. *Social Work, 44,* 455–468.

McMillen, J. C. (2004). Posttraumatic growth: What's it all about? *Psychological Inquiry, 15,* 48–52.

Mendola, R., Tennen, H., Affleck, G., McCann, L., & Fitzgerald, T. (1990). Appraisal and adaptation among women with impaired fertility. *Cognitive Therapy and Research, 14,* 79–93.

Mohr, D. C., Dick, L. P., Russo, D., Pinn, J., Boudewyn, A. C., Likosky, W., & Goodkin, D. E. (1999). The psychosocial impact of multiple sclerosis: Exploring the patient's perspective. *Health Psychology, 18,* 376–382.

Neimeyer, R. A. (2004). Fostering posttraumatic growth: A narrative elaboration. *Psychological Inquiry, 15,* 53–59.

Nolen-Hoeksema, S., & Davis, C. G. (2004). Theoretical and methodological issues in the assessment and interpretation of posttraumatic growth. *Psychological Inquiry, 15,* 60–64.

O'Leary, V. E., Alday, C. S., & Ickovics, J. R. (1998). Life change and posttraumatic growth. In R. G. Tedeschi, C. L. Park, & L. G. Calhoun (Eds.), *Posttraumatic growth: Positive change in the aftermath of crisis* (pp. 127–151). Mahwah, NJ: Erlbaum.

Pakenham, K. I. (2005). Benefit finding in multiple sclerosis and associations with positive and negative outcomes. *Health Psychology, 24,* 123–132.

Park, C. L. (2004). The notion of stress-related growth: Problems and prospects. *Psychological Inquiry, 15,* 69–76.

Park, C. L. (2005). Religion and meaning. In R. F. Paloutzian & C. L. Park (Eds.), *Handbook of the psychology of religion and spirituality* (pp. 295–314). New York: Guilford Press.

Park, C. L., Cohen, L. H., & Murch, R. (1996). Assessment and prediction of stress-related growth. *Journal of Personality, 64,* 71–105.

Park, C. L., & Fenster, J. R. (2004). Stress-related growth: Predictors and processes. *Journal of Social and Clinical Psychology, 23,* 195–215.

Park, C. L., & Folkman, S. (1997). Meaning in the context of stress and coping. *General Review of Psychology, 1,* 115–144.

Park, C. L., & Helgeson, V. S. (2006). Stress-related growth following highly stressful or traumatic life events: Current status and future directions. *Journal of Consulting and Clinical Psychology, 74,* 791–796.

Park, C. L., & Lechner, S. (2006). Measurement issues in assessing growth following stressful life experiences. In L. G. Calhoun & R. G. Tedeschi (Eds.), *Handbook of posttraumatic growth: Research and practice* (pp. 47–67). Mahwah, NJ: Erlbaum.

Roberts, K. J., Lepore, S. J., & Helgeson, V. S. (2005). Social-cognitive correlates of adjustment to prostate cancer. *Psycho-Oncology, 14,* 1–10.

Ross, M. R. (1989). Relation of implicit theories to the construction of personal histories. *Psychological Review, 2,* 341–357.

Sears, S. R., Stanton, A. L., & Danoff-Burg, S. (2003). The Yellow Brick Road and the Emerald City: Benefit finding, positive reappraisal coping, and posttraumatic growth in women with early-stage breast cancer. *Health Psychology, 22,* 487–497.

Segerstrom, S. C., Stanton, A. L., Alden, L. E., & Shortridge, B. E. (2003). A multidimensional structure for repetitive thought: What's on your mind, and how, and how much? *Journal of Personality and Social Psychology, 85,* 909–921.

Seligman, M. E. P., & Csikszentmihalyi, M. (2000). Positive psychology: An introduction. *American Psychologist, 55,* 5–14.

Siegel, K., & Schrimshaw, E. W. (2000). Perceiving benefits in adversity: Stress-related growth in women living with HIV/AIDS. *Social Science & Medicine, 51,* 1543–1554.

Sledge, W. H., Boydstun, J. A., & Rabe, A. J. (1980). Self-concept changes related to war captivity. *Archives of General Psychiatry, 37,* 430–443.

Stanton, A., Bower, J. E., & Low, C. A. (2006). Posttraumatic growth after cancer. In L. G. Calhoun & R. G. Tedeschi (Eds.), *Handbook of posttraumatic growth: Research and practice* (pp. 138–175). Mahwah, NJ: Erlbaum.

Suls, J., & Mullen, B. (1984). Social and temporal bases of self-evaluation in the elderly: Theory and evidence. *International Journal of Aging and Human Development, 18,* 111–120.

Taylor, S. E. (1983). Adjustment to threatening events: A theory of cognitive adaptation. *American Psychologist, 38,* 1161–1173.

Taylor, S. E. (1989). *Positive illusions: Creative self-deception and the healthy mind.* New York: Basic Books.

Taylor, S. E., & Brown, J. D. (1994). Positive illusions and well-being revisited: Separating fact from fiction. *Psychological Bulletin, 116,* 21–27.

Tedeschi, R. G., & Calhoun, L. (2004). Posttraumatic growth: Conceptual foundations and empirical evidence. *Psychological Inquiry, 15,* 1–15.

Tennen, H., & Affleck, G. (2002). Benefit-finding and benefit-reminding. In C. R. Snyder & S. J. Lopez (Eds.), *Handbook of positive psychology* (pp. 584–597). London: Oxford University Press.

Tennen, H., Affleck, G., Urrows, S., Higgins, P., & Mendola, R. (1992). Perceiving control, construing benefits, and daily processes in rheumatoid arthritis. *Canadian Journal of Behavioural Science, 24,* 186–203.

Thornton, A. A., & Perez, M. A. (2005). Posttraumatic growth in prostate cancer survivors and their partners. *Psycho-Oncology, 15,* 285–296.

Ullrich, P. M., & Lutgendorf, S. K. (2002). Journaling about stressful events: Effects of cognitive processing and emotional expression. *Annals of Behavioral Medicine, 24,* 244–250.

Updegraff, J. A., & Taylor, S. E. (2000). From vulnerability to growth: Positive and negative effects of stressful life events. In J. H. Harvey & E. Miller (Eds.), *Loss and trauma: General and close relationship perspectives* (pp. 3–28). Philadelphia: Brunner-Routledge.

Weinrib, A. Z., Rothrock, N. E., Johnsen, E. L., & Lutgendorf, S. K. (2006). The assessment and validity of stress-related growth in a community-based sample. *Journal of Consulting and Clinical Psychology, 74,* 851–858.

Weiss, T. (2002). Posttraumatic growth in women with breast cancer and their husbands: An inter-subjective validation study. *Journal of Psychosocial Oncology, 20,* 65–80.

Widows, M. R., Jacobsen, P. B., Booth-Jones, M., & Fields, K. K. (2005). Predictors of posttraumatic growth following bone marrow transplantation for cancer. *Health Psychology, 24,* 266–273.

Wilson, A. E., & Ross, M. (2001). From chump to champ: People's appraisals of their earlier and present selves. *Journal of Personality and Social Psychology, 80,* 572–584.

Wilson, A. E., & Ross, M. (2003). The identity function of autobiographical memory: Time is on our side. *Memory, 11,* 137–149.

Wortman, C. B. (2004). Posttraumatic growth: Progress and problems. *Psychological Inquiry, 15,* 81–90.

Yalom, I. (1980). *Existential psychotherapy.* New York: Basic Books

2

Assessing Positive Life Change: In Search of Meticulous Methods

Howard Tennen and Glenn Affleck

Until recently, we were convinced that the greatest challenge to the systematic study of people's claims of growth and benefits in the face of serious illness, disability, disaster, and loss was that investigators could not agree on how to think about these claims (Tennen & Affleck, 1998, 2002). We thought that reports of growth and benefits needed a conceptual home. So we reviewed the various views of growth and benefit finding in the literature, and we discovered that people's reports of growth and benefits have been viewed as maladaptive reality distortions, selective appraisals, coping strategies, an aspect of personality, a way of explaining characteristic hedonic levels, a reflection of people's implicit theories of change, a downward temporal comparison, and as an indicator of genuine change. Accordingly, we urged investigators to evaluate these conceptualizations of growth and benefit finding before attempting to improve their measurement. Now, after reviewing the past 5 years of research, we have concluded that the challenge of finding appropriate metrics for growth and benefit finding may be even more daunting than formulating a consensus for the conceptualization of these phenomena. Our goals in this chapter are to describe what we consider serious flaws in the way growth and benefit finding are currently measured and to offer a new assessment approach.

Do Growth and Benefit-Finding Scales Measure Growth and Benefit Finding?

The recent upsurge in research on posttraumatic growth and benefit finding has been hastened by the availability of scales and interview questions purporting to measure growth and benefit finding in the context of adversity. The three most widely used growth scales, the Posttraumatic Growth Inventory (PTGI; Tedeschi & Calhoun, 1996), the Stress-Related Growth Scale (SRGS; Park, Cohen, & Murch, 1996; see Armeli, Gunthert, & Cohen, 2001, for a revised version), and the Changes in Outlook Questionnaire (CiOQ; Joseph et al., 2005; Joseph, Williams, & Yule, 1993), as well as the two most widely used benefit-finding scales, the Benefit-Finding Scale (BFS; Mohr et al., 1999; see also Danoff-Burg & Revenson, 2005; Pakenham, 2005) and the Benefit-Finding Scale for Breast Cancer (BFS-C; Tomich & Helgeson, 2004, 2006; see also Carver & Antoni, 2004), are easy to administer and demonstrate good internal consistency. Scores on these scales typically, although not always, predict outcomes that we expect growth and benefit finding to predict, such as well-being and morbidity. Growth scores and benefit finding, in turn, are predicted by personal characteristics that we expect should predict growth and benefit finding following adversity, such as optimism and a sense of mastery (Tedeschi & Calhoun, 2004). These scales also have excellent face validity, and for this reason they are readily accepted by research participants, many of whom find that scale items map well onto their personal experience. Similarly, benefit finding measured by interview has strong face validity. For example, Affleck, Tennen, et al. (Affleck, Tennen, Croog, & Levine, 1987; Affleck, Tennen, & Rowe, 1991) asked research participants who had recently experienced a first heart attack or had a newborn requiring intensive care, "As difficult as it's been, have there been any benefits or gains that wouldn't have occurred if you hadn't experienced a heart attack/had a newborn in the NICU?" Armed with scales that have the trappings of psychometric excellence, and interview questions that seemingly measure benefit finding in a straightforward manner, investigators have examined the nomological network (Cronbach & Meehl, 1955) of posttraumatic growth (PTG), stress-related growth (SRG), and benefit finding (BF).

What Do PTG, SRG, and BF Scales and Interviews Require of Respondents?

Although research participants readily complete measures of PTG, SRG, and BF, and respond easily to interview questions regarding benefit finding, an examination of scale items raises serious concerns as to whether people can accurately portray the growth and the benefits they claim to have experienced. Table 2.1 presents sample items from each of the scales and interviews along with instructions to participants. Instructions for the PTGI ask participants to rate how much they have changed on each scale item as the result of the crisis they faced. For example, people are asked to report how much closer they feel to others as a consequence of their crisis. Similarly, the SRGS requires participants to evaluate how much they experienced each of the personal changes depicted in the scale as a result of their past year's most stressful event. As shown in Table 2.1, the other scales provide comparable instructions.

We find it instructive to consider the mental operations required to provide ratings for PTGI, SRGS, CiOQ, BFS, and BFS-C items. A response to each scale item requires the respondent to engage in five assessments. He or she must (a) evaluate his or her current standing on the dimension described in the item (e.g., a sense of closeness to others), (b) recall his or her previous standing on the same dimension, (c) compare the current and previous standings, (d) assess the degree of change, and (e) determine how much of that change can be attributed to the stressful encounter. Engaging in these five steps, the participant responds to each scale item. It is tempting to argue that research participants do not actually make such evaluations, but rather offer global impressions of personal change. However, if people simply offer their global impressions of change, they are not reporting stress-related change, which is precisely what we seek to mea-

Table 2.1. Instructions and Sample Items From Widely Used Growth and Benefit-Finding Scales and Interviews

Measure	Instructions and sample items
Posttraumatic Growth Inventory (PTGI; Tedeschi & Calhoun, 1996)	Indicate for each of the statements below the degree to which this change occurred in your life as a result of your crisis: A sense of closeness with others I'm more likely to change things that need changing Knowing I can handle difficulties
Stress-Related Growth Scale (SRGS; Park, Cohen, & Murch, 1996)	Rate how much you experienced each item below as a result of this year's most stressful event I learned to look at things in a more positive way I learned to take responsibility for what I do I feel freer to make my own decisions
Changes in Outlook Questionnaire (Joseph et al., 2005)	As a result of _____ I value my relationships much more now I'm a more understanding and tolerant person now I value other people more now
Benefit-Finding Scale (Mohr et al., 1999)	As a result of experiencing _____ I have become more respectful of others I am more compassionate toward others I am more motivated to succeed
Benefit-Finding in Breast Cancer Scale (Tomich & Helgeson, 2004)	Having had breast cancer . . . has made me more grateful for each day has led me to be more accepting of things has brought my family closer together
Interview	As difficult as it's been, have there been any benefits or gains that wouldn't have occurred if you hadn't experienced _____ ? (Affleck, Tennen, Croog, & Levine, 1987; Affleck, Tennen, & Rowe, 1991) In what ways, if any, has being HIV positive changed you as a person for the better or for the worse? (Updegraff, Taylor, Kemeny, & Wyatt, 2002) How has _____ changed you or affected you as a person? How has _____ changed or affected your relationships with other people? (Mohr et al., 1999)

Note. The Thriving Scale (Abraido-Lanza, Guier, & Colón, 1998), not included here, was derived from the PTGI and the SRGS.

sure. In other words, the best we can hope for is that individuals who complete scales measuring growth in the face of adversity are actually engaging in the five appraisals we propose. It may be equally tempting to assert that we should be interested only in perceived benefits rather than actual benefits. However, even investigators who insist that reality is irrelevant for benefit finding should be interested in differentiating individuals whose reported benefits map onto documented change from those for whom reported benefits are unrelated to documented change. Our suspicion, simply stated, is that people cannot accurately generate or manipulate the information required to faithfully report trauma- or stress-related growth or to report benefits that result from threatening encounters. We now review the evidence that supports our reservation.

RECALLING PERSONAL CHANGE. All published measures of stress- or trauma-related growth require respondents to recollect personal change over time, that is, to engage in assessments (a) through (d) mentioned previously. The implicit assumption is that people can recall personal change accurately. Yet there is little empirical support for this assumption. Indeed, the psychological literature demonstrates consistently that people are unable to recollect personal change accurately. We now summarize several key studies that demonstrate how recollections of personal change are flawed.

Costa and McCrae (1989; Herbst, McCrae, Costa, Feaganes, & Siegler, 2000) assessed the Big Five personality traits (i.e., Neuroticism, Extraversion, Openness, Conscientiousness, and Agreeableness) twice over 6 years. After the second assessment, participants were asked to report changes in their personalities over the 6 years. Perceived changes in personality were at best weak predictors of residualized change scores. Indeed, Costa and McCrae concluded, "It appears that self-perceived changes in personality are misperceptions" (p. 65). Similarly, Henry, Moffit, Caspi, Langley, and Silva (1994) collected 18 years of repeated measures of well-being and behavior from a large and well-characterized cohort, asking participants to recall how much they changed on the measured constructs. Retrospective reports of change showed poor agreement with prospective data documenting actual changes. More recently, Robins, Noftle, Trzesniewski, and Roberts (2005) reported the findings of a study that measured college students' personality 6 times over 4 years. After the Year 4 assessment, they measured perceived personality change. Most of these students believed that their personality had changed substantially in positive ways; from their reports, we might be led to infer that they experienced transition-to-college related growth. However, the correspondence between actual change measured prospectively and perceived change was, once again, quite modest.

Each of these studies revealed only modest concordance between recalled personal change and prospectively assessed change over 4 to 18 years. Perhaps people are better at recalling personal change over briefer periods of time. Although this is a reasonable speculation, the assertion that recall of personal change is not accurate over long periods makes current theorizing about posttraumatic growth suspect. Current theory asserts that growth is more likely to occur later in the coping process (Tedeschi & Calhoun, 2004). However, if people cannot recall change accurately over long periods of time, the limits of personal recall would make it difficult at best to measure growth later in the coping process.

There is also rather clear evidence that people cannot recall personal change accurately even over a few months. In a pivotal study, Wilson and Ross (2001) asked college students to rate their social skills, self-confidence, and life satisfaction in September and then again in November. Their September self-ratings were somewhat more favorable than their November ratings. But when these students were asked in November to describe themselves as they were in September on these same attributes, they rated their September self as inferior to their November self. In other words, they perceived improvement in the face of actual decline. Had Wilson and Ross asked their participants how much they had changed since September, they would almost surely have found evidence of growth when there was none.

More recently, Stone (2005) demonstrated how reports of symptom change may not reflect actual change. Patients with fibromyalgia recorded their fatigue several times a day during treatment. Later, they reported their symptom change from pretreatment to posttreatment. Remarkably, Stone found no difference in the trajectory of the daily reports of fatigue among patients who recalled that their fatigue had improved, those who reported no change, and those who recalled that their fatigue had worsened from pretreatment to posttreatment. Although the focus of this study was symptom change rather than personal change following trauma, Stone's findings demonstrate clearly the limits of recall even over relatively brief periods.

RECALLING INTERPERSONAL CHANGE. Although the evidence reviewed to this point reveals that people are unable to accurately report personal change, perhaps they are more accurate in reporting positive relationship changes. Fortunately, there is a well-developed literature on which to draw to answer this question.

In one of several studies of perceived growth in close relationships, Kirkpatrick and Hazan (1994) asked dating couples to assess the current quality of their relationship once a year for 4 years. In the 4th year, these couples were asked about the quality of their relationship in each of the previous years that they had participated in the study. As a group, couples recalled that the strength of their love had grown over time, just as participants in studies of posttraumatic growth report that their close relationships have deepened and grown. Yet, the prospective ratings Kirkpatrick and Hazan had collected revealed no increases in reported love and attachment. These findings are important for another reason. In the stress-related growth literature, even modest agreement regarding change between the participant and a significant other has been interpreted as evidence for the validity of the reported change. Such agreement is frequently interpreted as evidence for the accuracy of such reports. Kirkpatrick and Hazan's findings demonstrate that within-couple agreement about positive relationship change does not mean that such change actually occurred.

Kirkpatrick and Hazan's (1994) findings have received conceptual replication. Karney and Coombs (2000; see also Karney & Frye, 2002) found that wives in couples who had been followed for 10 years recalled their initial assessments of their marriages, made 10 years earlier, as worse than they actually were. Consequently, they reported that their marriages had improved. In fact, women held more negative appraisals of their marriage than they had 10 years earlier. Their reports of relationship growth were misguided not only in magnitude but also in direction.

Taken together, these studies of couples' recollections of relationship change present a formidable challenge for the assessment of posttraumatic growth. They also provide a clue as to how a sense of growth might emerge when none has occurred: People may rather easily come to believe they have grown by deprecating their past selves to bask in the glow of personal progress. This tendency to distance one's current self from a past self through deprecation of the past self (McFarland & Alvaro, 2000), or by temporally distancing the past self in response to motivational concerns (Ross & Wilson, 2002), or by making downward temporal comparisons (Albert, 1977) means that reports of growth or benefits in the aftermath of adversity cannot be taken at face value from scores on the PTGI, SRGS, CiOQ, BFS, BFS-C, or related measures. Evidence that partners manufacture improvement by rewriting their history as a couple suggests that we cannot rely on a partner's agreement with growth reports as a validity check.

ATTRIBUTING GROWTH TO A TRAUMATIC EXPERIENCE. Thus far, we have demonstrated that even if people are able to accurately evaluate their current standing on the dimensions described on posttraumatic growth and stress-related growth inventories, most do not reliably recall their previous (i.e., pre-event) standing on these dimensions. Whether this inaccurate recall is motivated by a desire to distance the current self from a past self or reflects memory decay, the evidence is clear: Recall of one's previous self is flawed. Without an accurate recollection of the pretrauma self, how can people realistically compare their current and previous standings on the dimensions assessed in traumatic growth and benefit-finding inventories, and how can they assess the degree of change correctly? Even if people were not burdened by these recall problems, to complete current measures of PTG, SRG, and BF, they would need to accurately engage in the fifth assessment we mentioned previously; that is, they must determine how much change can be attributed to the traumatic event itself. In other words, people must be able to accurately judge covariation or a contingency between the event and subsequent personal changes.

A good deal of evidence demonstrates how judgments of covariation or contingent relationships are biased through illusory correlation (Chapman, 1967), whereby the individual who expects a relationship between two variables tends to overestimate the magnitude of any relation that might exist, or even infer a relation when none exists. In other words, people have great difficulty detecting, let alone recalling, covariation. For example, Todd et al. (2005) compared people's questionnaire reports that they drank alcohol in response to negative affect—a contingent relationship—with real-time electronic diary data that actually captured negative affect and drinking as they occurred. The retrospective questionnaire-based accounts of "drinking to cope" showed a remarkably modest concordance with the association between negative mood and drinking as they were measured close to their real-time occurrence. Todd et al. conjectured that participants' implicit theories (Ross, 1989) of when people drink may have guided their retrospective reports but not their actual drinking patterns. Several investigators have conjectured that the same sorts of implicit theories are at work when people are asked to describe ways in which they have grown or the benefits they experienced in the face of adversity (Conway & Ross, 1984; Tennen & Affleck, 2002).

Consider someone in a three-wave longitudinal PTG, BF, or SRG study, a rare but desirable study design. The participant is asked at each time point to recall her most negative encounter or a particular negative event during the previous year. Although she is asked to rate the growth she experienced from that most negative event, she, like nearly all other study participants, also experienced other events during each wave that were somewhat less negative, but still potentially growth producing. Indeed, some of these other events were similar to those selected by other participants as their most negative event.

Now consider what participants need to do to appropriately complete the growth questionnaire. The following equation summarizes what is required to respond to each item:

$$\text{SRG} = (\text{Self } t+1 - \text{Self } t) - \Sigma(\text{Self } t+1 - \text{Self } t)$$

In this equation, the first parenthetical term represents the most negative event, and the second, less negative events. To accurately convey the amount of growth that occurred for each item, the respondent must first compare herself in the present with how she recalls being on that dimension prior to the event, and then estimate how much of that difference is due to the event rather than to a secular trend, a developmental change, or other nonstress related process. The respondent must also consider all other negative events of consequence and calculate how much positive change each event produced. The sum of that multiple event-related change then needs to be subtracted from the change subjectively attributed to the most negative event. That difference represents the scale item's stress-related growth attributable to the target event.

It is tempting to argue that these mental gymnastics are unnecessary, but if individuals who complete measures of PTG, BF, or SRG are not engaging in these cognitive processes, we wonder just how they derive their responses. Might they simply be recalling how much they have changed without consideration of the negative event? That would be unfortunate, because investigators would not have an indicator of PTG, BF, or SRG. Alternatively, participants may consider the most negative event, but ignore other negative events that might have prompted growth. By doing this, they are not following the scale's instructions. Our point is that although research participants complete measures of PTG, SRG, and BF, we should not interpret their compliance as evidence that they have engaged in the mental processes these scales demand. We have known for a half century that people cannot combine such complex information (Meehl, 1957). Measures of PTG, SRG, and BF are not exceptions to this rule.

Influence of Popular Culture on Assessment

One possible explanation for the difficulty people have in accurately conducting the five previously mentioned assessments is that popular culture emphasizes the idea of growth following adversity. Although Wortman (2004) and others have warned about the risks of having the concept of posttraumatic growth embraced by the popular culture, there is ample evidence that the notion of growth following adversity has already infused popular culture (Tennen & Affleck, 2005). This infusion, in turn, has fortified people's implicit theories regarding this phenomenon (see chap. 1, this volume). The American Psychological Association (APA) has contributed to the popularization of growth in the aftermath of adversity through its Road to Resilience campaign, which offers the public inspiring vignettes depicting people who have experienced PTG along with encouraging reminders to regularly reassess one's own growth following an adverse experience by using their online version of the PTGI.

Ross (1989) argued convincingly that people maintain personal theories about how personal change occurs and that these theories may lead people to overestimate the amount of change that has occurred. He also noted that the more widely a theory of change is embraced in a culture, the more likely it is that most people will accept that theory as an expectation and as an explanation of changes in their own lives. Western culture has long held the premise that people gain wisdom and more productive lives in the aftermath of trauma. That premise is echoed and magnified through our daily exposure to popular media proffering poignant stories about individuals claiming personal growth in response to adversity, and through Web sites such as APA's Road to Resilience that encourage people who have been victimized to look for signs of posttraumatic growth. These forces of popular culture create a genuine challenge to investigators trying to measure and understand posttraumatic growth.

Summary

Our review of the literature documenting the significant limitations in people's capacity to recall personal change leads us to doubt that people can accurately generate, manipulate, or reconstruct the information required to faithfully report posttraumatic growth. Recall decay aside, people may be motivated to experience or claim personal progress. However, even among those relatively few people with near perfect recall and no motivational impetus, the challenge of detecting and recalling trauma-related change (i.e., change that takes into account developmental trajectories unrelated to any particular event) is formidable. We must conclude that in view of the cognitive demands they require from respondents, current measures of PTG and BF do not and cannot adequately measure growth in the aftermath of adversity.

Can Growth and Benefit-Finding Scales Test Theories About How Growth Happens?

Retrospective assessment of PTG and BF not only fails to measure growth but also fails to provide a mechanism for testing how growth happens. We illustrate this problem, which we view as impeding the advancement of theory, by turning briefly to two well-accepted conceptualizations of how posttraumatic growth happens. Consider first the plausible hypothesis that the more stressful a life situation is, the more potential it provides for growth or benefit finding (Cadell, Regehr, & Hemsworth, 2003). Indeed, this hypothesis guides investigators interested in PTG and BF to study people who have encountered serious illness (Lechner, Carver, Antoni, Weaver, & Phillips, 2006; Widows, Jacobsen, Booth-Jones, & Fields, 2005), disability (McGrath & Linley, 2006), significant personal loss (Nolen-Hoeksema & Davis, 2002; Safer, Bonanno, & Field, 2001), disasters (McMillen, Smith, & Fisher, 1997), and other misfortunes, rather than studying individuals facing everyday trials and tribulations. More stressful life circumstances require more cognitive processing, which in turn provides the opportunity for personal growth or benefit finding.

This line of thinking is plausible and worthy of empirical investigation. However, reliance on retrospective reports of growth and benefit finding makes fair tests impossible. This is because, just as people deprecate their past selves to enhance themselves in the present, people also regularly exaggerate in retrospect the stressfulness of life encounters as a way to enhance their current selves. Schacter (2001) provided convincing evidence to support his conclusion that "exaggerating the difficulty of past experiences is another way people enhance [their current status]" (p. 152). The problem is that in the context of retrospective assessment of PTG, SRG, and BF, the notion that more threatening events hold the potential for more growth maps directly onto the dynamics of self-enhancing strategies. Theory asserts that more stressful encounters should generate more opportunities for growth, so that greater adversity should lead to reports of more growth or benefits. However, convergent evidence that people's recollections are created in part as a self-enhancement strategy leads to the same prediction: Retrospective reports of greater past adversity should be associated with more self-reported personal growth. This may not occur because adversity is the wellspring of growth, but rather because a greater desire to enhance one's current self will produce both reports of growth and recollections of greater adversity.

Another interesting conceptualization is that growth is strengthened over the course of dealing with a chronic stressor. A variation of this formulation is that growth or benefit finding tends to emerge later in the coping process (Janoff-Bulman & Frantz, 1997; Pakenham, 2005; Park, 1998). This is another reasonable formulation of how growth or benefit finding should occur, one that seems well-suited for empirical investigation. However, the universal use of retrospective indicators of PTG, SRG, and BF in the research literature has made it impossible to test this thesis in a straightforward manner. If people are inclined to distance their current self from their pretrauma self (Libby & Eibach, 2002), retrospective reports of growth will produce greater growth over time as individuals feel the need to create a sense of personal progress (Schacter, 2001).

We selected these two conceptualizations of personal growth following threatening encounters because they are plausible, straightforward, and, if not restrained by our commitment to retrospective assessment, quite testable. However, the study of PTG, SRG, and BF has hampered testing such hypotheses by uncritically accepting retrospective reports of the stressful encounters themselves and the change that followed. Schacter (2001) referred to the tendency to exaggerate past difficulties and deprecate past selves as a revisionist bias. We have been remiss in accepting such revisionism as faithful depictions of past events and personal growth as it occurred.

Can Growth and Benefit-Finding Scales Detect a Special Private Experience of Growth?

As we discussed previously, reports in which couples show agreement with each other's growth ratings can be completely contradicted by the couples' own prospective reports (Karney & Frye, 2002). However, some researchers claim that reports of growth need not even be consistent between the participant and his or her friend or partner. These researchers claim that many of the items included in the various questionnaires measuring PTG, SRG, and BF capture "private experiences" that are unlikely to be noticed, even by significant others. For example, appreciating the value of one's own life or being more grateful for each day may not be qualities that others would notice, and may not emerge in everyday discussion. If this is so, even modest concordance would conceivably signal the validity of growth reports provided retrospectively. However, evidence from diverse sources points to stress-related growth experiences as being quite public.

There is good reason to believe that research participants' growth experiences are often discussed with others. Indeed, Harvey, Barnett and Overstreet (2004) have suggested that one way that people adapt to threatening events is by developing a personal narrative that they then communicate to close others. But it is Swann's (1983, 1987) theoretical formulations and experimental studies on self-verification that offer the best reasons to take issue with the premise that growth experiences are private and that we can therefore expect no more than modest agreement between participants and their coinformants. Swann demonstrated convincingly that people seek out others in their lives who see them as they see themselves, and that they assemble their social networks so that they regularly encounter others who support their self-views. Indeed, Swann interprets the available evidence as demonstrating that people exclude from their everyday lives individuals who will not confirm their views of themselves.

We believe that these interpersonal dynamics of self-verification are even more entrenched following a life crisis or potentially traumatic experience. As Swann (1983, 1987) notes, when people's identities are threatened, their attempts to self-verify intensify. Janoff-Bulman (1992) has elegantly articulated how traumatic encounters threaten assumptions about the self. Taken together, theory and evidence suggest that traumatic encounters are important opportunities for individuals to gather people into their social environment who will support their sense of positive change, while distancing themselves from those who may not endorse the change. Because people "actively create self-confirmatory environments" (Swann, 1983, p. 60), particularly when the self is threatened, we find it difficult to understand how an informant selected by a research participant in a study of PTG, SRG, or BF might provide adequate criteria against which to judge the accuracy of the participant's reports of growth.

Why Assessing the Veracity of Growth Is Important

It may seem as though we have put excessive emphasis on measuring actual growth and verifiable benefits. Investigators whose conceptual perspective leads them to view PTG, SRG, and BF as positive illusions, or as coping strategies, or as manifestations of downward temporal comparisons (see MacFarland & Alvaro, 2000; Nolen-Hoeksema & Davis, 2004) may argue that they are interested in only the adaptive value of growth and benefit reports rather than their veracity.

There are at least two reasons why investigators who do not view reports of PTG, SRG, and BF as reflections of genuine change should nonetheless be interested in whether such change has occurred. First, some formulations of growth that do not view growth and benefit reports as valid nonetheless demand repeated measures of participants' status on various growth dimensions. For example, to evaluate whether PTG is a deprecation of one's previous self, an investigator must have an indicator of the previous and current self on the dimension of interest. Similarly, an investigator working from the perspective of temporal comparison theory (Albert, 1977) hypothesizes that when efforts to reduce negative discrepancies between the past and the present are unsuccessful, their research participants will construct positive changes. This formulation requires indicators of participants' views of the self on more than one occasion.

Second, an important aspect of evaluating whether retrospective reports of growth or benefits represent coping strategies, selective appraisals, or positive illusions is to demonstrate that these retrospective reports predict behavior, emotional experience, well-being, or health, independent of measured growth or benefits. Indeed, such a demonstration would seem to make a strong case for the role of coping in adjustment to threatening events, and the power of positive illusions.

There is already fascinating evidence that, in some circumstances, recalled experience is a better predictor of subsequent behavior than is actual experience measured in real time. For example, Kahneman, Fredrickson, Schreiber, and Redelmeier (1993) found that individuals who had participated in an ice submersion task were more willing to repeat the trial they remembered as less painful than to repeat the trial that online (i.e., real-time) measures suggested were less painful, even after the researchers explained the difference between the two. Similarly, Wirtz, Kruger, Scollon, and Diener (2003) found that remembered experience of spring break rather than online experience predicted participants' desire to take a similar vacation in the future.

However, for theorists and investigators who believe that recalled growth—as a coping strategy, a selective evaluation, or a positive illusion—is important in its own right as an indicator of adaptation to threatening events and/or a predictor of well-being and health, we offer the following challenge. Just as Kahneman et al. (1993) and Wirtz et al. (2003) demonstrated that recalled experience rather than measured experience predicts people's willingness and interest in repeating an experience, investigators of PTG, SRG, and BF should design their studies in a way that allows them to demonstrate that recalled growth and benefits predict adaptational outcomes of interest beyond the predictive value of measured growth and benefits. Such a strategy would have several significant advantages. First, it would guide the assessment of growth and benefit finding. If, echoing the findings of Kahneman et al. and Wirtz et al., recalled growth and recalled benefits, as they are now measured, predict well-being, biological indicators of health, illness symptoms, mortality, and other outcomes of interest, whereas measured growth and measured benefits do not predict these outcomes, current measurement strategies would receive strong support. We can imagine, for example, that recalled growth but not measured growth might generate positive affect. Carver and Scheier (1990) have demonstrated that only information about change over time (i.e., a sense of progress) gives rise to positive affect. Recalled growth rather than measured growth would almost surely reinforce a sense of personal progress.

A second advantage of turning to indicators of measured growth is that it would help position PTG, SRG, and BF within a conceptual context, something that is sorely needed. If recalled growth and recalled benefits are relatively independent of measured growth and measured benefits and if most people recalled more growth than they experienced, PTG, SRG, and BF could be studied effectively as positive illusions.

A third advantage of including indicators of measured growth as well as recalled growth in studies of PTG, SRG, and BF is that it allows for the documentation of individual differences in the concordance between recalled growth and measured growth. This would generate interest in moderators of that association. For example, might people who generate redemptive sequences in their life narratives (Pals & McAdams, 2004) show a more modest relationship between recalled and measured growth than individuals who do not produce these narrative sequences? Similarly, might individuals with a stronger growth orientation (Dykman, 1998) generate less concordance between recalled and measured growth and benefits than their less growth-oriented counterparts? Might those who hold "incremental" self-views show less concordance between recalled and measured growth and benefits than those who maintain "entity" self-views (Dweck, 1999)? We see considerable promise in such moderation studies.

Finally, including indicators of measured as well as of recalled growth and benefits in studies of PTG, SRG, and BF would allow investigators to make head-to-head comparisons between various conceptualizations of trauma-related growth and benefit finding. For example, the position that growth reports represent genuine positive changes (Epel, McEwen, & Ickovics, 1998; Tedeschi & Calhoun, 1995) would predict strong concordance between measured and recalled growth, whereas the positive illusion perspective would predict less concordance and perhaps noteworthy individual differences in concordance. Carefully designed studies could also determine whether growth requires a deprecation of a former self and whether research participants who report growth are making downward temporal comparisons. These potential advantages of a recalled-measured growth design hold the promise of generating new knowledge, testing competing theories, and vitalizing this most promising yet vulnerable field of inquiry.

The Response Shift Conundrum

Throughout this chapter, we have underscored the significant limitations of retrospective assessments of growth and benefit finding. These limitations have led us to endorse the prospective tracking of growth and benefits. However, this sort of prospective tracking is not without its critics. We now turn our attention to these criticisms, specifically the concept of "response shift" (Sprangers & Schwartz, 1999).

Consider a prospective study of SRG that is conducted in a way that is consistent with our proposed recalled-measured growth design, that is, a fully prospective design with repeated measures of participants' current status on various dimensions from which growth will be calculated by the investigator.

Now imagine a participant who is completing our proposed current status version of the SRGS for the first time. She is asked to rate her faith in God, and she rates herself as 2 on a 0 to 4 scale. Six months later, and after a near fatal automobile accident, she participates in the second wave of the prospective study. She again rates her faith in God, and again she rates herself as 2 on the 0 to 4 scale. The investigator then asks this participant to retrospectively rate the strength of her faith in God as it was 6 months earlier. She rates her previous faith in God as 1 on the same scale.

An autobiographical memory theorist would surmise that this participant was rewriting her personal history to create a sense of positive change. But another interpretation of this pattern of ratings is that this participant's comparison state—her reference point—changed since her traumatic experience. Specifically, she may have come to realize from her car crash that her initial reference point was too low. She now appreciates just how much faith in God is possible and how much room there is for improvement on this personal attribute. In other words, her previous sense of what *4,* the endpoint of our rating scale, means has changed. This phenomenon is referred to as response shift, and the participant's retrospective judgment is known as the *then-test.* Sprangers and Schwartz (1999) and others (Aiken, 1986; Aiken & West, 1990) would assert that the then-test is more valid than the initial prospective rating of current status, and they would endorse a comparison of the participant's rating during the second wave of the study with her then-test rating to eliminate response shift effects.

Although intuitively appealing, there are several reasons to interpret with caution a response shift and then-test approach to the measurement of PTG, SRG, and BF. First, longitudinal factor analyses of data from several studies reveal that people change their priorities when faced with a deteriorating condition, and that their focus shifts from physical functioning to well-being (Norman, 2003). How such priority shifts affect response shifts is not clear. Second, there is evidence that more variance in the then-test is attributable to recall bias than to a recalibration of standards (Schwartz, Sprangers, Carey, & Reed, 2004). Findings such as this favor the repeated assessment of participants' current status. Finally, the retrospective judgment involved in the then-test requires individuals to recall a previous state and then adjust their rating on the basis of the new reference point. Yet the evidence we reviewed throughout this chapter indicates that people are quite biased in recalling their previous states (e.g., see Wilson & Ross, 2001).

Norman (2003) referred to this debate between the autobiographical memory perspective and the response shift perspective as "an interesting conundrum." We agree, although we believe that the available evidence favors the prospective repeated assessment of people's current status to document growth and benefit finding. Most relevant to our discussion is that neither the autobiographical memory nor the response shift perspective supports the current PTG, SRG, BF retrospective methodology of asking people how much they have changed and how much of that change is attributable to a particular threatening encounter. In view of the overwhelming evidence against such assessment methods, we believe the burden is now on investigators who use them to defend their methods with supporting data.

Toward Meticulous Methods: A Proposal

We summarized converging evidence from numerous studies demonstrating that people are inclined to create a sense of growth when they recall personal change; they rewrite their relationship histories to create a sense of progress and they frequently deprecate a former self as a way to view the current self in a more positive light. We also demonstrated how it is improbable that research participants accurately complete existing measures of PTG, SRG, and BF. To do so, they would need to compare their current and previous standing on each scale item, assess the degree of change, and then determine how much of that change is event related. What we know about inaccuracies and bias in the detection of change, and especially in the detection of contingent change, makes it difficult to argue that people can engage in the mental operations required to complete the existing measures in the way they were meant to be completed. Finally, we explained how Western tradition, popular culture, and even a major professional organization have promoted the notion that people grow from major threatening encounters, and this has almost surely influenced most people's implicit theories of change in the context of adversity. We believe that when considered together, these problems pose a genuine challenge for current indicators of PTG, SRG, and BF. We now propose an approach to the measurement of growth and benefit finding that we believe addresses this challenge.

Our proposed approach involves changes in study design and changes in construct measurement. Our design recommendation is straightforward: We urge investigators to turn to prospective or nearly prospective study designs to examine the predictors, temporal dynamics, and consequences of PTG, SRG, and BF. We are certainly not the first to suggest the application of prospective, longitudinal designs in this area of inquiry (Linley & Joseph, 2004; Nolen-Hoeksema & Davis, 2004; Tedeschi & Calhoun, 2004; Tennen & Affleck, 2002). Although fully prospective designs may be difficult to implement, longitudinal and nearly prospective studies are feasible and would allow investigators to assess growth and benefit finding moving forward rather than looking back. Individuals at high risk for threatening medical events and those being tested for potentially life-threatening illnesses would be ideal cohorts from which to select a sample from among those subsequently afflicted (S. Lechner, personal communication, September 15, 2006). Individuals with a terminally ill loved one might likewise create a cohort from which to select a sample to prospectively examine growth in response to bereavement (Davis, Nolen-Hoeksema, & Larson, 1998). Individuals who recently faced an unanticipated major medical threat (Affleck et al., 1987, 1991), or who recently experienced a disaster (McMillen et al., 1997) offer other opportunities for the study of PTG, SRG, and BF. Although not without their limitations, studies of these or related populations would be a great advance over the cross-sectional or two-wave longitudinal designs that now are used in nearly all current studies.

Although it would be a strong start, prospective or nearly prospective studies will not address all the concerns we raised in this chapter unless such studies also include indicators of measured growth in addition to recalled growth. Measured growth requires the investigator to compute positive and negative changes in various theory-relevant dimensions by tracking over time each participant's current status on those dimensions. This measurement approach allows investigators to do what they do well: create indicators of participants' current status and calculate change directly by examining over several time points the trajectory of participants' current state. Moreover, this approach leaves to participants what only they can do: provide reports of their current status vis-à-vis their behavior, affective state, and appraisals of their social world. It relieves them from making judgments that they are incapable of making accurately, from engaging in mental processes that require them to recall, gather, and organize information about their past selves and speculate how that differs from their current selves, and from offering opinions based on the subjective assessment of covariation. Table 2.2 contrasts existing indicators of growth and benefit finding with indicators that assess current status.

Thus far, we have emphasized how to measure growth and benefits. An equally important issue is the domains of change that are measured. Whereas most published measures of PTG, SRG, and BF focus on subjective aspects of growth, Carver and Scheier (2003) and Aldwin (1994) asserted that people can emerge from stressful and even traumatic experiences with new skills and greater knowledge. These aspects of growth are ideally suited for performance indicators. Indeed, we know of no other area of psychological inquiry in which the gold standard for assessing change in a skill is to ask people whether their skill level changed since the previous assessment (see Tennen, Affleck, & Tennen, 2002). As Westen and Weinberger (2004) stated, "In most areas of psychology we measure skills or aptitudes rather than asking individuals to self-report them" (p. 600). Similarly, the field of achievement testing would be in a sorry state if the standard approach involved asking people to rate on a 5-point scale how much more knowledge they have now compared with the last time they were evaluated. We urge investigators to consider implementing performance indicators when theory and/or the nature of the stressful encounter lead the investigator to anticipate changes in skills and knowledge. Performance indicators, like the current status items we propose for measuring subjective aspects of growth, would leave to the investigator the task of calculating change over time.

Future Directions

Current conceptualizations of PTG, SRG, and BF create considerable measurement challenges. Yet without fully prospective designs that assess both recalled and measured growth, we will surely have more of what now characterizes this area of inquiry: a myriad of post hoc explanations for a provocative phenomenon. Continuing the current retrospective approach in the study of growth and benefits will have predictable consequences: Ultimately, investigators and theorists will begin to pick up their marbles to play elsewhere. As they do, studies of PTG, SRG, and BF will at first migrate to more marginal publications and then eventually will stop being the focus of systematic investigation. This would be a most unfortunate fate for such a provocative and promising area of psychological inquiry.

Table 2.2. Comparison of Current and Proposed Item Content From Widely Used Growth and Benefit-Finding Scales

Measure	Current instructions and sample items	Proposed instructions and sample items
Posttraumatic Growth Inventory (Tedeschi & Calhoun, 1996)	Indicate for each of the statements below the degree to which this change occurred in your life as a result of your crisis: A sense of closeness with others I'm more likely to change things that need changing Knowing I can handle difficulties	Indicate how well each of the statements below describes you: I have a sense of closeness with others I change things that need changing I know I can handle difficulties
Stress-Related Growth Inventory (Park, Cohen, & Murch, 1996)	Rate how much you experienced each item below as a result of this year's most stressful event: I learned to look at things in a more positive way I learned to take responsibility for what I do I feel freer to make my own decisions	Indicate how well each of the statements below describes you: I look at things in a positive way I take responsibility for what I do I feel free to make my own decisions
Changes in Outlook Questionnaire (Joseph et al., 2005)	As a result of _____ I value my relationships much more now I'm a more understanding and tolerant person now I value other people more now	Indicate how well each of the statements below describes you: I value my relationships I'm an understanding and tolerant person I value other people
Benefit Finding Scale (Mohr et al., 1999)	As a result of experiencing _____ I have become more respectful of others I am more compassionate toward others I am more motivated to succeed	Indicate how well each of the statements below describes you: I am respectful of others I am compassionate toward others I am motivated to succeed
Benefit Finding in Breast Cancer Scale (Tomich & Helgeson, 2004)	Having had breast cancer . . . has made me more grateful for each day has led me to be more accepting of things has brought my family closer together	Indicate how well each of the statements below describes you: I am grateful for each day I am accepting of things I am close to my family

References

Abraido-Lanza, A. F., Guier, C., & Colón, R. M. (1998). Psychological thriving among Latinas with chronic illness. *Journal of Social Issues, 54,* 405–424.

Affleck, G., Tennen, H., Croog, S., & Levine, S. (1987). Causal attributions, perceived benefits, and morbidity after a heart attack: An 8 year study. *Journal of Consulting and Clinical Psychology, 55,* 29–35.

Affleck, G., Tennen, H., & Rowe, J. (1991). *Infants in crisis: How parents cope with newborn intensive care and its aftermath.* New York: Springer-Verlag.

Aiken, L. S. (1986). Retrospective self-reports by clients differ from original reports: Implications for the evaluation of drug treatment programs. *The International Journal of the Addictions, 21,* 767–788.

Aiken, L. S., & West, S. G. (1990). Invalidity of true experiments: Self-report pretest biases. *Evaluation Review, 14,* 374–390.

Albert, S. (1977). Temporal comparison theory. *Psychological Review, 84,* 485–503.

Aldwin, C. M. (1994). *Stress, coping, and development: An integrative perspective.* New York: Guilford Press.

Armeli, S., Gunthert, K. C., & Cohen, L. H. (2001). Stressor appraisals, coping, and post-event outcomes: The dimensionality and antecedents of stress-related growth. *Journal of Social and Clinical Psychology, 20,* 366–395.

Cadell, S., Regehr, C., & Hemsworth, D. (2003). Factors contributing to posttraumatic growth: A proposed structural equation model. *American Journal of Orthopsychiatry, 73,* 279–287.

Carver, C. S., & Antoni, M. H. (2004). Finding benefit in breast cancer during the year after diagnosis predicts better adjustment 5 to 8 years after diagnosis. *Health Psychology, 23,* 595–598.

Carver, C. S., & Scheier, M. F. (1990). Origins and functions of positive and negative affect: A control-process view. *Psychological Review, 97,* 19–35.

Carver, C. S., & Scheier, M. F. (2003). Three human strengths. In L. G. Aspinwall & U. M. Staudinger (Eds.), *A psychology of human strengths: Fundamental questions and future directions for a positive psychology* (pp. 87–102). Washington, DC: American Psychological Association.

Chapman, L. J. (1967). Illusory correlation in observational report. *Journal of Verbal Learning and Verbal Behavior, 6,* 151–156.

Conway, M., & Ross, M. (1984). Getting what you want by revising what you had. *Journal of Personality and Social Psychology, 47,* 738–748.

Costa, P. T., Jr., & McCrae, R. R. (1989). Personality continuity and the changes of adult life. In M. Storandt & G. R. VandenBos (Eds.), *The adult years: Continuity and change* (Vol. 8, pp. 41–77). Washington, DC: American Psychological Association.

Cronbach, L., & Meehl, P. (1955). Construct validity in psychological tests. *Psychological Bulletin, 52,* 281–302.

Danoff-Burg, S., & Revenson, T. (2005). Benefit-finding among patients with rheumatoid arthritis: Positive effects on interpersonal relationships. *Journal of Behavioral Medicine, 28,* 91–103.

Davis, C. G., Nolen-Hoeksema, S., & Larson, J. (1998). Making sense of loss and growing from the experience: Two construals of meaning. *Journal of Personality and Social Psychology, 75,* 561–574.

Dweck, C. S. (1999). *Self-theories: Their role in motivation, personality, and development.* Philadelphia: Taylor & Francis.

Dykman, B. M. (1998). Integrating cognitive and motivational factors in depression: Initial tests of a goal-orientation approach. *Journal of Personality and Social Psychology, 74,* 139–158.

Epel, E. S., McEwen, B. S., & Ickovics, J. R. (1998). Embodying psychological thriving: Physical thriving in response to stress. *Journal of Social Issues, 54,* 301–322.

Harvey, J. H., Barnett, K., & Overstreet, A. (2004). Trauma growth and other outcomes attendant to loss. *Psychological Inquiry, 15,* 26–29.

Henry, B., Moffitt, T. E., Caspi, A., Langley, J., & Silva, P. A. (1994). On the 'remembrance of things past': A longitudinal evaluation of the retrospective method. *Psychological Assessment, 6,* 92–101.

Herbst, J. H., McCrae, R. R., Costa, P. T., Jr., Feaganes, J. R., & Siegler, I. C. (2000). Self-perceptions of stability and change in personality at midlife: The UNC alumni heart study. *Assessment, 7,* 379–388.

Janoff-Bulman, R. (1992). *Shattered assumptions*. New York: Free Press.

Janoff-Bulman, R., & Frantz, C. M. (1997). The impact of trauma on meaning: From meaningless world to meaningful life. In M. Power & C. R. Brewin (Eds.), *The transformation of meaning in psychological therapies* (pp. 91–106). New York: Wiley.

Joseph, S., Linley, P. A., Andrews, L., Harris, G., Howle, B., Woodward, C., & Shevlin, M. (2005). Assessing positive and negative changes in the aftermath of adversity: Psychometric evaluation of the Changes in Outlook Questionnaire. *Psychological Assessment, 17,* 70–80.

Joseph, S., Williams, R., & Yule, W. (1993). Changes in outlook following disaster: The preliminary development of a measure to assess positive and negative responses. *Journal of Traumatic Stress, 6,* 271–279.

Kahneman, D., Fredrickson, B. L., Schreiber, C. A., & Redelmeier, D. A. (1993). When more pain is preferred to less: Adding a better end. *Psychological Science, 4,* 401–405.

Karney, B. R., & Coombs, R. H. (2000). Memory bias in long-term close relationships: Consistency or improvement? *Personality and Social Psychology Bulletin, 26,* 959–970.

Karney, B. R., & Frye, N. E. (2002). "But we've been getting better lately": Comparing prospective and retrospective views of relationship development. *Journal of Personality and Social Psychology, 82,* 222–238.

Kirkpatrick, L. A., & Hazan, C. (1994). Attachment styles and close relationships: A four-year prospective study. *Personal Relationships, 1,* 123–142.

Lechner, S. C., Carver, C. S., Antoni, M. H., Weaver, K. E., & Phillips, K. M. (2006). Curvilinear associations between benefit finding and psychosocial adjustment to breast cancer. *Journal of Consulting and Clinical Psychology, 74,* 828–840.

Libby, L. K., & Eibach, R. P. (2002). Looking back in time: Self-concept change affects visual perspective in autobiographical memory. *Journal of Personality and Social Psychology, 82,* 167–179.

Linley, P. A., & Joseph, S. (2004). Positive change following trauma and adversity: A review. *Journal of Traumatic Stress, 17,* 11–21.

McFarland, C., & Alvaro, C. (2000). The impact of motivation on temporal comparisons: Coping with traumatic events by perceiving personal growth. *Journal of Personality and Social Psychology, 79,* 327–343.

McGrath, J. C., & Linley, P. A. (2006). Post-traumatic growth in acquired brain injury: A preliminary small scale study. *Brain Injury, 20,* 767–773.

McMillen, J. C., Smith, E. M., & Fisher, R. H. (1997). Perceived benefit and mental health after three types of disaster. *Journal of Consulting and Clinical Psychology, 65,* 733–739.

Meehl, P. E. (1957). When shall we use our heads instead of the formula? *Journal of Counseling Psychology, 4,* 268–273.

Mohr, D. C., Dick, L. P., Russo, J. P., Boudewyn, A. C., Likosky, W., & Goodkin, D. E. (1999). The psychological impact of multiple sclerosis: Exploring the patient's perspective. *Health Psychology, 18,* 376–382.

Nolen-Hoeksema, S., & Davis, C. G. (2002). Positive responses to loss: Perceiving benefits and growth. In C. R. Snyder & S. Lopez (Eds.), *Handbook of positive psychology* (pp. 598–607). New York: Oxford University Press.

Nolen-Hoeksema, S., & Davis, C. G. (2004). Theoretical and methodological issues in the assessment and interpretation of posttraumatic growth. *Psychological Inquiry, 15,* 60–64.

Norman, G. (2003). Hi! How are you? Response shift, implicit theories and differing epistemologies. *Quality of Life Research, 12,* 239–249.

Pakenham, K. I. (2005). Benefit finding in multiple sclerosis and associations with positive and negative outcomes. *Health Psychology, 24,* 123–132.

Pals, J. L., & McAdams, D. P. (2004). The transformed self: A narrative understanding of posttraumatic growth. *Psychological Inquiry, 15,* 65–69.

Park, C. L. (1998). Implications of posttraumatic growth for individuals. In R. G. Tedeschi, C. L. Park, & L. G. Calhoun (Eds.), *Posttraumatic growth: Positive change in the aftermath of crisis* (pp. 153–178). Mahwah, NJ: Erlbaum.

Park, C. L., Cohen, L. H., & Murch, R. L. (1996). Assessment and prediction of stress-related growth. *Journal of Personality, 64,* 71–105.

Robins, R. W., Noftle, E. E., Trzesniewski, K. H., & Roberts, B. W. (2005). Do people know how their personality has changed? Correlates of perceived and actual personality change in young adulthood. *Journal of Personality, 73,* 489–521.

Ross, M. (1989). The relation of implicit theories to the construction of personal histories. *Psychological Review, 96,* 341–357.

Ross, M., & Wilson, A. E. (2002). It feels like yesterday: Self-esteem, valence of personal past experiences, and judgments of subjective distance. *Journal of Personality and Social Psychology, 82,* 792–803.

Safer, M. A., Bonanno, G. A., & Field, N. P. (2001). "It was never that bad": Biased recall of grief and long-term adjustment to the death of a spouse. *Memory, 9,* 195–204.

Schacter, D. L. (2001). *The seven sins of memory: How the mind forgets and remembers.* New York: Houghton Mifflin.

Schwartz, C. E., Sprangers, M. A. G., Carey, A., & Reed, G. (2004). Exploring response shift in longitudinal data. *Psychology and Health, 19,* 51–69.

Sprangers, M. A. G., & Schwartz, C. E. (1999). Integrating response shift into health-related quality of life research: A theoretical model. *Social Science & Medicine, 48,* 1507–1515.

Stone, A. A. (2005, April). *Real-time ePRO data collected using eDiaries: Comparisons to recall-based measures of change.* Paper presented at the Drug Information Association conference on Benefits and Challenges with ePRO, Arlington, VA.

Swann, W. B., Jr. (1983). Self-verification: Bringing social reality into harmony with the self. In J. Suls & A. G. Greenwald (Eds.), *Social psychological perspectives on the self* (pp. 33–66). Hillsdale, NJ: Erlbaum.

Swann, W. B., Jr. (1987). Identity negotiation: Where two roads meet. *Journal of Personality and Social Psychology, 53,* 1038–1051.

Tedeschi, R., & Calhoun, L. G. (1995). *Trauma & transformation: Growing in the aftermath of suffering.* Thousand Oaks, CA: Sage.

Tedeschi, R., & Calhoun, L. G. (1996). The Posttraumatic Growth Inventory: Measuring the positive legacy of trauma. *Journal of Traumatic Stress, 9,* 455–471.

Tedeschi, R., & Calhoun, L. G. (2004). Posttraumatic growth: Conceptual foundations and empirical evidence. *Psychological Inquiry, 15,* 1–18.

Tennen, H., & Affleck, G. (1998). Personality and transformation in the face of adversity. In R. G. Tedeschi, C. L. Park, & L. G. Calhoun (Eds.), *Posttraumatic growth: Positive changes in the aftermath of crisis* (pp. 65–98). Hillsdale, NJ: Erlbaum.

Tennen, H., & Affleck, G. (2002). Benefit-finding and benefit-reminding. In C. R. Snyder & S. J. Lopez (Eds.), *Handbook of positive psychology* (pp. 584–597). New York: Oxford University Press.

Tennen, H., & Affleck, G. (2005, May). *Positive change following adversity: In search of novel theories, meticulous methods and precise analytic strategies.* Paper presented at the American Psychological Association conference on Perspectives on Positive Life Changes, Benefit Finding and Growth Following Illness, Storrs, CT.

Tennen, H., Affleck, G., & Tennen, R. (2002). Clipped feathers: The theory and measurement of hope. *Psychological Inquiry, 14,* 163–169.

Todd, M., Armeli, S., Tennen, H., Carney, M. A., Ball, S. A., Kranzler, H. R., & Affleck, G. (2005). Drinking to cope: A comparison of questionnaire and electronic diary reports. *Journal of Studies on Alcohol, 66,* 1121–1129.

Tomich, P. L., & Helgeson, V. S. (2004). Is finding something good in the bad always good? Benefit finding among women with breast cancer. *Health Psychology, 23,* 16–23.

Tomich, P. L., & Helgeson, V. S. (2006). Breast cancer recurrence and cognitive adaptation theory: Are there limits? *Journal of Consulting and Clinical Psychology, 74,* 980–987.

Updegraff, J. A., Taylor, S. E., Kemeny, M. E., & Wyatt, G. E. (2002). Positive and negative effects of HIV infection in women with low socioeconomic resources. *Personality and Social Psychology Bulletin, 28,* 382–394.

Westen, D., & Weinberger, J. (2004). When clinical description becomes statistical prediction. *American Psychologist, 59,* 595–613.

Widows, M. R., Jacobsen, P. B., Booth-Jones, M., & Fields, K. K. (2005). Predictors of posttraumatic growth following bone marrow transplantation for cancer. *Health Psychology, 24,* 266–273.

Wilson, A. E., & Ross, M. (2001). From chump to champ: People's appraisals of their earlier and present selves. *Journal of Personality and Social Psychology, 80,* 572–584.

Wirtz, D., Kruger, J., Scollon, C. N., & Diener, E. (2003). What to do on spring break? The role of predicted, online, and remembered experience in future choice. *Psychological Science, 14,* 520–524.

Wortman, C. B. (2004). Posttraumatic growth: Progress and problems. *Psychological Inquiry, 15,* 81–90.

3 _____

Challenges in Studying Positive Change After Adversity: Illustrations From Research on Breast Cancer

*Charles S. Carver, Suzanne C. Lechner,
and Michael H. Antoni*

Many people initially assumed that the ability to find benefits from an illness would contribute to better adjustment to the illness, and much research has supported that view. In persons with various cancers, for example, links have emerged between concurrent benefit finding and lower distress (Fife, 1995; Ho, Chan, & Ho, 2004; Katz, Flasher, Cacciapaglia, & Nelson, 2001; Taylor, Lichtman, & Wood, 1984; Urcuyo, Boyers, Carver, & Antoni, 2005; Vickberg, Bovbjerg, DuHamel, Currie, & Redd, 2000; Vickberg et al., 2001), higher self-esteem, less anxiety (Lewis, 1989), greater well-being (Carpenter, Brockopp, & Andrykowski, 1999; Curbow, Somerfield, Baker, Wingard, & Legro, 1993; Urcuyo et al., 2005), more positive mood (Carver & Antoni, 2004; Katz et al., 2001; Sears, Stanton, & Danoff-Burg, 2003; Tomich & Helgeson, 2002), and higher current life satisfaction and estimates of future life satisfaction (Curbow et al., 1993).

Yet a number of studies of women treated for breast cancer have obtained findings that differ from these. In some cases, no relation emerged between benefit finding and distress or well-being (Antoni et al., 2001; Cordova, Cunningham, Carlson, & Andrykowski, 2001; Curbow et al., 1993; Fromm, Andrykowski, & Hunt, 1996; Schulz & Mohamed, 2004; Sears et al., 2003; Tomich & Helgeson, 2002; Widows, Jacobsen, Booth-Jones, & Fields, 2005). In at least one case, benefit finding early in the cancer experience related to higher distress and reports of poorer quality of life later on (Tomich & Helgeson, 2004).

These puzzling inconsistencies generated much comment among researchers interested in benefit finding (for reviews, see Stanton, Bower, & Low, 2006; see also chap. 10, this volume). What might account for the inconsistency?

Curvilinear Associations?

We recently addressed this question, conceptually and empirically (Lechner, Carver, Antoni, Weaver, & Phillips, 2006), pursuing a line of thought that had first been developed in an earlier study (Lechner, Zakowski, Antoni, Greenhawt, & Block, 2003). Specifically, we considered the possibility that benefit finding might not always be related in a linear fashion to other aspects of psychosocial well-being; the relation might be curvilinear.

We know from our experiences with breast cancer patients in previous studies that women differ quite dramatically in how they react to diagnosis and initial treatment. For some women, the immediate reaction is that it is a major life crisis. Other women see the disease as just one more of life's adversities (we leave aside for now the question of whether this reaction simply defers the issue, which the women take up again later on). Given these impressions, and the curvilinear idea suggested by Lechner et al. (2003), we posed the following possibility: Perhaps there are subsets of women who respond differently to the stressor of breast cancer, such that relations between benefit finding and other outcomes were sometimes obscured by the composition of a given sample.

How might this occur? Consider the possible existence of three groups of patients (see Figure 3.1). As was just suggested, some women may fail to experience breast cancer as a crisis (Group 1). With no sense of crisis, these women are likely to have low distress. With no sense of crisis, there is no particular reason to expect benefit finding, either. The other two groups do experience the event as a crisis, but they respond to it differently. We hypothesized that the experience of breast cancer leads some women (Group 2) to experience mostly benefit finding (with less distress), and leads others (Group 3) to experience mostly distress (with less benefit finding). This divergence of reactions would yield an inverse relation between outcomes, but only in the latter two groups. To the extent that Group 1 is also represented in the data set, that linear relationship would be disrupted. Indeed, if all three of these groups were in a given sample, an accurate graphical representation of their responses would show a curvilinear relation between benefit finding and other psychosocial outcomes. Relatively low distress would relate both to low benefit finding (Group 1) and to high benefit finding (Group 2); higher distress would relate to intermediate levels of benefit finding.

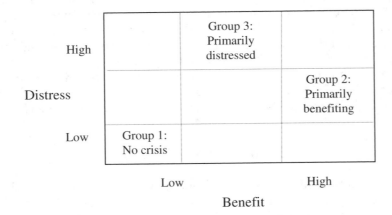

Figure 3.1.   Hypothesized reaction patterns among breast cancer patients.

Evidence of Nonlinear Relations

We examined this possibility by reanalyzing data from two samples that had previously been studied in other ways by the University of Miami's psycho-oncology research group. We conducted several analyses on these samples, using the data we had available on both short-term and long-term well-being. Thus, we were able to look at the possibility of curvilinear relations at two different stages of the cancer experience.

Women in the first study had participated in a natural history study examining adjustment to breast cancer. They were initially assessed at 3, 6, or 12 months following surgery. The participants were 230 early-stage breast cancer patients recruited through medical practices in the Miami area and through the local American Cancer Society office (see Lechner et al., 2006, for details of sample characteristics). Of the starting sample, 101 (44%) were located and reassessed between 5 and 8 years postsurgery. Of the 101 in the follow-up, 5 had not fully completed the initial benefit-finding measure; they were omitted from the analyses, yielding a final sample for the follow-up of 96.

Benefit finding was measured in the initial study using 17 items with the stem "Having had breast cancer . . ." and ending with a benefit that might plausibly follow a cancer experience (Tomich & Helgeson, 2004). The items pertained to family and social relations, life priorities, spirituality, career goals, self-control, and acceptance of life circumstances. Respondents indicated the extent to which they agreed that they had experienced each benefit as a result of having had breast cancer. They could also indicate whether an item was not applicable; "not applicable" responses were dropped, and the average was computed from the remaining responses. The same items were used at follow-up, with slight changes in the response options.

A variety of other measures were also collected at each assessment, including self-ratings of quality of life, emotional distress, depressive symptoms, and social disruption. These were then related to the measure of benefit finding as a predictor, both as a linear effect and as a quadratic effect (i.e., benefit finding centered, then squared).

Early benefit finding in this study meant benefits reported at either 3, 6, or 12 months postsurgery (women had been assessed at one of those three times, in roughly equal numbers). As in the initial report of these data (Urcuyo et al., 2005), there were linear relations of benefit finding with quality of life, depression, and negative affect. In addition, benefit finding related in a curvilinear way to concurrent quality of life but not to the other outcomes.

Associations at follow-up (i.e., 5–8 years after surgery) were more numerous (see Figure 3.2). As had been reported by Carver and Antoni (2004), benefit finding was related in a linear fashion to quality of life, positive affect, negative affect, and social disruption. These effects were qualified by quadratic relations between benefit finding and quality of life (as in the earlier assessment), and also between benefit finding and positive affect, negative affect, depression symptoms, and the index of social disruption.

Was this pattern of quadratic associations a fluke? Could it be replicated? To gain more information about these questions, we turned to a second sample of 136 women who had been recruited 2 to 8 weeks after surgery for a psychosocial

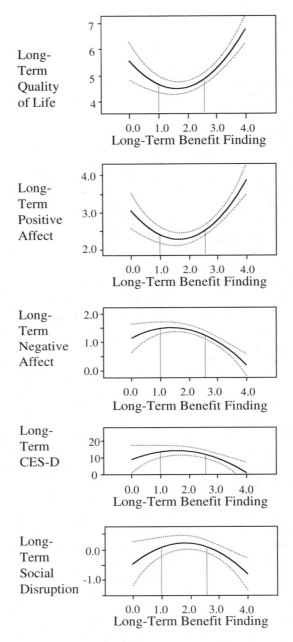

Figure 3.2. Quadratic relations of concurrent benefit finding to rated quality of life, positive affect, negative affect, depressive symptoms, and social disruption at long-term follow-up, 5 to 8 years postsurgery. Dotted lines represent 95% confidence intervals. CES-D = Center for Epidemiological Studies Depression Scale. Reprinted from "Curvilinear Associations Between Benefit Finding and Psychosocial Adjustment to Breast Cancer," by S. C. Lechner, C. S. Carver, M. H. Antoni, K. E. Weaver, and K. M. Phillips, 2006, *Journal of Consulting and Clinical Psychology, 74,* p. 832. Copyright 2006 by the American Psychological Association.

intervention study (Antoni et al., 2001). They were assessed several times during that study. Five years after their surgery, 74 of the women underwent another assessment. The measures completed were much the same as in the other study, with the addition of the Impact of Event Scale (Horowitz, Wilner, & Alvarez, 1979), which measures unwanted intrusion of thoughts and images about a particular stressor—in this case breast cancer—and efforts to avoid those thoughts.

In this sample, all participants were assessed within the first 2 months after surgery. This sample thus was far more homogeneous in that respect than the first sample. Participants were also assessed substantially earlier in the cancer experience than were most of the participants in the first sample. In the initial data, there had not been significant linear associations between benefit finding and other outcomes. However, there were significant quadratic relationships between benefit finding and social disruption, thought intrusion, and thought avoidance, and marginal relationships with respect to distress and quality of life (see Figure 3.3).

In the follow-up data (5 years later), only positive affect had a linear association with benefit finding. However, this linear effect was qualified by a significant curvilinear relationship. Two other curvilinear associations approached significance. As Figure 3.4 shows, the quadratic relationship between benefit finding and perceived quality of life that had been observed earlier was replicated at long-term follow-up. There was no quadratic effect for negative affect or depressive symptoms, but the effect for social disruption approached significance.

What Differentiates Regions of the Curve?

To explore the meaning of the various quadratic effects, we divided each sample into segments based on benefit-finding scores. We did so on the basis of areas where the slope of the line varied appreciably, as in the use of the scree test in factor analysis. The vertical lines in Figures 3.2 through 3.4 indicate the points at which the sample was split. The three groups were uneven in size, with the low benefit group being consistently smallest. In the first sample, the low benefit group was only 6% of the initial sample and 9% of the sample at follow-up. In the second sample, the low benefit group was 19% of the initial sample and 21% at follow-up. After splitting the sample into groups, we compared the groups with each other with respect to other variables in the data set, to try to help interpret the curvilinear effects. Of particular interest was how women for whom well-being coincided with high benefit finding differed from those for whom well-being coincided with low benefit finding.

The latter group, the group we earlier suggested did not experience the cancer as a crisis, can be characterized only tentatively because many of the findings distinguishing them from the others were ephemeral, and were not replicated across samples. In various analyses, these women had less advanced disease (i.e., lower stage and fewer positive nodes), were less likely to be exposed to chemotherapy, and reported being less concerned about damage to their body. They appeared to be engaged in less psychological work surrounding the breast cancer experience, as they also reported less examining of their feelings, less reframing, less religious coping, and (in one sample) less active coping. Our

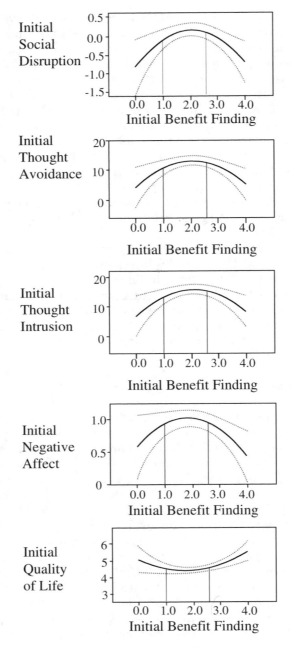

Figure 3.3. Quadratic relations of concurrent benefit finding to perceived quality of life, negative affect, social disruption, and thought intrusion at initial assessment, 2 months postsurgery. Dotted lines represent 95% confidence intervals. Reprinted from "Curvilinear Associations Between Benefit Finding and Psychosocial Adjustment to Breast Cancer," by S. C. Lechner, C. S. Carver, M. H. Antoni, K. E. Weaver, and K. M. Phillips, 2006, *Journal of Consulting and Clinical Psychology, 74,* p. 836. Copyright 2006 by the American Psychological Association.

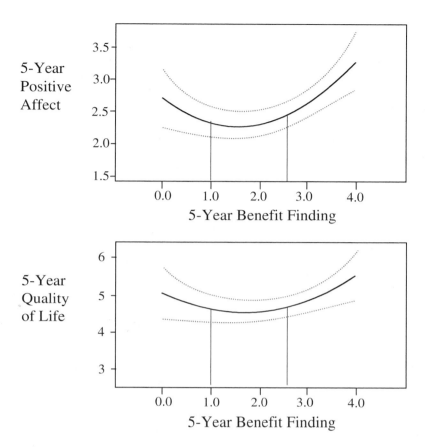

Figure 3.4. Quadratic relations of concurrent benefit finding to perceived quality of life and positive affect at long-term follow-up, 5 years postsurgery. Dotted lines represent 95% confidence intervals. Reprinted from "Curvilinear Associations Between Benefit Finding and Psychosocial Adjustment to Breast Cancer," by S. C. Lechner, C. S. Carver, M. H. Antoni, K. E. Weaver, and K. M. Phillips, 2006, *Journal of Consulting and Clinical Psychology, 74,* p. 836. Copyright 2006 by the American Psychological Association.

inference is that, being less threatened, they may have been less inclined to search for benefits. A degree of life threat may be a necessary condition for the growth process to unfold in persons with major illness (Tedeschi & Calhoun, 2004). Thus, there is at least some support for our initial view of this group.

When the other two groups were compared with each other, in contrast, the picture was quite intuitive. Women in the intermediate range of benefit finding had worse psychosocial profiles. They had higher levels of intrusive thoughts about breast cancer (and reported more effort to avoid such thoughts), greater distress and social disruption, and lower self-reported quality of life than the women who reported greater benefit. Those who reported greater benefit and higher well-being were higher in dispositional optimism, and reported more use of coping strategies such as positive reframing, acceptance, and, quite consistently, religious coping (cf. Park, Cohen, & Murch, 1996). It is also noteworthy that the coping differences between these groups were consistently restricted to these particular aspects of coping. If one considered only these two groups, higher levels of benefit finding appear to be one element in a more general picture of greater psychosocial well-being.

The picture we have presented thus far is essentially one of three kinds of people (or three profiles of tendencies). However, it has also been argued that benefit finding emerges over time and self-examination (Frazier, Conlon, & Glaser, 2001; Tedeschi & Calhoun, 2004). Did benefit finding evolve over time in these two samples of cancer patients? We were not able to find much evidence of such a process. Indeed, benefit finding was relatively stable across time. In the second sample, for example, the test–retest correlation for benefit finding across 5 years was .58. It may have been the case that important changes were taking place in the weeks immediately after diagnosis and surgery that we were unable to observe. Because we did not assess the women immediately at diagnosis, we are unable to know this with certainty.

Nonetheless, the data we have examined are consistent with a view in which different people take different orientations to their experiences, involving differing balances of benefit and distress. This echoes, with respect to benefit finding, a point we have made elsewhere with respect to the aftermath of breast cancer more generally. That is, we have found evidence of a great deal of stability in psychosocial well-being across the period of treatment and for many years thereafter (Carver et al., 2005). The findings appear to indicate a pervasive role for personality and perhaps a stable social context in subjective well-being among breast cancer survivors. It may be the case that there is a similar role for personality and social context with respect to benefit finding after serious illness.

Methodological Issues for Future Work

We began this examination of curvilinear associations because of inconsistency in reports of how benefit finding relates to other aspects of psychosocial well-being after treatment for a major illness. We mentioned that inconsistency in the first place because we were considering a particular criterion for deciding whether a reported benefit was indeed a benefit. The criterion in question was the existence of a systematic association with other indices of well-being.

We believe the results described in the previous section make a fairly persuasive case that the same event happening to different people will generate a sense of crisis in some people but not in others. Furthermore, given a sense of crisis, some people will have an experience that is generally dominated by distress rather than benefits, whereas others will have an experience that is generally dominated by benefits rather than distress. We make no claim that these results indicate that benefit finding reduces distress (the effects we reviewed were all cross-sectional).

These results have potentially important methodological implications for future research on these phenomena. Most simply, they show that linear models, as are typically used in studies in this area, do not always provide a complete picture of the relationships among these variables. Our own prior analyses of some of these data, in which only linear effects were tested, clearly missed part of the picture (Antoni et al., 2001; Carver & Antoni, 2004; Urcuyo et al., 2005).

Another methodological issue also follows from this point. If the pattern of a quadratic relationship between benefit finding and other outcomes generalizes more broadly, it means that the sort of linear associations that are observed between benefit finding and other outcomes will depend on quirks of a particular sample, even if the true underlying (curvilinear) relationship is constant. That is, if a given sample happens to incorporate a larger proportion of persons falling toward one end of this relationship, positive relations will be observed between benefit finding and well-being (as reported by Urcuyo et al., 2005). If the sample happens to have a larger proportion of persons falling toward the other end, inverse relations will be observed. If neither of these happens, there will be no relationship (as reported by Antoni et al., 2001). This is an important issue to keep in mind in future studies of benefit finding.

It is hard to know exactly what to do about this issue, however, beyond looking religiously at quadratic components of the relationship. That is, there is a nagging conceptual issue hidden in the methodological issue. The conceptual issue concerns exactly what we are trying to study. It might be argued that the portion of the distribution who do not experience the event as a crisis do not really belong in the analyses. After all, we think we are studying reactions to traumatic or threatening events. If a subset of persons fail to experience the event in that way, their reactions do not reflect responses to the situation we thought we were studying.

On the other hand, it could be argued that even if a person's response to the event were total indifference, it would be just as legitimate as any other response (Stroebe, Schut, & Stroebe, 2005; Wortman & Silver, 1989). That, indeed, would be the person's actual construal of the situation and response to it. The issue here is analogous to the one faced in life event research concerning the objective reality of an event versus the individual construal of the event. What dictates the person's reactions to the event appears to be the person's unique construal of it. Indeed, that construal already is part of the person's reaction to the event.

Clinical Implications

As noted previously, the work described here does not permit the inference that benefit finding has a causal influence on the other outcome variables. However, the findings do suggest that the experience of benefit finding is one element of a more general sense of well-being in a person who is actively engaged in the attempt to deal with a serious health threat. More precisely, this appears to be true if, and only if, the person is actually experiencing the health threat as a serious adversity. This pattern appears to have some clinical implications.

It seems reasonable to suggest from these findings that strategies aimed at fostering benefit from a health threat may be helpful for people who are already experiencing the event as a serious threat. As Tedeschi and Calhoun (2004;

see also Calhoun & Tedeschi, 1999) have noted, interventions aimed at promoting benefit finding are scarce, but some interventions contain techniques that seem to promote benefit finding as one pathway to better outcomes. For example, cognitive restructuring can be used to increase positive reframing and decrease pessimistic appraisals (Beck, 1981). Expressive writing (Smyth, Stone, Hurewitz, & Kaell, 1999; Stanton et al., 2002; Ullrich & Lutgendorf, 2002) and supportive expressive therapy techniques (Spiegel, Bloom, Kramer, & Gottheil, 1989) may also increase the degree to which people process emotions surrounding the illness, which may promote benefit finding. The very consistent association of religious coping with high levels of benefit finding suggests that approaches addressing the use of religion as a coping strategy among persons with a religious commitment may also promote benefit finding.

On the other hand, the findings also seem to have an implication with respect to those breast cancer patients who are not reporting either benefit or distress. Specifically, some of these women may not be experiencing the cancer diagnosis and treatment as a crisis. Intervening with these women to facilitate benefit finding may have little impact on their psychosocial adjustment; indeed, it might potentially be disruptive. Such types of interventions thus may not be beneficial for them. In sum, we believe that those who are in distress remain the target for change.

Future Directions

What do we see as important directions for future work? The question that remains most salient to us is what differentiates the three regions of the curve obtained in these studies. There appear to be different reaction patterns, but we were less successful in determining their origins than in revealing their existence. One direction for the future, then, would be to explore further the reasons why the confrontation with a potentially fatal disease leads some people to react mostly with disruption of various aspects of their well-being, others to react mostly by finding benefits from the experience, and yet others to be essentially unreactive.

References

Antoni, M. H., Lehman, J. M., Kilbourn, K. M., Boyers, A. E., Culver, J. L., Alferi, S. M., et al. (2001). Cognitive–behavioral stress management intervention decreases the prevalence of depression and enhances benefit finding among women under treatment for early-stage breast cancer. *Health Psychology, 20,* 20–32.

Beck, A. T. (1981). *Cognitive therapy and the emotional disorders.* New York: International Universities Press.

Calhoun, L. G., & Tedeschi, R. G. (1999). *Facilitating posttraumatic growth: A clinician's guide.* Mahwah, NJ: Erlbaum.

Carpenter, J. S., Brockopp, D. Y., & Andrykowski, M. A. (1999). Self-transformation as a factor in the self-esteem and well-being of breast cancer survivors. *Journal of Advanced Nursing, 29,* 1402–1411.

Carver, C. S., & Antoni, M. H. (2004). Finding benefit in breast cancer during the year after diagnosis predicts better adjustment 5 to 8 years after diagnosis. *Health Psychology, 23,* 595–598.

Carver, C. S., Smith, R. G., Antoni, M. H., Petronis, V. M., Weiss, S., & Derhagopian, R. P. (2005). Optimistic personality and psychosocial well-being during treatment predict psychosocial well-being among long-term survivors of breast cancer. *Health Psychology, 24,* 508–516.

Cordova, M. J., Cunningham, L. L. C., Carlson, C. R., & Andrykowski, M. A. (2001). Posttraumatic growth following breast cancer: A controlled comparison study. *Health Psychology, 20,* 176–185.

Curbow, B., Somerfield, M. R., Baker, F., Wingard, J. R., & Legro, M. W. (1993). Personal changes, dispositional optimism, and psychological adjustment to bone marrow transplantation. *Journal of Behavioral Medicine, 16,* 423–443.

Fife, B. L. (1995). The measurement of meaning in illness. *Social Science and Medicine, 40,* 1021–1028.

Frazier, P., Conlon, A., & Glaser, T. (2001). Positive and negative life changes following sexual assault. *Journal of Consulting and Clinical Psychology, 69,* 1048–1055.

Fromm, K., Andrykowski, M. A., & Hunt, J. (1996). Positive and negative psychosocial sequelae of bone marrow transplantation: Implications for quality of life assessment. *Journal of Behavioral Medicine, 19,* 221–240.

Ho, S. M., Chan, C. L. W., & Ho, R. T. H. (2004). Posttraumatic growth in Chinese cancer survivors. *Psycho-Oncology, 13,* 377–389.

Horowitz, M., Wilner, N., & Alvarez, W. (1979). Impact of Event Scale: A measure of subjective stress. *Psychosomatic Medicine, 41,* 209–218.

Katz, R. C., Flasher, L., Cacciapaglia, H., & Nelson, S. (2001). The psychosocial impact of cancer and lupus: A cross-validational study that extends the generality of "benefit-finding" in patients with chronic disease. *Journal of Behavioral Medicine, 24,* 561–571.

Lechner, S. C., Carver, C. S., Antoni, M. H., Weaver, K. E., & Phillips. K. M. (2006). Curvilinear associations between benefit finding and psychosocial adjustment to breast cancer. *Journal of Consulting and Clinical Psychology, 74,* 828–840.

Lechner, S. C., Zakowski, S., Antoni, M. H., Greenhawt, M., & Block, P. (2003). Do sociodemographic and disease-related variables influence benefit-finding in cancer patients? *Psycho-Oncology, 11,* 1–9.

Lewis, F. M. (1989). Attributions of control, experienced meaning, and psychosocial well-being in patients with advanced cancer. *Journal of Psychosocial Oncology, 7,* 105–119.

Park, C. L., Cohen, L. H., & Murch, R. L. (1996). Assessment and prediction of stress-related growth. *Journal of Personality, 64,* 71–105.

Schulz, U., & Mohamed, N. E. (2004). Turning the tide: Benefit finding after cancer surgery. *Social Science and Medicine, 59,* 653–662.

Sears, S. R., Stanton, A. L., & Danoff-Burg, S. (2003). The Yellow Brick Road and the Emerald City: Benefit finding, positive reappraisal coping, and posttraumatic growth in women with early-stage breast cancer. *Health Psychology, 22,* 487–497.

Smyth, J. M., Stone, A. A., Hurewitz, A., & Kaell, A. (1999). Effects of writing about stressful experiences on symptom reduction in patients with asthma or rheumatoid arthritis: A randomized trial. *Journal of the American Medical Association, 281,* 1304–1309.

Spiegel, D., Bloom, G. C., Kramer, J. S., & Gottheil, E. (1989). Effect of psychosocial treatment on survival of patients with metastatic breast cancer. *The Lancet, 2,* 888–891.

Stanton, A. L., Bower, J. E., & Low, C. A. (2006). Posttraumatic growth after cancer. In L. G. Calhoun & R. G. Tedeschi (Eds.), *Handbook of posttraumatic growth: Research and practice* (pp. 138–175). Mahwah, NJ: Erlbaum.

Stanton, A. L., Danoff-Burg, S., Sworowski, L. A., Collins, C. A., Branstetter, A. D., Rodriguez-Hanley, A., et al. (2002). Randomized, controlled trial of written emotional expression and benefit finding in breast cancer patients. *Journal of Clinical Oncology, 20,* 4160–4168.

Stroebe, M. S., Schut, H., & Stroebe, W. (2005). Attachment in coping with bereavement: A theoretical integration. *Review of General Psychology, 9,* 48–66.

Taylor, S. E., Lichtman, R. R., & Wood, J. V. (1984). Attributions, beliefs about control, and adjustment to breast cancer. *Journal of Personality and Social Psychology, 46,* 489–502.

Tedeschi, R. G., & Calhoun, L. G. (2004). Posttraumatic growth: Conceptual foundations and empirical evidence. *Psychological Inquiry, 15,* 1–18.

Tomich, P. L., & Helgeson, V. S. (2002). Five years later: A cross-sectional comparison of breast cancer survivors with healthy women. *Psycho-Oncology, 11,* 154–169.

Tomich, P. L., & Helgeson, V. S. (2004). Is finding something good in the bad always good? Benefit finding among women with breast cancer. *Health Psychology, 23,* 16–23.

Ullrich, P. M., & Lutgendorf, S. K. (2002). Journaling about stressful events: Effects of cognitive processing and emotional expression. *Annals of Behavioral Medicine, 24,* 244–250.

Urcuyo, K. R., Boyers, A. E., Carver, C. S., & Antoni, M. H. (2005). Finding benefit in breast cancer: Relations with personality, coping, and concurrent well-being. *Psychology and Health, 20,* 175–192.

Vickberg, S. M. J., Bovbjerg, D. H., DuHamel, K. N., Currie, V., & Redd, W. H. (2000). Intrusive thoughts and psychological distress among breast cancer survivors: Global meaning as a possible protective factor. *Behavioral Medicine, 25,* 152–160.

Vickberg, S. M. J., DuHamel, K. N., Smith, M. Y., Manne, S. L., Papadopoulos, E. B., & Redd, W. H. (2001). Global meaning and psychological adjustment among survivors of bone marrow transplant. *Psycho-Oncology, 10,* 29–39.

Widows, M. R., Jacobsen, P. B., Booth-Jones, M., & Fields, K. K. (2005). Predictors of posttraumatic growth following bone marrow transplantation for cancer. *Health Psychology, 24,* 266–273.

Wortman, C., & Silver, R. (1989). The myths of coping with loss. *Journal of Consulting and Clinical Psychology, 57,* 349–357.

Part II

Developmental Issues

4

Benefit Finding Among Children and Adolescents With Diabetes

Vicki S. Helgeson, Lindsey Lopez,
and Constance Mennella

Although growth and benefit finding have been studied extensively among adults, there is little research on this topic among children and adolescents. In this chapter, we address four questions about benefit finding and growth among children. First, do children construe benefits from adversity? To the extent that benefit finding is an abstract cognitive skill, one may expect little benefit finding among younger children and increases in benefit finding with age. Second, if benefit finding occurs in children, are the kinds of benefits that children construe from adversity the same as those documented among adults? Third, what is the source of these benefits? Do benefits emerge from characteristics of the child or the stressor, or from the social environment? Finally, what are the implications of benefit finding or growth for well-being among children?

We address these four questions by reviewing the sparse literature that exists on benefit finding and growth among children and adolescents. We also incorporate data from an ongoing study of adolescents with diabetes into this discussion. We conclude the chapter by outlining a set of directions for future research.

Do Children Construe Benefits From Adversity?

In this section we examine the extent to which previous research has shown that children and adolescents construe benefits from adversity. Then, we present data from our study of adolescents with diabetes. Finally, we synthesize our findings with previous research.

We, the chapter authors, acknowledge the support of grant R01 DK60586 from the National Institutes of Health to conduct this work and the support of the Pediatric Clinical and Translational Research Center at Children's Hospital (GCRC Grant 5MO1 RR00084). We are grateful to the hospital clinic staff for their support, to Pamela Snyder for overseeing the day-to-day aspects of this project, and to Laura Viccaro for her editorial comments on this work. We also appreciate the assistance of all the Carnegie Mellon research assistants who conducted these interviews and to the children and their parents for their cooperation.

Existing Literature

The large body of literature on vulnerability and resilience among children shows that some children adapt better to stressful events than others (see Aldwin & Sutton, 1998, for a review). Resilience is not the same as benefit finding or growth, however. Resilience reflects positive adjustment to traumatic or adverse life events, whereas growth represents transformation and change (Kilmer, 2006; Lepore & Revenson, 2006). Far fewer studies explicitly examine benefits or areas of growth in children following adversity. We located 14 such studies. Quantitative indicators of growth were reported in 11 of them, as shown in Table 4.1.

The majority of these studies examined growth among children by adapting one of the most widely used adult inventories, the Posttraumatic Growth Inventory (PTGI; Tedeschi & Calhoun, 1996). Studies of children and adolescents typically have modified the PTGI by altering item wording to increase comprehensibility for children and/or by changing the response scale. For example, Cryder, Kilmer, Tedeschi, and Calhoun (2006) developed the PTGI for children (PTGI-C) by altering the wording of the PTGI items and reducing the response scale from 6 to 4 points. The PTGI-C was administered to children ages 6 to 15 years who had been evacuated or displaced from their homes by Hurricane Floyd. The authors found a moderate amount of growth, as indicated by the mean of 65.11 (*SD* = 11.87) on a scale that ranged from 21 to 84.

Using a somewhat older sample (ages 8–25 years), Yaskowich (2005) administered the PTGI-C (i.e., the original 6-point response scale) to youth and young adults who had been diagnosed with cancer between 2 and 14 years ago. The author compared participants' responses with adult norms from the PTGI (Tedeschi & Calhoun, 1996). She concluded that children with cancer experience growth similarly to adults, as indicated by the fact that 48% had scores that were at or above the adult mean score. The mean score was 69.4 (*SD* = 24.12) on a scale that ranged from 21 to 126, indicating a small amount of growth. The most common domain of growth was in the area of relationships.

Ickovics et al. (2006) modified the PTGI for use with 14- to 19-year-old urban adolescent girls (*N* = 328) by rewording items to facilitate comprehension, changing the response scale to a 3-point format (i.e., 0 = *no change*, 1 = *a little change*, and 2 = *a lot of change*), and omitting the two spiritual growth items. Participants were asked to indicate the hardest thing you ever had to deal with. Means for the four subscales ranged from 1.16 to 1.87 (*SD*s = .21–.59), again suggesting that some growth had occurred. The highest amount of growth was in the appreciation of life domain, and the lowest amount of growth was in the relationships domain.

A large study of Israeli adolescents (Grades 7–9; *N* = 2,999) found a much smaller amount of growth in connection with exposure to terror (Laufer & Solomon, 2006). The researchers modified the PTGI for these adolescents by translating the original version into Hebrew, changing the response scale to a 4-point format (i.e., 1 = *no change*, 4 = *significant change*), and adding 12 items that reflected domains that were particularly important to Israeli adolescents (i.e., 8 responsibility items and 4 connection-to-homeland items). The

Table 4.1. Quantitative Assessment of Growth

Study	Mean age (SD)	Age range	Growth mean (SD)	Range	No. of items	Response scale	Stressor
Barakat, Alderfer, and Kazak (2006)	14.70 (SD = 2.4)	11–19	2.80 (SD = 2.2)	1–9	9	0–1	Cancer
Cryder, Kilmer, Tedeschi, & Calhoun (2006)	9.54 (SD = 2.64)	6–15	65.11 (SD = 11.87)	21–84	21	1–4	Hurricane Floyd
Helgeson, Lopez, and Mennella (this chap.)	12.10 (SD = .77)	10–14	2.73–3.67 (SD = .64–.89)	1–5	15	1–5	Adolescents with diabetes
Ickovics et al. (2006)	17.24 (SD = 1.49)	14–19	1.16–1.87 (SD = .21–.59)	0–57	19	0–3	Hardest thing ever had to deal with
Kazak, Stuber, Barakat, and Meeske (1996)	12.58 (SD = 3.54)	6–19	2.70 (no SD)	1–9	9	0–1	Cancer
Laufer and Solomon (2006)	—	13–16	2.04 (SD = .67)	1–4	33	1–4	Exposure to terror
Milam, Ritt-Olson, Tan, Unger, and Nezami (2005)	13.54 (SD = .52)	Grade 8	3.64 (SD = .79)	1–5	11	1–5[a]	September 11th terrorist attacks
Milam, Ritt-Olson, and Unger (2004)	15.80 (SD = 1.52)	Grades 9–12	3.56 (SD = .71)	1–5	16	1–5[a]	Most traumatic event
Pakenham and Bursnall (2006)	15.60 (SD = 3.97)	10–24	45.17 (SD = 12)	18–90	18	1–5	Carers of parents with MS
Park (2006)	—	15–18	3.65 (SD = .52)	1–5	16	1–5[a]	Critical negative event
Phipps, Long, and Ogden (2007)	12.35 (SD = 3.4)	7–18	37.35 (SD = 7.8)	10–50	10	1–5	Cancer
Yaskowich (2005)	16.10 (SD = 3.36)	8–25	69.40 (SD = 24.12)	21–126	21	1–6	Cancer

[a]For this response scale, 1 = *high negative change*; 3 = *no change*; 5 = *high positive change*.

scale mean was 2.04 (SD = .67), suggesting that respondents experienced only mild growth.

Three studies made a significant change to the response scale of the PTGI and detected small amounts of growth. Milam, Ritt-Olson, and Unger (2004) asked Hispanic adolescents (N = 435) in Grades 9 through 12 (M = 15.8 years) to recall the most traumatic event they had experienced in the past 3 years. For each of 16 items (i.e., a modification of some of the original PTGI items plus some new items), they indicated whether they had experienced a negative or positive change (i.e., 1 = highly negative change, 3 = no change, and 5 = highly positive change). The mean of 3.56 (SD = .71) revealed only a small amount of growth. Using the same response scale for 11 of the items in another study, Milam et al. examined the frequency of growth among 514 eighth graders 8 to 9 months following the September 11th terrorist attacks (Milam, Ritt-Olson, Tan, Unger, & Nezami, 2005). The mean score was 3.64 (SD = .79), again indicating a small amount of positive change. Using the 16-item version of the scale, S. Park (2006) examined an ethnically diverse group of adolescents ages 15 to 18 years with respect to a "critical negative event" in their lives. The overall mean of 3.65 (SD = .52) indicated a small amount of growth. The majority of the sample (60%) averaged a 3, indicating no change, 28% showed some growth (4 or 5 on the scale), and 12% reported negative changes (1 or 2 on the scale).

Five groups of researchers designed their own measures of growth for children. One group developed the Impact of Traumatic Stressors Interview Schedule for adolescents (mean age = 12.58 years [SD = 3.54]) who had undergone treatment for cancer (Kazak, Stuber, Barakat, & Meeske, 1996). The interview included a series of questions about whether respondents felt they had changed because of the experience. Of nine possible domains (e.g., relationships with others, performance in school), adolescents noted 2.7 changes for the better and less than 1 change for the worse. In a second study of childhood cancer survivors ages 11 to 19 years, the same scale (now titled the Perceptions of Changes in Self scale) was used (Barakat, Alderfer, & Kazak, 2006). The number of improvements on the 9-item scale was used as an indicator of growth. The majority of respondents (85%) reported an improvement in at least one of the nine domains whereas a minority (32%) reported four or more areas of improvement. The average number of changes was 2.8 (SD = 2.2). The most common domain of improvement was "how I think about my life," identified by just over half (53%) of respondents.

One group of researchers developed a growth measure based on adult versions of other benefit-finding scales (e.g., see Tomich & Helgeson, 2004) and used it with children ages 7 to 18 years who had cancer (Phipps, Long, & Ogden, 2007). The 10-item scale emphasized increases in personal strength and improved relationships. The average score was 37.35 (SD = 7.8) on a scale that ranged from 10 to 50, indicating a moderate amount of growth.

A third group of investigators developed their own measure of growth and administered it to children of a parent who had multiple sclerosis (MS; Pakenham & Bursnall, 2006). Children ages 10 to 25 years responded to the 18-item instrument in regard to the benefits of caregiving. The average scale response was 45.17 (SD = 12) (with a range of 18–90), which reflected a modest amount of growth. No information was provided on which items were endorsed more strongly than others.

A fourth group asked older adolescents (ages 16–22 years), who had experienced the death of a family member or friend in the past 2 months, which of seven possible benefits, derived from pilot-testing, had occurred (Oltjenbruns, 1991). The most commonly checked items were "have a deeper appreciation of life" (74%) and "show greater caring for loved ones" (67%). Of the 93 participants, only 1 reported no benefits and 3 did not answer the question. This study provides substantial support for the existence of growth among older adolescents and young adults and suggests that previously identified domains of growth among adults are common among this age group.

One final study did not directly assess growth but determined the extent to which it occurred from a qualitative analysis of interview notes from children ages 7 to 18 years who had experienced road traffic accidents. Just under half (42%) of the children spontaneously reported some aspect of growth, most often in the domain of appreciation of life (Salter & Stallard, 2004).

Taken collectively, it is difficult to determine from this small set of studies whether children and adolescents engage in benefit finding and experience growth to the extent that has been documented among adults. The issue remains unresolved for several reasons. First, none of these studies asked participants to describe ways in which they had benefited or grown from a stressful life event (with the exception of Salter & Stallard, 2004). In the majority of cases, they were asked to complete a growth inventory with the domains of growth specified by adults. Items used with adults were adapted in terms of comprehensibility but not in terms of content. Thus, the question remains as to whether these domains represent the domains of growth that pervade the lives of children and adolescents who face stressful life events. Second, the previous set of studies typically enrolled a heterogeneous age range of children and adolescents, making it unclear how age is related to growth. One study examined children who were ages 6 to 15 years (Cryder et al., 2006), two examined children ages 7 to 18 years (Phipps et al., 2007; Salter & Stallard, 2004), and other studies examined a group of people that included children, adolescents, and young adults (ages 10–24 years in Pakenham & Bursnall, 2006; ages 8–25 years in Yaskowich, 2005). To further explore these issues, we conducted a study of children with diabetes who were of a relatively homogeneous age range, and examined the extent of growth, in part, by having them identify the benefits themselves. We view these data as preliminary, however, as they have not been previously published.

Growth Among Adolescents With Diabetes

We enrolled 132 adolescents with diabetes (i.e., 70 girls, 62 boys) ages 10 to 14 years (M = 12 years) into a longitudinal study that involved annual interviews over a period of 5 years (see Helgeson, Viccaro, Becker, Escobar, & Siminerio, 2006, for details on recruitment and demographic characteristics). During the second annual interview (T2), we asked them to rate the overall effect of the illness on their lives in terms of positivity and negativity and to identify ways in which they may have benefited from their illness. From these open-ended responses, we created a closed-ended growth inventory that we administered the following year (T3).

Table 4.2. Frequencies of Responses to Perceived Illness Effects Item

Response	T2 diabetes (%)	T3 diabetes (%)	Breast cancer survivors (%)
1 (*all bad*)	1.6	2.4	2.2
2 (*mostly bad*)	5.6	5.6	4.9
3 (*some bad/good*)	69.0	70.2	23.5
4 (*mostly good*)	21.4	18.5	38.8
5 (*all good*)	2.4	3.2	30.6

Note. T2 = second annual interview; T3 = third annual interview; M for T2 diabetes = 3.17; M for T3 diabetes = 3.15; M for breast cancer survivors = 3.91; N for T2 diabetes = 126; N for T3 diabetes = 124; N for breast cancer survivors = 183.

OVERALL EFFECTS OF ILLNESS. At both T2 and T3, children were asked to think about the ways that diabetes affects their lives and to rate, using a 5-point scale, whether it has an overall good effect or a bad effect. As shown in Table 4.2, the average response was just above 3 at both assessments, indicating that the majority of respondents perceived the illness as having both good and bad effects. These findings are consistent with the mean level of benefits reported by Milam et al. (2004, 2005) when they used a response scale that ranged from negative to positive changes. However, the average score in our study and Milam's studies is lower than the average score found in a large group ($n = 240$) of 10-year disease-free breast cancer survivors who we recently interviewed. As shown in Table 4.2, the mean for the breast cancer survivors is substantially higher and skewed toward the positive side of the scale.

DOMAINS OF BENEFITS. We wanted to learn more about the areas in which adolescents with diabetes derived benefits. Therefore, we followed the T2 question with the following: "I want you to think about what might be good about diabetes. If someone your age was diagnosed with diabetes, what would you tell him or her was good about having diabetes, if anything?" Open-ended responses were coded into the nine categories shown in Table 4.3 by two independent raters. Inter-rater reliability was high (kappa = .90, $p < .01$). A third rater resolved the inconsistencies.

The most frequent response was in a category that we called "diabetes perks." These included responses such as missing school to go to the doctor and getting out of class to test blood sugar. The next most frequent response was "good health practices," which reflected behaviors in which respondents engaged to maintain or improve their health, such as eating a healthy diet and exercising. "Meet new people" was the third most frequently mentioned category, which reflected the opportunity to meet peers with diabetes, for example by attending diabetes camp. The fourth most frequent response was "more responsible," which reflected the idea that managing diabetes made a person more responsible. Only one respondent identified enhanced relationships as a benefit from diabetes. Just over one-quarter of respondents said that they could not name anything good about having diabetes. The majority of participants identified only one benefit (64%), but the number of benefits identified ranged from 0 to 4.

Table 4.3.   Domains of Benefits Identified at T2

Benefit	*N*	%
Diabetes perks (e.g., "eat stuff in class"; "get out of school")	37	29
Good health practices (e.g., "diet—watch what you eat"; "keeps weight on track")	34	27
Meet new people (e.g., "get to go to diabetes camp"; "a chance to meet a lot of new friends")	21	17
More responsible (e.g., "made me a more responsible person"; "makes you more mature")	13	10
Increased attention (e.g., "everybody's interested in you"; "get a lot more attention")	10	8
Understand body (e.g., "learn a lot about your body"; "realize how different parts of body work")	8	6
Improved relationships (e.g., "find out who your true friends are")	1	1
Miscellaneous	3	2
Could not name anything	33	26

Note.   Percentages add up to more than 100% because respondents could identify more than one benefit. T2 = second annual interview.

CREATION OF SCALE. We used the responses to the previously mentioned open-ended question to create a closed-ended Adolescent Benefit-Finding Scale (AD-BFS) that we administered at the next wave of assessment (T3). The scale consisted of 17 items, each of which was rated on a 5-point scale. Sample items included "Diabetes has made me a more responsible person" and "Diabetes has helped me to have a healthy diet." The overall internal consistency of the scale was .84. We examined whether the scale was unidimensional with principal component analysis followed by varimax rotation. Using the eigenvalue greater than 1.0 criterion, four factors emerged. One factor represented improved relationships, a second factor represented diabetes perks, a third factor reflected personal strength (e.g., being a more responsible person), and a fourth factor represented health benefits (e.g., exercise). We discarded two items because their content was less specific than the other items and they cross-loaded on multiple factors; that is, they did not fall neatly into a domain either empirically or conceptually.

The remaining 15 items that compose each of the four benefit-finding subscales are shown in Table 4.4. The correlations among the subscales ranged from moderate to null, supporting our decision to distinguish them. The Personal Strength subscale was related to the Health, Relationships, and Perks subscales ($r = .49$, $p < .001$; $r = .52$, $p < .001$; $r = .22$, $p < .05$). The Relationship subscale was related to the Health and Perks subscales ($r = .28$, $p < .001$; $r = .22$, $p < .05$), but the Health subscale was unrelated to the Perks subscale.

There also were significant differences in the level of benefits across the four domains as determined by a repeated measures analysis of variance, $F(3, 123) = 48.49$, $p < .001$. Within-subject contrasts revealed that all subscales differed significantly from one another at $p < .001$. As shown in the last column of Table 4.4, personal strengths were endorsed more than health benefits,

Table 4.4. Adolescent With Diabetes Benefit-Finding Scale

Subscale name	Alpha	Mean	SD
Personal Strength	.76	3.67	.64
Diabetes has made me a responsible person.			
Diabetes has made me a mature person.			
Diabetes has taught me to deal better with problems.			
Diabetes has made me a strong person.			
Health	.62	3.39	.71
Diabetes has helped me to keep my weight under control.			
Diabetes has helped me to have a healthy diet.			
Diabetes has helped me to exercise.			
Relationships	.78	3.13	.78
Diabetes has made me close to my family.			
Diabetes has helped me to determine who my true friends are.			
Diabetes has taught me that I can count on other people if I need help.			
Diabetes has made me close to my friends.			
Diabetes has taught me that other people care about me.			
Perks	.67	2.73	.89
Diabetes allows me to eat snacks in class when my sugar is low.			
Diabetes allows me to get special treatment.			
Diabetes gives me an excuse to get out of things.			

which were endorsed more than improved relationships, which in turn were endorsed more than perks. All means indicate a modest amount of growth.

Summary

In sum, when asked whether there was anything positive about diabetes, about three quarters of respondents identified a benefit. The vast majority identified only one benefit, and a sizeable number of participants were unable to identify a benefit, which is inconsistent with the finding reported by Oltjenbruns (1991). However, he interviewed a sample of older adolescents (ages 16–22 years). It is not clear whether our findings are related to the age of the children we interviewed or to the illness that we examined. Regardless, these findings call into question the practice of adapting item content generated by adults into scales for children and adolescents.

We also noticed several additional issues that warrant comment. First, participants who were unable to identify a benefit at T2 did not necessarily have a lower score on the T3 growth inventory. Second, respondents typically reported that the effects of diabetes on their lives were mixed, consisting of both positive and negative effects, consistent with the literature among adults.

The nature of the benefits adolescents with diabetes identified differed in a number of important ways from the benefits noted in the adult literature. The most frequent category of benefits was Perks. Perks were side benefits of having to take care of the illness, such as getting out of class and being able to eat snacks in school. Although perks may be a benefit from diabetes in literal terms, perks are not the kind of benefit that Tedeschi and Calhoun (1995) had in mind when they articulated their theory of posttraumatic growth following adversity. Perks do not reflect a way in which a person has grown following trauma. The Perks category may be unique to children and adolescents. Note that younger children were more likely than older ones to identify perks as a diabetes benefit. Although perks were the most frequent response named in response to the open-ended question, the Perks subscale received the lowest endorsement of the four benefit-finding subscales.

The second most frequently articulated category of benefits was "good health practices." This is a category of growth that is missing from typical adult inventories but has been noted as a serious omission in that literature (see chap. 6, this volume). In a study of women with breast cancer, Sears, Stanton, and Danoff-Burg (2003) observed that health benefits were commonly identified in response to an open-ended benefit-finding question. In our current research with 10-year survivors of breast cancer, we found that 47% of them identified changes in health behaviors as a long-lasting benefit of having been diagnosed and treated for breast cancer. Future research with children and adults should include this domain of benefits, at least when the stressful event involves a health threat.

There are several categories of benefits found in the adult literature that were rarely mentioned by adolescents with diabetes in response to the open-ended question. "Improved relationships" is a commonly cited benefit in the adult literature. It was the most common domain of growth in Yaskowich's (2005) study of children ages 8 to 25 years who had had cancer but the least common domain of growth in the Ickovics et al. (2006) study of urban adolescents ages 14 to 19 years who responded to a range of stressors. The adolescents in our study rarely mentioned improved relationships as a benefit of diabetes. The only category that emerged relevant to relationships was "meet new people." The opportunity to expand one's social network may be more salient to adolescents than the opportunity to improve existing relationships. In addition, peer relationships may be more relevant to adolescents than family relationships (Holmbeck et al., 2000), and, at that stage of life, peer relationships are in a state of flux. For many adolescents, it is possible that current relationships did not exist at the time the stressor occurred (i.e., when they were diagnosed). In those cases, adolescents would have difficulty reporting changes in relationships. Thus, relationship change may be an area of growth more relevant to adults than adolescents.

Adolescents also may be more focused on the potential for their illness to have negative rather than positive effects on relationships. Adhering to the diabetes regimen forces adolescents to behave differently from their peers at a time when they want to fit in. Any stressful life event has the potential to set adolescents apart from their peers. A healthy adolescent is concerned with being rejected by peers. These fears may be intensified among adolescents with a chronic illness, such as diabetes. Thus, it may be important to distinguish the effects of illness on peer versus other relationships when studying children and adolescents.

A common domain of growth in the adult literature is enhanced feelings of personal strength. A kind of personal strength noted by adolescents with diabetes was the "more responsible" domain. Adolescents with diabetes have to engage in a number of self-care behaviors on a regular basis, which includes monitoring diet, testing blood sugar, and administering insulin multiple times a day. Tending to all of these behaviors has the potential to make one a more responsible person. It is not clear from our data, however, how prominent this domain of growth is. Although only 10% of respondents spontaneously articulated this benefit, the Personal Strength subscale was the most highly endorsed on the AD-BFS. There are several possible explanations for this discrepancy. One possibility is that personal strength is something adolescents with diabetes perceive but fail to articulate when asked an open-ended question. Alternatively, personal strength may not be something that adolescents with diabetes perceive as a benefit from their illness, but they endorse it on a questionnaire because of demand characteristics. Adolescents may be familiar with the idea of gaining strength from adversity because social network members (e.g., parents, physicians) have told them that they are stronger for having had to face diabetes. We will return to this point later in the chapter.

None of the respondents gave responses that would fit into the commonly assessed domains of appreciation of life or spirituality noted among adults. Several studies of children suggested that appreciation of life was a common domain of growth. Ickovics et al. (2006) found the highest amount of growth in the appreciation of life domain. Oltjenbruns (1991) found that appreciation of life was the most commonly reported benefit of the seven assessed. Salter and Stallard (2004) found that appreciation of life was the most common spontaneous response. And Barakat et al. (2006) found that the most common area of positive change was the way adolescents thought about their life. Appreciation of life may not be a salient benefit of diabetes. Although diabetes can pose a life threat, the threat is typically not imminent. That is, the costs of not taking care of diabetes on a regular basis are more likely to be realized in adulthood in terms of damage to eyes, kidneys, nerves, and blood vessels (The Diabetes Control and Complications Trial Research Group, 1993). These costs may not be readily apparent to youth with diabetes. Appreciation of life also may be a less common form of growth from diabetes because the majority of participants experienced illness onset many years earlier. Adolescents in this study were diagnosed with diabetes between 1 and 13 years earlier when first enrolled in this study. In fact, 43% of adolescents were unable to recall life before diabetes. There may need to be a more definitive adverse event in recent memory for appreciation of life to occur.

We conclude that the benefits that children and adolescents identify, at least in response to diabetes, are not the ones reflected in adult inventories. To the extent that these findings generalize across other childhood illnesses or stressful events, adapting adult inventories for use with adolescents may be misleading. Adolescents identify benefits that are more concrete than those identified by adults. This may be due to their cognitive level of development. With age comes an increase in abstract thinking. Next, we examine the link of age to growth.

Relationship Between Age and Growth

Existing Literature

It is not clear that growth increases with age. Of six studies that examined the relation between age and benefit finding, two found a positive relation (Milam et al., 2004; Salter & Stallard, 2004), one found a negative relation (Laufer & Solomon, 2006), and three found no relation (Barakat et al., 2006; Pakenham & Bursnall, 2006; Phipps et al., 2007).

Adolescents With Diabetes

Age was not related to whether someone identified a benefit of diabetes or to the number of benefits identified. However, age was related to the kind of benefit identified. Children who identified perks were younger ($M = 12.86$, $SD = .64$) than children who did not ($M = 13.27$, $SD = .80$), $t(125) = 2.78$, $p < .01$. By contrast, children who identified health benefits were older ($M = 13.51$, $SD = .87$) than children who did not ($M = 13.02$, $SD = .71$), $t(125) = -3.27$, $p = .01$. When asked about the effects of diabetes on one's life (the question in Table 4.2), age was not related to T2 responses but was related to T3 responses: Older participants perceived the illness as having more negative effects, $r = -.22$, $p < .05$. Age was not related to the AD-BFS.

We found little evidence that age is related to more growth. Instead, we found that older adolescents were more likely to perceive their illness in negative rather than in positive terms. This is not due to older adolescents having experienced the illness for a longer time, because age is unrelated to length of illness in this sample. Older adolescents may be more bothered by having to take care of their illness on a daily basis. They may be especially likely to perceive the illness as intruding on their independence and interfering with peer relationships. As these youth move into older adolescence, some of the negative effects may dissipate and opportunities for growth could emerge. We found that age was related to the kinds of benefits identified, with younger adolescents identifying perks and older adolescents noting positive effects on health. The nature of benefits perceived may further change with age. We anticipate that categories of growth will become more abstract as adolescents get older, reflective of those found on adult inventories.

Origins of Benefit Finding

One question that the adult literature on benefit finding has failed to embrace is the source of benefits or growth. Is the propensity to derive benefits from adversity a dispositional characteristic? Are there characteristics of the stressful life event such as severity and recency that affect children's tendency to derive benefits? How does the social environment contribute to stress-related growth among children? We address each of these questions in the sections that follow.

Resilient Personality

A variety of personality characteristics that imply resilience have been linked to benefit finding among adults, including optimism, religiosity, and the tendency to engage in positive reappraisal (Helgeson, Reynolds, & Tomich, 2006). Despite these findings, studies of benefit finding among adolescents and children have rarely examined the role of personality. Two studies examined optimism, both finding that those higher in optimism tended to report more benefits (Milam et al., 2005; Phipps et al., 2007). The latter study also found a positive relation between benefit finding and self-esteem. Three studies (Laufer & Solomon, 2006; Milam et al., 2004, 2005) found that children and adolescents who identified with a religion or who considered themselves to be more religious reported more benefits. Two studies examined the relation of self-efficacy to growth, one finding no relation (Yaskowich, 2005) and one finding that growth was related to self-efficacy in regard to coping (Cryder et al., 2006).

We had two variables in the study of adolescents with diabetes that were relevant to the construct of a resilient personality. Higher self-worth was related to perceiving more positive effects of diabetes (see Table 4.2) at T2, $r = .32$, $p < .001$, and T3, $r = .35$, $p < .001$. Higher self-worth also was related to higher scores on the AD-BFS, $r = .33$, $p < .001$. Second, we measured self-efficacy with respect to diabetes (i.e., confidence that one could adhere to the diabetes regimen). Diabetes self-efficacy was related to perceiving more positive effects of the illness at T2, $r = .22$, $p < .05$, and marginally at T3, $r = .17$, $p < .10$, but was not related to the AD-BFS. Although there are few data that bear on this question, the data that do exist are consistent with the possibility that the ability to derive benefits from trauma is part of a constellation of resilient personality characteristics in children.

Characteristics of the Stressor

The possibility also exists that the stressful life event inspires growth. Some stressors may be more beneficial than others, and some features of the stressor, such as how long ago it occurred and how severe it is, may activate growth.

DURATION OF STRESSOR. Tedeschi and Calhoun's (1995) theory of post-traumatic growth seems to suggest that growth takes time to occur. That is, people need time to process the event, consider its impact on their lives, and find ways of altering their lives for the better after the event has occurred. An alternative view of growth is that people report benefits in response to distress (C. L. Park & Helgeson, 2006). To the extent that people are more distressed when an event first occurs, one may observe higher benefit scores when one is more proximal to the stressor. The meta-analytic review of the adult literature revealed no relation between time since event and growth. Among children, only three studies examined this relation. Two studies found no relation (Barakat et al., 2006; Milam et al., 2004), and the third found that more benefits were reported when a shorter time since the event had passed (Phipps et al., 2007). However, in the latter study, time since diagnosis was confounded with age at diagnosis (i.e., longer time since diagnosis equaled younger age at diagnosis), and younger age at diagnosis was associated with fewer benefits. Barakat et al. (2006) also found that younger age at cancer diagnosis was associated with less growth.

We examined the extent to which length of illness was associated with benefits in adolescents with diabetes. Length of illness was not associated with whether someone identified a benefit, the number of benefits identified in response to the open-ended question, the overall effects of the illness on one's life question, or AD-BFS scores.

THREAT SEVERITY. A second characteristic of the stressor that could be related to benefit finding is threat severity. The meta-analytic review of the adult literature showed that both perceived threat severity and objective threat severity were related to more growth (Helgeson, Reynolds, & Tomich, 2006). Three studies of children support this finding. In one study of adolescents with cancer, those who perceived greater threat reported more benefits (Barakat et al., 2006). In another study of children with cancer, more cognitive and physical impairments and perceptions of more severe disease were related to more growth (Yaskowich, 2005). In the study of Israeli youth, growth scores were associated with objective threat severity (i.e., experiencing more terror incidents) and subjective threat severity (i.e., greater fear during terror incidents; Laufer & Solomon, 2006). However, S. Park (2006) found no relation between growth and the severity of stressors adolescents reported. In the study of child caregivers, Pakenham and Bursnall (2006) found equivocal support; benefits were unrelated to parent functional impairment or perceived stress of having to care for a parent, but more benefits were reported when the parent had an additional disability beyond MS. We did not have a measure of perceived threat in our study. One could consider metabolic control to indicate the severity of the illness, or at least the current state of the illness. However, metabolic control was unrelated to any of our measures of benefit finding.

Social Environment

Researchers have rarely examined the extent to which the social environment contributes to growth (see chap. 8, this volume). As with the adult literature, studies of benefit finding among children and adolescents have rarely examined the role of social support. Two studies noted a positive relation. Yaskowich (2005) found that total social support predicted more benefit finding, but noted that no single source of social support (e.g., parents, friends, teachers, classmates) was a significant predictor. Milam et al. (2005) found that greater discussion of the event with network members was associated with more benefit finding. Although this is not a direct measure of social support, it may suggest that the use of social support can lead to growth. In fact, Pakenham and Bursnall (2006) found that benefit finding was related to seeking support but was unrelated to the number of support providers or support satisfaction. S. Park (2006) found no relation between growth and social resources, which included community and neighborhood involvement and religion.

There are a number of reasons why social support could contribute to growth. First, the link may be direct in that support network members could identify possible positive outcomes from a stressful life event. In the case of children, parents may point out personal strengths gained or improvements in relationships as a way to help their children cope with stressful events. A study of parents of teenage girls with diabetes showed that parents perceive that their children benefit from the illness, most notably by becoming more responsible (Mellin, Neumark-Sztainer, & Patterson, 2004). As children are repeatedly exposed to these suggestions of growth, they may come to recognize events or qualities that confirm growth. That is, parents may suggest areas of growth that could be adopted and internalized by the child. To address this issue, we developed a Parental Facilitation of Benefits scale in our study of children with diabetes and administered it at T3. Sample items included, "How often do your parents point out the positive aspects of diabetes?"; "How often do your parents tell you that you are a stronger person for having diabetes?"; and "How often do your parents tell you that you are actually healthier because of your diabetes?" Parent support for benefit finding was not related to the overall effects of the illness question but was related to higher scores on the AD-BFS, $r = .48, p < .001$.

Second, children who live in an overall supportive environment might be more likely to have the resources to construe benefits from adversity. Thus, we examined the link between benefit finding and perceptions of general parent support. Parent support was not related to the overall effects of the illness but was related to higher scores on the AD-BFS, $r = .28, p < .001$.

Finally, parents might provide a role model for deriving benefits from adversity. To the extent that children learn to do the same, parent and child growth should be correlated. In our study of children with diabetes, we administered a benefit-finding scale to parents, which reflected their ability to derive personal benefits from having a child with diabetes. We found no relation between parents' personal growth and children's personal growth. Yaskowich (2005) also compared both parent and child reports of growth and found no relation. She argued that benefit finding might be an internal experience to which other people do not have access. In fact, she noted that less than half of the children in her study were aware of their parents' personal growth.

Whether adolescents perceived the illness as having an overall positive or negative effect on their lives was not related to parent facilitation of benefits or overall parental support. However, there was a strong relation between parent facilitation of benefits and adolescents' AD-BFS scores, and a modest relation between general parent support and adolescents' AD-BFS scores. There was no relation between parents' and adolescents' personal growth. Thus, the link between the social environment and adolescent growth may be more explicit than implicit. That is, parents may be a source of children's growth to the extent that they articulate ways in which the child has grown from the illness. It is interesting to note that the relation between parent benefit-finding support and adolescent benefit finding became stronger with age and longer length of illness. With time, adolescents have more opportunities to be exposed to their parents' ideas and more time to internalize those ideas. Future research should aim to determine whether parent facilitation of benefit finding leads adolescents to internalize those benefits.

Relation of Benefit Finding to Health Outcomes

As noted at the outset of the chapter, the meta-analytic review of the adult literature (Helgeson, Reynolds, & Tomich, 2006) revealed that benefit finding was related to some health outcomes but not to others and that the relations that did emerge were not always consistent. Here we review the literature on benefit finding and well-being in children and then report on the relations we found in our own data on children with diabetes.

Existing Literature

Of the 14 studies of children and adolescents, 8 measured well-being and found relations to benefit finding to be inconsistent. Two studies showed no relations of benefit finding to distress. A study of Hispanic adolescents coping with a stressful event revealed no relation linking benefit finding to depression (Milam et al., 2004), and a study of child survivors of a traffic accident showed no relation of benefit finding to PTSD classification (Salter & Stallard, 2004). A study of children with cancer showed that benefit finding was not related to posttraumatic stress or health-related quality of life, but was related to reduced anxiety (Phipps et al., 2007). Two studies showed that benefit finding was related to greater posttraumatic stress: a study of adolescents with a history of cancer (Barakat et al., 2006) and a study of adolescents exposed to terror (Laufer & Solomon, 2006).

Finally, three studies showed benefit finding to be related to less distress. A study of adolescents after the September 11th terrorist attacks showed that benefit finding was associated with less anxiety and less depression (Milam et al., 2005). A prospective study of adolescents found that growth predicted a decline in distress when controlling for pre-event levels (Ickovics et al., 2006). And a third study of child caregivers to parents with MS showed that benefit finding was related to less psychological distress (Pakenham & Bursnall, 2006). However, when a larger number of child caregivers were examined, that relation disappeared (Pakenham, Chiu, Bursnall, & Cannon, 2007). Yet, benefit finding was related to greater positive affect in both samples. Two studies also linked benefit finding to lower substance use (Milam et al., 2004, 2005). Thus, like the adult literature, the relation of benefit finding to health outcomes is mixed.

Adolescents With Diabetes

We examined the relation of benefit finding to psychological and physical health among adolescents with diabetes. Whether or not someone identified a benefit at T2 was not related to any of the health outcomes we assessed (i.e., depressive symptoms, anxiety, anger, self-care behavior, and metabolic control). However, identifying more benefits was related to more depressive symptoms, $r = .19$, $p < .05$, more anger, $r = .19$, $p < .05$, and worse self-care behavior, $r = -.19$, $p < .05$.

The overall effects question that we administered at T2 and T3 was related to several health outcomes. As shown in the first column of Table 4.5,

Table 4.5. Relation of Growth Scales to Health Outcomes

Health outcomes	T2 positive effects	T3 positive effects	AD-BFS total	AD-BFS Strength	AD-BFS Health	AD-BFS Relationships	AD-BFS Perks
Depression	-.25**	-.26**	-.13	-.19*	-.12	-.07	.02
Anxiety	-.18*	-.16†	.02	.01	.09	-.01	.00
Anger	-.03	-.26**	-.06	-.08	-.13	-.03	.06
Self-care	.12	.20*	.12	.14	.20*	.08	-.12
Metabolic control	.05	-.17†	-.11	-.12	-.10	-.09	.02

Note. T2 = second annual interview; T3 = third annual interview; AD-BFS = Adolescent Benefit-Finding Scale.
†p < .10. *p < .05. **p < .01. ***p < .001.

perceived positive effects were related to fewer depressive symptoms and less anxiety at T2. Relations were stronger at T3: Perceived positive effects were related to fewer depressive symptoms, less anger, better self-care, and, marginally, to less anxiety and better metabolic control. However, the AD-BFS was not related to any outcome at T3 (see Table 4.5). When specific subscales were examined, personal strength was related to less depression, and the Health subscale was related to better self-care. The Relationships subscale and the Perks subscale were not related to any of the outcomes. In summary, within the same study, we found different relations of benefit finding to outcomes, depending on the specific measures used.

Summary

We noted at the outset of the chapter that findings regarding the links of benefits to health in the adult literature are mixed. Our findings regarding the relation of benefits to health among children and adolescents also were mixed. We measured benefits in a variety of ways and obtained a variety of findings. Whether or not someone identified a benefit of diabetes was not related to any health outcome, although identifying more benefits was associated with more distress (i.e., depressive symptoms and anger) and worse self-care. By contrast, perceiving the illness in positive terms was related to good health outcomes (i.e., less distress and better self-care). Finally, benefit-finding inventory scores were not related to any outcome.

In some ways, these results are not surprising, because we found only modest overlap among our measures of benefit finding. Sears et al. (2003) also examined benefit finding from a variety of perspectives and found that their measures tapped distinct but related constructs. The modest relation we found between the perceived illness effects question and the benefit-finding scale is consistent with Thornton's (2002) point that finding benefits does not imply the absence of negative stressor effects. The inconsistent relations of benefit finding to health outcomes in this study may reflect the idea that deriving benefits from adversity is accompanied by positive as well as negative changes.

Although the benefit-finding inventory that we created was not associated with any health outcomes, it was correlated with a personality characteristic that is often conceptualized as an outcome: high self-esteem. This finding is consistent with the results from the recent meta-analytic review of benefit finding among adults (Helgeson, Reynolds, & Tomich, 2006) that showed that benefit-finding scales were most strongly related to positive affect outcomes, including high self-esteem. These findings underscore the possibility that deriving benefits from adversity may be an outcome in and of itself that is distinct from other psychological health outcomes that focus on negative sequelae.

Overall Summary and Conclusions

The results from our study concur with the existing literature that children and adolescents derive some benefits from adversity. Although the magnitude or number of benefits differed across studies, most children found some benefits from the stressful life events they experienced. We found that more than 75% of adolescents with diabetes were able to identify at least one benefit from their illness. However, it is perhaps more interesting that a quarter of respondents were unable to identify a benefit. The young age of our respondents is a likely contributor to the lower than expected reports of growth. With age comes an increase in abstract thinking, an increase in life experiences, and more future-oriented thinking. The literature is unclear as to whether age is associated with growth reports. It was not in our study, although we had a restricted age range. We suggest that future research examine indicators of cognitive maturity rather than relying on age alone as an indicator of maturity (Wysocki et al., 1996).

Our findings highlight not only that children and adolescents are less likely to report benefits from adversity but also that the benefits they do report are not the same as those reported by adults. The domains of benefits identified by the adolescents in our study differed from those examined in previous studies. One way in which our research differs from much of the previous literature is that we provided adolescents with the opportunity to identify the domain of growth. Consistent with other studies, adolescents with diabetes frequently endorsed items suggesting some kind of personal growth. However, unlike previous research, adolescents with diabetes were unlikely to identify growth in the areas of appreciation of life and enhanced relationships. We suggest that future research with children and adolescents allow participants to discuss areas of growth in a more unstructured manner before administering any kind of growth inventory. We need to know more about the domains of growth and the benefits of stressors that are perceived by youth.

One issue that we examined in this chapter that has not been examined in past research is the source of benefit finding. Consistent with research among adults, we found strong evidence that the ability to derive benefits from adversity may be part of a constellation of resilient personality characteristics. However, we also found that the social environment may play an important role in growth. Among adolescents with diabetes, we found that those individuals whose parents provided support for benefit finding were more likely to report growth. We also found that this relation was stronger for older adolescents and adolescents who had had the illness for some time. Furthermore, general parental support was associated with higher growth scores. The process by which parents facilitate benefit finding needs to be explored in future research. How much exposure to benefits is needed before children begin to internalize them? And, are they truly internalizing the benefits or just mimicking what parents have said?

The relation of benefit finding to health is mixed in the adult literature, child literature, and in the study we presented. The inconsistencies across studies and across benefit-finding measures have led researchers to call into question the validity of growth measures (C. L. Park & Helgeson, 2006). Children's reports of benefits suffer from some of the same problems as those of adults. Reports of benefit finding may be artificially inflated because of demand characteristics (e.g., see Nolen-Hoeksema & Davis, 2004; Tomich & Helgeson, 2004). That is, people assume that they are supposed to have benefited when provided with a list of possible benefits contained on typical inventories. The old adage, "What doesn't kill you makes you stronger," is part of Western culture. However, children who face a stressful event might be less familiar with this idea and, therefore, less vulnerable to these demand characteristics. One way to deal with the response bias issue is to ask open-ended questions about change. When we did this, we found that a sizeable number of respondents (26%) reported no growth. In addition, adolescents tended to generate more superficial benefits, such as perks, rather than areas of growth, such as personal strength.

One way to address response bias is to administer a set of neutral items and ask respondents whether the domain changed for the better or the worse. It interesting to note that the two studies of children that used this kind of response scale (Barakat et al., 2006; Milam et al., 2004, 2005) found much smaller indications of growth. Using a scale in which one end represents negative change and the other positive change is not without problems, however. This response scale assumes that a person cannot experience both positive and negative change within the same domain. This is clearly problematic as the majority of children with diabetes said the illness was associated with both positive and negative effects.

There are arguments as to why children might be more or less vulnerable to the demand characteristic to report more growth than actually experienced. On the one hand, children are known to be especially concerned with adult approval, making them more vulnerable to demand characteristics in the presence of adults. On the other hand, children may be less familiar with the idea of benefiting from adversity and, thus, less susceptible to this particular demand characteristic.

One piece of evidence from our study of children with diabetes suggests that children are less vulnerable than adults to this response bias. When we factor analyzed the growth inventory, we obtained four distinct domains of benefits. Although distinct domains of benefits are reflected in the content of adult inventories, many studies have failed to empirically identify distinct domains through factor analysis and instead use a unidimensional scale (e.g., see Tomich & Helgeson, 2004). This has led researchers to be concerned that there is a response bias leading people to endorse all benefits or none, without paying attention to the distinctions among the domains. That our participants distinguished among domains gives some credibility to the idea that they were considering the unique effects of diabetes on their lives.

Before concluding, we must note that some unique aspects of our study may make our findings difficult to reconcile with previous research. Because diabetes is a chronic illness, adolescents may be unlikely to identify more abstract domains, such as religion or life appreciation, because they do not view their illness as a life-changing event but, rather, as an ongoing stressor with which they must live.

However, chronicity probably interacts with severity. An acute stressor that is severe, such as the death of a parent, may be more likely to lead to life changes than a chronic stressor that is less severe, such as asthma or diabetes. A stressful event that is high in threat severity and chronic, such as cancer, may lead to the most change.

We interviewed adolescents who had been diagnosed with diabetes between 1 and 13 years earlier. Although the disease diagnosis may have been a traumatic event, it is difficult to know whether participants perceive diabetes in this way years later. Some participants were diagnosed with diabetes when they were young and could not recall a time when they did not have diabetes. For those participants, it may have been especially difficult to make judgments about the impact that diabetes had had on their lives. A similar concern has been raised by other studies. Two studies of children with cancer showed that those who had been diagnosed at an earlier age reported low levels of growth (Barakat et al., 2006; Phipps et al., 2007). Similarly, the adolescents with diabetes in our study who had had the disease for a longer period of time were less likely to name health benefits. If adolescents cannot compare their situations pre- and postdiabetes, it will be difficult to notice a change in behavior. Areas of benefit finding such as personal strength and perks may have been more salient to the adolescents in our study because they can derive these by comparison with peers. Getting out of school and eating snacks are activities that are likely to be salient to adolescents because they distinguish them from their peer group.

Future Directions

Taken collectively, the findings from this review raise more questions than provide definitive answers. There is clearly a need for more research on benefit finding among children and adolescents. Future research should continue to explore benefit finding with qualitative measures rather than relying on inventories of benefits that may be less relevant to children's lives. Future research also should measure aspects of personality that are relevant to benefit finding, to get a better indication of what aspect of this process can be attributed to personality variables and what aspect of it is driven by the situation, the traumatic event. Future research should examine how the different dimensions of stressful life events, such as chronicity and controllability affect growth.

People may be more likely to derive benefits from events that they perceive as uncontrollable. As such, future research should continue to explore how the social environment contributes to benefit finding. If researchers regard deriving benefits from adversity as a positive outcome, it is important to know how this process evolves during childhood and adolescence.

References

Aldwin, C. M., & Sutton, K. J. (1998). A developmental perspective on posttraumatic growth. In R. G. Tedeschi, C. L. Park, & L. G. Calhoun (Eds.), *Posttraumatic growth: Positive changes in the aftermath of crisis* (pp. 43–63). Mahwah, NJ: Erlbaum.

Barakat, L. P., Alderfer, M. A., & Kazak, A. E. (2006). Posttraumatic growth in adolescent survivors of cancer and their mothers and fathers. *Journal of Pediatric Psychology, 31*, 413–419.

Cryder, C. H., Kilmer, R. P., Tedeschi, R. G., & Calhoun, L. G. (2006). An exploratory study of posttraumatic growth in children following a natural disaster. *American Journal of Orthopsychiatry, 76*, 65–69.

Diabetes Control and Complications Trial Research Group. (1993). The effect of intensive treatment of diabetes on the development and progression of long-term complications in insulin-dependent diabetes mellitus. *The New England Journal of Medicine, 329*, 977–986.

Helgeson, V. S., Reynolds, K. A., & Tomich, P. L. (2006). A meta-analytic review of benefit finding and growth. *Journal of Consulting and Clinical Psychology, 74,* 797–816.

Helgeson, V. S., Viccaro, L., Becker, D., Escobar, O., & Siminerio, L. (2006). Diet of adolescents with and without diabetes: Trading candy for potato chips? *Diabetes Care, 29,* 982–987.

Holmbeck, G. N., Colder, C., Shapera, W., Westhoven, V., Kenealy, L., & Updegrove, A. (2000). Working with adolescents: Guides from developmental psychology. In P. C. Kendall (Ed.), *Child and adolescent therapy: Cognitive behavioral procedures* (2nd ed., pp. 334–385). New York: Guilford Press.

Ickovics, J. R., Meade, C. S., Kershaw, T. S., Milan, S., Lewis, J. B., & Ethier, K. A. (2006). Urban teens: Trauma, posttraumatic growth, and emotional distress among female adolescents. *Journal of Consulting and Clinical Psychology, 74,* 841–850.

Kazak, A. E., Stuber, M. L., Barakat, L. P., & Meeske, K. (1996). Assessing posttraumatic stress related to medical illness and treatment: The impact of traumatic stressors interview schedule (ITSIS). *Families, Systems, & Health, 14,* 365–380.

Kilmer, R. (2006). Resilience and posttraumatic growth in children. In L. G. Calhoun & R. G. Tedeschi (Eds.), *Handbook of posttraumatic growth: Research and practice* (pp. 264–288). Mahwah, NJ: Erlbaum.

Laufer, A., & Solomon, Z. (2006). Posttraumatic symptoms and posttraumatic growth among Israeli youth exposed to terror incidents. *Journal of Social and Clinical Psychology, 25,* 429–447.

Lepore, S., & Revenson, T. (2006). Relationships between posttraumatic growth and resilience: Recovery, resistance, and reconfiguration. In L. G. Calhoun & R. G. Tedeschi (Eds.), *Handbook of posttraumatic growth: Research and practice* (pp. 24–46). Mahwah, NJ: Erlbaum.

Mellin, A. E., Neumark-Sztainer, D., & Patterson, J. M. (2004). Parenting adolescent girls with Type 1 diabetes: Parents' perspectives. *Journal of Pediatric Psychology, 29,* 221–230.

Milam, J. E., Ritt-Olson, A., Tan, S., Unger, J. B., & Nezami, E. (2005). The September 11th, 2001 terrorist attacks and reports of posttraumatic growth among a multi-ethnic sample of adolescents. *Traumatology, 11,* 233–246.

Milam, J. E., Ritt-Olson, A., & Unger, J. B. (2004). Posttraumatic growth among adolescents. *Journal of Adolescent Research, 19,* 192–204.

Nolen-Hoeksema, S., & Davis, C. G. (2004). Theoretical and methodological issues in the assessment and interpretation of posttraumatic growth. *Psychological Inquiry, 15,* 60–65.

Oltjenbruns, K. A. (1991). Positive outcomes of adolescents' experience with grief. *Journal of Adolescent Research, 6,* 43–53.

Pakenham, K. I., & Bursnall, S. (2006). Relations between social support, appraisal and coping and both positive and negative outcomes for children of a parent with multiple sclerosis and comparisons with children of healthy parents. *Clinical Rehabilitation, 20,* 709–723.

Pakenham, K. I., Chiu, J., Bursnall, S., & Cannon, T. (2007). Relations between social support, appraisal and coping and both positive and negative outcomes in young carers. *Journal of Health Psychology, 12,* 89–102.

Park, C. L., & Helgeson, V. S. (2006). Growth following highly stressful events: Current status and future directions. *Journal of Consulting and Clinical Psychology, 74,* 791–796.

Park, S. (2006). *Exposure to community violence and aggressive beliefs in adolescents: Role of posttraumatic growth and developmental resources.* Unpublished doctoral dissertation, Fuller Theological Seminary, Pasadena, CA.

Phipps, S., Long, A. M., & Ogden, J. (2007). Benefit finding scale for children: Preliminary findings from a childhood cancer population. *Journal of Pediatric Psychology, 32,* 1264–1271.

Salter, E., & Stallard, P. (2004). Posttraumatic growth in child survivors of a road traffic accident. *Journal of Traumatic Stress, 17,* 335–340.

Sears, S. R., Stanton, A. L., & Danoff-Burg, S. (2003). The Yellow Brick Road and the Emerald City: Benefit finding, positive reappraisal coping and posttraumatic growth in women with early-stage breast cancer. *Health Psychology, 22,* 487–497.

Tedeschi, R. G., & Calhoun, L. G. (1995). *Trauma and transformation: Growing in the aftermath of suffering.* Thousand Oaks, CA: Sage.

Tedeschi, R. G., & Calhoun, L. G. (1996). The Posttraumatic Growth Inventory: Measuring the positive legacy of trauma. *Journal of Traumatic Stress, 9,* 455–471.

Thornton, A. A. (2002). Perceiving benefits in the cancer experience. *Journal of Clinical Psychology in Medical Settings, 9,* 153–165.

Tomich, P. L., & Helgeson, V. S. (2004). Is finding something good in the bad always good? Benefit finding among women with breast cancer. *Health Psychology, 23,* 16–23.

Wysocki, T., Taylor, A., Hough, B. S., Linscheid, T. R., Yeates, K. O., & Naglieri, J. A. (1996). Deviation from developmentally appropriate self-care autonomy: Association with diabetes outcomes. *Diabetes Care, 19,* 119–125.

Yaskowich, K. M. (2005). *Posttraumatic growth in children and adolescents with cancer.* Unpublished doctoral dissertation, University of Calgary, Calgary, Alberta, Canada.

5

Life Span Developmental Perspectives on Stress-Related Growth

Carolyn M. Aldwin, Michael R. Levenson, and Linda Kelly

Stress-related growth (SRG) addresses positive change in psychological and biological processes, and therefore it is inherently a developmental topic. Much of the research in this area has been conducted by health psychology researchers and clinicians, often in disease-related contexts, and usually does not include a developmental focus. However, many of the issues that are currently being debated about the nature, duration, and extent of change echo similar debates in the field of life span developmental psychology (see Aldwin & Levenson, 2004). Thus, we believe that the fields of health psychology and SRG may benefit from a life span developmental perspective, which is the primary purpose of this chapter. Specifically, pediatric behavioral medicine studies often need to focus on the developmental level and skills of patients. Similarly, older adults are likely to be the participants in studies of patients with chronic illnesses, such as heart disease and cancer. Understanding the processes of adult development and the factors that promote it, even in the context of chronic or life-threatening illness, may have both scientific and practical applications. Older adults are generally the ones facing chronic illnesses, and understanding the developmental tasks that they face, and how illness complicates these tasks, may help in promoting SRG in later life.

To that end, we provide a brief synopsis of different approaches to conceptualizing change in adulthood and then link the concept of SRG to these different developmental perspectives on positive development. Specifically, we frame our discussion in terms of the dialectic between loss and growth, as well as review some of the literature on whether SRG processes change with age. We also examine the personal and contextual issues which moderate this phenomenon. Unlike some of the other chapters in this book, we do not focus on a particular illness but rather on the importance of loss for development, especially within the context of major illness. As noted by Moos and Schaefer (1984), a major task facing those with chronic illness is coping with loss of specific physical capacities or a positive, youthful self-image. Sometimes, the severity of the illness results in the loss of work or relationships, or precludes future possibilities for what Hooker and McAdams (2003) called "desirable possible selves." Eventually, loss of life itself may need to be faced.

Our contention is that adult development, and SRG in particular, often stems from coping with loss; thus, this process can be seen in multiple disease contexts. Understanding this process in general may help to inform the process of SRG with specific illnesses.

Perspectives on Change in Adulthood

A Brief Primer on Life Span Developmental Theories

Traditional debates in life span developmental theory have involved hypotheses based on two models of development, ontogenetic and sociogenic change (see Levenson & Crumpler, 1996). Briefly, ontogenetic developmental theories argue that there are systematic changes within individuals that reflect inherent developmental, or age-related, processes. Early proponents of this theory, such as Erikson (1950) and Kohlberg (1984), argued that developmental stages reflect discontinuous or qualitative shifts that are sequential, irreversible, invariant, and universal. That is, these stages build on one another in the same manner in all individuals regardless of culture or gender. Erikson posited eight stages, each of which involves a developmental dialectic. Three of these occur in adulthood: intimacy versus isolation in young adulthood, generativity versus stagnation in midlife, and ego integrity versus despair in late life. The struggle with these developmental dialectics formed the background for transitions through stages, with the resolution of each forming the context for the next.

Similarly, Kohlberg (1984) argued that a set of stages informed the development of moral reasoning, which not all individuals traversed in adulthood but which nonetheless formed the developmental matrix. Most individuals remain at Stage 4, the conventional or social conformity stage, but there are three additional postconventional stages in adulthood: social contract, principled, and moral transcendence (Kohlberg, 1984; Kohlberg & Ryncarz, 1990).

Sociologists such as Neugarten (1969) and Dannefer (1984) criticized the ontogenetic approach, arguing that change in adulthood follows the sociocultural patterning of social roles, and that there was no inherent sequence of stages. This sociogenic or life course development approach argued that there were no developmental stages in adulthood but that there were simply changes that varied as a function of the age-graded relinquishment and acquisition of social roles that were informed by one's gender, social status, and culture. Thus, people change, not because of inherent developmental processes but as a function of taking on parenting roles and relinquishing child roles, taking on worker roles and relinquishing student roles, and so forth. The behaviors exhibited in these roles are governed by social mores. Furthermore, there may be cohort differences in life experiences, and it is not possible to determine from cross-sectional studies whether any age-related differences reflect developmental or cohort influences. For example, a developmental explanation of lower levels of depressive symptoms in older adults might be that their greater life experience leads to better mental health than younger adults. A cohort explanation would be that younger cohorts may report more depressive symptoms, either because of a decrease in stigmatization of mental illness across cohorts or because younger cohorts are genuinely more distressed (see Twenge, 2000).

Thus, in many ways, a life course perspective (LCP) takes a diametrically opposed approach to that taken by ontogenetic theories. Instead of universal goals, LCP focuses on individual differences in preferred goal outcomes. Change is seen as probabilistic rather than inevitable, and plastic rather than irreversible. Individual trajectories are emphasized over sequential stages, and change is seen as quantitative (i.e., gradual and continuous), rather than qualitative or sudden shifts in organization (see Lerner, 2002). For contemporary views of the LCP, see Elder and Shanahan (2006) and Settersten (2006).

There have been various attempts at reconciling these two views, the most notable of which is developmental systems theory (DST; Ford & Lerner, 1992; Lerner, Theokas, & Jelicic, 2005). Proponents of DST have argued that development did occur in adulthood but that it was influenced by a variety of biological, personal, and social factors. DST adopts the hallmark of plasticity and probability of change and set the stage for the empirical examination of individual trajectories. However, unlike the earlier theories, DST does not posit an ultimate goal or telos, but argues that goals varied by personal predilection and sociocultural influence. Nonetheless, most developmental theories focus on gains in positive characteristics, such as mastery and integrity (Ryff, 1989). In fact, many of the SRG-related changes in values, social relations, coping and mastery, turning points, and spiritual development (see Tedeschi & Calhoun, 2004) are similar to those posited by developmental theorists. Thus, in the next sections we review the similarities and differences between SRG and life span developmental theories.

VALUES. Whereas early developmental theorists such as Buhler, Massarik, and Bugental (1968) sought to develop a life span perspective focused on values, more recent theorists have emphasized changes in goal structure. Brandstädter (1999) described this as a change from assimilative to accommodative goals such that individuals shift from seeking to change their external circumstances to seeking to change themselves to accommodate the loss of control brought about by stressful demands such as illness. In the SRG literature, value changes are more generally framed as changes in priorities (e.g., the importance of family or health), as well as a greater appreciation of life. However, changes in the importance of family and health with age are well documented in the life span developmental literature (see Parker & Aldwin, 1995), and a greater appreciation of life is a hallmark of gerotranscendence theory (Tornstam, 1994), which is described in greater detail later in this chapter.

SOCIAL RELATIONS. A series of studies by Carstensen and her colleagues (see Carstensen, Mikels, & Mather, 2006, for a review) demonstrated that older adults are less likely to seek out new or extended social networks than are younger adults, but are more likely to focus on close relationships. However, Carstensen showed that this finding was not limited to aging per se but to a greater sense of mortality, as she and her colleagues found the same pattern among patients with AIDS. Thus, it is not surprising that the SRG literature also shows an enhanced sense of personal closeness with significant others (see Linley & Joseph, 2004, for a review).

COPING AND MASTERY. As yet, there is little consensus as to whether and how coping and mastery change with age. An early review of aging and sense of control (Lachman, 1986) found little evidence for age-related changes in general control, but found instead domain-specific changes often related to health (see also Skaff, 2007). The emerging consensus in the coping literature is that older adults, in the absence of cognitive deficits, do not show any decrement in coping with age. Instead, older adults may show conservation of resources in their coping efforts, but they still cope in effective ways (Aldwin, Sutton, & Lachman, 1996). One hallmark of SRG is a greater sense of personal mastery. There is some suggestion that mastery increases from young adulthood to midlife (see McCrae et al., 1999; Parker & Aldwin, 1997). Although McCrae et al. (1999) hypothesized that this increase in mastery was genetic in nature, given that it occurs worldwide, a more parsimonious explanation is that young adults face many challenges and normative stressors in assuming adult roles in careers and families, which in turn leads to increases in mastery. Levenson, Aldwin, and Cupertino (2001) argued elsewhere that adult development occurs through the process of coping with loss and stress, demonstrating how intricately intertwined the two areas are.

TURNING POINTS. The recognition of turning points in individuals' lives is an essential component of life course theory (see Elder & Shanahan, 2006; Settersten, 2006; Wethington, Kessler, & Pixley, 2004). Indeed, the existence of turning points is a sine qua non for understanding the plasticity and stochastic nature of life course development. The recognition of turning points grew out of studies of highly stressed children, most of whom successfully navigated the transition to adulthood, despite being exposed to parents who were mentally ill, poverty, the death of a parent, and so forth (see Werner & Smith, 2001). Often, turning points in these children's development allowed them to change the course of their developmental trajectories. One such turning point for many is military service (Elder & Clipp, 1989; Laub & Sampson, 2005); for others, it may be mentoring and opportunities provided by a caring adult (Werner & Smith, 2001). For life course theorists, these turning points are often discussed in terms of opportunities afforded by social structures, such as the military or community colleges (Settersten, 2005), but from an SRG perspective, idiosyncratic individual life events often form the context for turning points (McAdams & Bowman, 2001). Nonetheless, turning points are major points of overlap between SRG and life course theories.

SPIRITUAL DEVELOPMENT. Whether religiousness or spirituality increases with age remains unknown. Fowler's (1981) stages of faith model, which posits increasing social and ethical awareness similar to Kohlberg (1984), provides one possible life span approach to religiousness, but relatively few studies have used this model (Leak, 2003). Cross-sectional research has found that older adults are more religious on many dimensions of religiousness than younger adults, from religious attendance to religious or spiritual experience (Idler, 2006).

A handful of theorists have suggested that spirituality increases in late life (Tornstam, 1994; Vaillant, 2002), but the few longitudinal studies that exist yield contradictory results and strongly suggest that there is not a simple, linear increase.

For example, Wink and Dillon (2002), using data from the Intergenerational Study, found a nonlinear pattern of decreases in religiousness in midlife and increases later in life. Using growth mixture models on data from the Terman sample, McCullough, Enders, Brion, and Jain (2005) found three patterns in "religious consumption." One was increase until midlife followed by decrease (40% of the sample), another was a low level followed by decrease (41%), and the third was a high level followed by an increase in later life (19%). Furthermore, individual differences in life course patterns of religiousness increase with age, as is the case with other phenomena in life span development (Krause, 2006; Wink & Dillon, 2002). There are also clear period and cohort effects in religiousness (Idler, 2006). To our knowledge, however, none of these studies sought to explain change in religiousness as a function of stress or trauma. Nonetheless, several studies have shown that religiousness and religious coping are strong predictors of SRG (see Shaw, Joseph, & Linley, 2005, for a review). Thus, if older adults are becoming more religious, then it is possible that this would promote SRG in later life.

In summary, many similarities exist between SRG and classical and current theories of adult development. However, most of these theories are incremental; that is, they posit a gain or an increase in some characteristic (Levenson & Crumpler, 1996). It is our contention that loss processes are also an essential component of adult development, and, as such, form an even stronger link between SRG and adult development.

Loss and Self-Directed Development

One of the most important new developments in life span development theory is the idea of self-directed development (Brandstädter, 1999). According to this model, individuals set particular goals and then take steps to achieve those goals. The model emphasizes that development is intentional and involves self-regulation in the service of goals (Greve, Rothermund, & Wentura, 2005). This is relevant to SRG in two ways. First, Burt and Katz (1987), in a study of perceived benefits of stress among rape victims, found that enhanced self-directed activity was a major dimension of growth. This suggests that individuals who are able to perceive benefits of stress may have developed a tool to enhance their future development.

Second, Levenson et al. (2001) argued that adult development involves loss as well as gains. Whereas Baltes (1987) specified that development consists of a balance between losses and gains, and life course theory argues that development consists of relinquishment, or loss, of roles and acquisition of others, Levenson et al. argued that adult development, conceptualized in terms of wisdom, occurs through the loss of barriers to the development of positive characteristics. McKee and Barber (1999) argued that a major barrier to the development of wisdom is the existence of personal illusions. For example, addicts falsely believe that they can control their addiction or minimize its ill effects. Perspicacity, central to wisdom, involves the ability to see through illusions.

Personal stress or trauma is widely thought to shatter one's assumptions about the world (Janoff-Bulman, 2004). Assumptions about the world and one's place in it are among those illusions thought to be shattered by trauma (Epstein, 1991). In particular, serious illness often challenges assumptions about one's invulnerability and self-concept. It changes beliefs about what is important in life as well as one's social environment. It can clarify priorities, and reveal "real" friends versus fair weather friends. Levenson et al. (2001) argued that the loss of these types of self-limiting assumptions is essential to the development of wisdom, as is the loss of negative characteristics such as hostility, impatience, self-centeredness, greed, and so forth.

In some circumstances, stressful life events may result from these self-limiting assumptions or negative characteristics. For example, a woman in one of our studies who had experienced parental divorce was determined to maintain her marriage by being what she thought was the perfect wife. Unfortunately, she was not aware that her idea of perfection was not shared by her husband, and she was consequently severely traumatized by her divorce. Similarly, Caspi, Elder, and Bem (1987) showed that individuals who had temper tantrums in childhood often grew up to be hostile adults, which led to limited educational and occupational attainment, and presumably greater exposure to stressful life events, such as being fired and divorced. Presumably, these types of events would provide the opportunity for self-examination and the determination to modulate one's behavior and lose negative characteristics and self-limiting assumptions. Thus, stress constitutes a context for the development of wisdom in adulthood, depending on how individuals cope with it (Aldwin, 2007).

In summary, there are numerous points of correspondence between theories of SRG and life span developmental theory. Many of the constructs that are thought to develop from undergoing trauma or major stressful life events are similar to constructs integral to development in adulthood. How individuals cope with stress is thought to be central to both SRG and the development of higher stages of adult development, including wisdom. The second half of this chapter focuses on empirical studies from the general literature and from our studies that tested different aspects of this theory. We also present a new approach to SRG (see Appendix 5.1).

Empirical Studies of Aging, Adult Development, and Stress-Related Growth

There are only a handful of studies that examine whether SRG varies with age. In this section, we review this literature and then present studies from our own research.

Are There Age-Related Differences in Stress-Related Growth?

There is conflicting evidence that SRG differs across adult age groups. Some studies have found no relationships between age at the time of the occurrence of the event and growth from that event in stressors as diverse as crime victimization (Collins, Taylor, & Skokan, 1990) and the Dresden bombings (Maercker & Herrle, 2003). A handful of studies have found that younger adults are more likely to report SRG in studies of cancer survivors (Sears, Stanton, & Danoff-Burg, 2003), war refugees (Powell, Rosner, Butollo, Tedeschi, & Calhoun, 2003), and bereaved parents (Polatinsky & Esprey, 2003). Similar results were found in a longitudinal and prospective study of bereavement by C. Davis, Nolen-Hoeksema, and Larson (1998). Younger respondents were more likely to report finding something positive from their experience than older respondents, but there were no age differences in making sense of the loss. However, studies have found SRG in later life (Lieberman, 1992; Park, Mills-Baxter, & Fenster, 2005). Thus, these findings should not imply that SRG does not occur in the elderly, but rather that young adults may be more likely to report growth when compared with older adults.

There is also evidence that age influences the type of SRG. For example, Curbow, Somerfield, Baker, Wingard, and Legro (1993) found age differences in the type of SRG experienced by long-term survivors of bone marrow transplants. Younger survivors more frequently redirected their lives, whereas older survivors were more likely to place more value on family relationships and to take more time for themselves.

Findings regarding age from investigations of different types of stressors have also been mixed. Evaluating significant life experiences of a volunteer sample that ranged in age from 30 to 60 years old, Finkel and Jacobsen (1977) found that participants who were in their 20s at the time of the event were more likely to convert their stress into "strens" (their term for SRG), compared with older age-at-event participants. Aldwin et al. (1996) found different results from three distinct samples. In one sample, drawn from a health maintenance organization (i.e., HMO), those who had experienced a low point in their young adulthood were more likely to have derived tangible advantages from their low point compared with those who had experienced a low point in later life. However, in the other two samples in this study (i.e., men from the Normative Aging Study [NAS] and college alumni from the Davis Longitudinal Study [DLS]), no age differences were found.

Stanton, Bower, and Low (2006) reviewed 19 studies of the correlations between age and SRG among cancer patients. In most (i.e., 12) of the studies, there were no significant correlations with age. In nine of the studies, younger individuals were more likely to report SRG. Both cohort and developmental factors may explain this difference. From a cohort perspective, younger adults may be more familiar with constructs in positive psychology and thus be more likely to report SRG (Manne et al., 2004). Developmentally, cancer and other chronic illnesses become more normative with age and thus may be less distressing (Salmon, Manzi, & Valori, 1996). Indeed, to the extent that SRG is related to the severity of the stressor, the lower levels of distress exhibited by older adults may also mitigate the development of SRG. However, Kurtz, Wyatt, and Kurtz's (1995) observation of a more positive philosophical or spiritual stance in older women with cancer highlights the observation that different types of SRG may show varying relationships with age.

In summary, there appears to be a weak, inverse relationship between age and SRG (Linley & Joseph, 2004). Tedeschi and Calhoun (2004) posited that younger people might be more open to learning and changing than are older people. This greater openness may also be a function of the type of stressors experienced with age; younger individuals may face stressors for which benefits are easier to identify (i.e., career change) than those experienced by older adults (Aldwin et al., 1996). Carver (1998) made a similar supposition, that growth can take place only in circumstances that are malleable enough to permit gain. Finally, young adults also have more time to effect positive changes. However, nearly all of the studies that have examined the differential effect of age on growth are cross-sectional and thus confound age with cohort effects. Furthermore, SRG can clearly occur throughout the life span; studies that examine different dimensions of SRG find that some types are positively associated with age.

If SRG is related to developmental factors, and the hypothesized outcomes are in many ways similar to those posited as higher stages of adult development, why would young people be more likely to exhibit SRG? An alternative interpretation is that there are individual differences in the ability of individuals to perceive benefits of stress, or, more precisely, to use the opportunities afforded by stressful life changes or transition points. Thus, these individual differences in cross-sectional analyses may obscure any age-related change in SRG. For example, younger individuals are more likely to receive higher levels of education than older adults; if education is associated with a greater ability to develop SRG, then cross-sectional studies may show that younger individuals are more likely to develop SRG. However, in the absence of longitudinal studies, it is not possible to say whether SRG changes with age.

The interrelationships between age, stress, coping, wisdom, and SRG have been major foci of our studies for the past few years; in the rest of this chapter we review those studies as well as some new data in support of the theoretical model which has been guiding our research. As depicted in Figure 5.1, loss may lead to two different trajectories. Along the resilience trajectory, loss can lead to SRG in the presence of resilience factors, such as intelligence, positive social support, and positive coping strategies, which include problem-focused coping and self-regulatory abilities. In turn, SRG can lead to wisdom, which may lead to better adaptation to chronic illness in later life. In the vulnerability trajectory, loss combined with vulnerability factors such as neuroticism, poor social support, low resource levels, and negative coping strategies (e.g., escapism, drug and alcohol abuse, wishful thinking) may lead to greater exposure to future stressful life events. This subsequently may lead to the development of chronic illnesses in midlife, which in turn may lead to poorer adaptation in late life.

It is important to note, however, that these trajectories are only probabilistic; other life events or chronic illness in midlife may lead to turning points. Positive coping with these turning points may lead to SRG and, consequently, the development of greater resilience. Thus, the process of coping with loss can lead to a greater vulnerability to the development of chronic illness. However, chronic illness itself can constitute a turning point, which may allow individuals to develop greater resilience. For example, an individual who uses food to cope with loss may develop a weight problem, leading to glucose intolerance and perhaps diabetes in midlife. However, this person may perceive this as a wake-up call, and make dramatic lifestyle changes, resulting in better weight control,

Resilience Trajectory

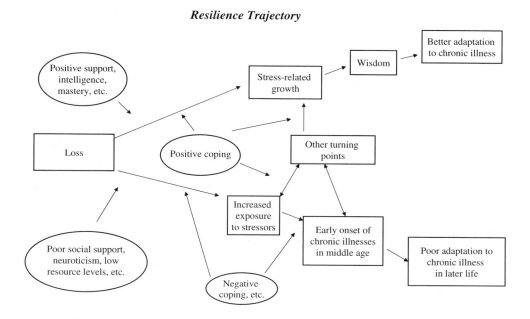

Figure 5.1. Vulnerability and resilience trajectories.

Vulnerability Trajectory

self-confidence, and so forth. Thus, a life span perspective on development and adaptation results in a complex model involving both short- and long-term outcomes, in which illness can be seen both as an outcome of the stress and coping process and as a stressor which may constitute an opportunity for SRG.

Stress-Related Growth and Positive Adaptation in Later Life

To date, no study has tested all of the hypothesized pathways in Figure 5.1, detailing the relationships among loss, coping, SRG, and wisdom. However, we conducted several studies that tested parts of the model; these are reviewed here.

LOSS, COPING, AND WISDOM. Schwarzwaelder (2004) examined the relationship between loss, coping, and wisdom in a sample of college students. As part of that project, we developed the Practical Knowledge Scale, a self-report measure of wisdom which parallels the five dimensions of wisdom proposed by Baltes and Staudinger (2000): factual knowledge, procedural knowledge, life span contextualism, values relativism, and uncertainty management. In this student sample, we found only four factors: factual knowledge; values relativism; uncertainty management; and a factor we called "social knowledge," the social aspect of procedural knowledge (i.e., knowing whom to go to for information or help in achieving one's goals; see Schwarzwaelder, Shiraishi, Levenson, & Aldwin, 2004). Serious loss in early life, typically bereavement, was only loosely linked to wisdom. Only social knowledge was higher in individuals who experienced serious losses.

Schwarzwaelder also assessed wisdom using the Adult Self-Transcendence Inventory (ASTI; Levenson, Jennings, Aldwin, & Shiraishi, 2005). The ASTI taps a construct similar to gerotranscendence (Tornstam, 1994), which refers to a shift in metaperspective, usually in later life. This shift reflects a decreased dependence on external factors (e.g., social roles, status, possessions) for self-definition (see also James, 1890/1981). This may lead to feeling more joyful, calmer, and less hostile toward others; feeling closer to both past and future generations; and being appreciative of the "small" things in life. As mentioned earlier, Levenson et al. (2001) hypothesized that loss plays a major role in the development of this perspective.

Schwarzwaelder (2004) found an interesting three-way interaction between loss, coping, and control beliefs. Individuals who reported a loss and who had high control beliefs and flexible coping strategies reported higher levels of self-transcendence, whereas individuals who experienced a loss and who had low control beliefs and inflexible coping strategies reported the lowest levels of self-transcendence. In other words, loss presents an opportunity: How one copes along with one's control beliefs affect whether there are positive outcomes to this stressor. This finding is consistent with a growing number of studies that suggest that how one copes with a stressor is a more important determinant of SRG than the occurrence of the stressor or trauma itself (see Aldwin, 2007, for a review).

STRESS-RELATED GROWTH, VALUES, AND WISDOM. Values as well as coping may be associated with wisdom and SRG. Le and Levenson (2005) found that values promoting competition (i.e., vertical individualism) were inversely associated with self-transcendence, but that egalitarian stances were positively associated with self-transcendence in a sample of university students. In a sample of immigrants from Vietnam, South Asia, and Central Europe, Boeninger, Le, and Aldwin (2005) found four types of SRG: tangible self-enrichment, emotional self-enrichment, enhanced life experience, and self-transformation. The best predictor of these different dimensions of SRG was the use of positive coping strategies, with religious coping most related to self-transformation. However, deficiency related values, those focusing on self-protectiveness and materialism, were inversely related to gaining life experience and self-transformation.

COMBAT, STRESS-RELATED GROWTH, AND WISDOM. Aldwin, Levenson, and Spiro (1994) examined the relationships among combat, positive and negative military experiences (primarily during World War II and the Korean War), and symptoms of posttraumatic stress disorder (PTSD) in later life among the men in the NAS. We expected to see a nonlinear relationship between combat exposure and positive military experiences; we found instead a linear relationship: The more combat experienced, the more individuals were likely to report positive experiences. Furthermore, perceiving positive experiences was related to lower levels of PTSD symptoms. A follow-up study (Aldwin & Levenson, 2005) using a British sample of older army veterans, the Chelsea Pensioners, found that the Positive Military Experiences Scale (Aldwin et al., 1994) factored into three subscales that were quite similar to SRG: increased coping and mastery skills, values, and enhanced life experiences. These factors seemed to protect both physical and mental health, at least for those veterans with lower amounts of combat exposure.

Jennings, Aldwin, Levenson, Spiro, and Mroczek (2006) examined the role of SRG from military experience and combat exposure in the development of wisdom in the men from the NAS. As mentioned earlier, in 1988, the men in the NAS reported on the positive and negative experiences of their military service during World War II and the Korean War. Then, in 2001, they completed the ASTI. Jennings et al. found that SRG positively predicted both self-transcendence and alienation scores 13 years later; these scores were partially mediated by positive coping strategies. Furthermore, individuals with moderate levels of combat exposure reported the highest levels of self-transcendence, whereas those with moderate and high combat levels reported the highest alienation levels.

AGING, COPING, AND STRESS-RELATED GROWTH. A major purpose of the DLS was to develop a systematic understanding of SRG by developing a series of questions derived from coding previous exploratory interviews (for preliminary results, see Aldwin et al., 1996). Different dimensions of SRG included changes in values, tangible gain, emotional gain, ability to take advantage of a situation, and learning about one's own vulnerabilities (see Appendix 5.1). Kelly (2006) examined the measurement model in the DLS using data collected in 2001, and developed an SRG measurement model which was a good fit to the data, $\chi^2 = 5.68$, ns, CFI = .996, RMSEA = .039. It is surprising that vulnerabilities loaded positively on the SRG latent factor, suggesting that confronting the truth about oneself aids the development of SRG.

For the purposes of this chapter, we examined the relationships among age, loss, coping, and SRG, using 749 men and women from this data set who had experienced a major low point in the previous 5 years (M = 42.40 years). Figure 5.2 presents the model we developed. As predicted, appraisals of harm or loss were related to SRG (β = .13). It is interesting to note that age was indeed negatively related to SRG (β = −.14). However, it was also significantly related to positive coping (β = .19), which in turn was strongly positively related to SRG (β = .71). Thus, the indirect effect of age on coping was β = .136, and the total effect was positive (β = .009). In other words, *ceteris paribus,* older individuals were less likely to report SRG. However, to the extent that they engaged in positive coping, older adults were likely to report more SRG. In contrast, harm or loss was negatively related to positive coping (β = −.05). Nevertheless, this effect was not enough to offset its positive effect on SRG, and the total effect of harm or loss on SRG was positive (β = .091).

One interpretation of these results is that there are individual differences in the effect of both age and loss on SRG. Although, in general, older adults are less likely to report SRG to the extent that some older individuals use positive coping strategies, they still have the possibility of deriving benefits from their stressors. Conversely, problems that involve harm or loss are slightly less likely to evoke the use of positive coping strategies, but still afford the possibility of SRG. Taken together with earlier studies (Jennings et al., 2006), this pattern of results suggests that the ability to perceive benefits from stress may result in higher levels of wisdom in later life.

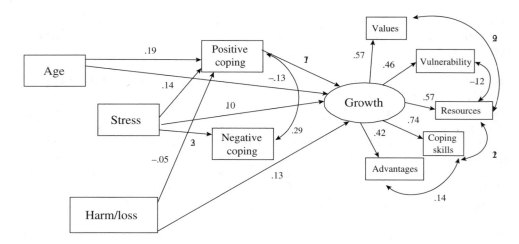

Figure 5.2. Structural equation model showing direct and indirect effects of age on stress-related growth (SRG) via coping processes. The model was a good fit to the data, CMIN/DF = 4.34, CFI = .931, RMSEA = .068.

Future Directions

SRG is inherently a developmental phenomenon, and many of its tenets bear a striking similarity to life span theories of development. For example, the hypothesized outcomes of SRG are similar to the higher stages of adult development. Although older adults may be less likely to report some types of SRG, other types of SRG may increase with age, especially the valuing of close relationships, a finding which is consistent with life span developmental theories. The incidence and prevalence of severe and chronic illnesses in later life, as well as the losses experienced in these contexts, may also promote SRG, even in later life, depending on how individuals cope with the illness. There are some intriguing suggestions that SRG earlier in life may be related to the development of wisdom in later life. Future research should specifically examine the differences between younger and older adults in the development of SRG and more explicitly link the theories and measures of adult development in stressful contexts, especially with regard to severe and chronic illnesses. In particular, longitudinal studies are needed that examine changes in SRG over time in both older and younger samples. For example, are younger individuals more likely to develop SRG in relation to a chronic illness, such as cancer, than are older individuals? If so, is this a function of education, or perhaps a function of differences in developmental constructs such as a sense of time until death? Older individuals may be more acutely aware of a lack of time and thus may feel that making changes is a futile exercise. On the one hand, the greater emotional complexity of older adults may make them more likely to maintain a positive stance even in the face of serious challenges such as cancer (cf. M. C. Davis, Zautra, Johnson, Murray, & Okvat, 2007) and thus they may be more likely to develop SRG. On the other hand, different facets of SRG may be more probable or appropriate in different age groups. Thus, much research is needed to disentangle the relationships among stress, age, adult development, and SRG. The important point is that development in adulthood and, by implication, SRG, may involve the loss of outmoded assumptions, coping strategies, or aspects of the self, and not just the development of new capacities and perspectives.

The artist Ruth St. Denis once wrote, "I stand willingly in the way of storms, that all my dead leaves may swirl away and be lost" (cited in Douglas-Klotz, 2005, p. 146). Thus, the "storms" or stressors of life, including chronic illnesses, however painful, may be just what are needed to rid oneself of negative aspects of the self. Given the high frequency of chronic illnesses in late life, more research is needed on how these illnesses may promote development in older adults.

Appendix 5.1: Stress-Related Growth Items

Were you able to turn any part of the situation to your advantage? (Circle all that apply.)

0. No
1. Yes, emotional well-being (e.g., pride, satisfaction).
2. Yes, tangible advantage/gain (including new coping skills).
3. Yes, developed new philosophy/attitude toward life.
4. Yes, other (please explain) _____

The following statements reflect some of the things people learn from going through a low point. Please indicate the extent to which you have learned the following things.

	Not at all	A little	Somewhat	A lot
1. Family is very important to me.	0	1	2	3
2. Religion/spirituality is very important to me.	0	1	2	3
3. Taking care of myself is very important to me.	0	1	2	3
4. I had positive psychological resources (e.g., ability to cope).	0	1	2	3
5. I had positive physical resources (e.g., physical stamina).	0	1	2	3
6. I had positive social resources (e.g., good friends, neighbors, family).	0	1	2	3
7. There were some things about myself with which I was not happy.	0	1	2	3
8. I could stand on my own two feet.	0	1	2	3
9. My health prevented me from doing as much as I would have liked.	0	1	2	3
10. Many people weren't as helpful as I would have liked.	0	1	2	3
11. New skills (e.g., I learned how to manage doctors.)	0	1	2	3
12. New, positive attitudes toward life.	0	1	2	3
13. There are some situations that I can't do anything about.	0	1	2	3
14. My longstanding values were a resource I could draw upon.	0	1	2	3
15. Other (please specify) _____	0	1	2	3

Were there any long-term effects? (Circle only one.)
0. None.
1. Yes, primarily positive effects.
2. Yes, primarily negative effects.
3. Yes, both positive and negative effects.

IF YES, what type of long-term effect(s)? (Circle all that apply.)
1. Emotional well-being (e.g., pride, satisfaction).
2. Emotional vulnerability (e.g., ashamed, disappointed).
3. Tangible advantage/gain (including new coping skills).
4. Tangible harm/loss.
5. Developed new philosophy/outlook on life.
6. Reinforced old philosophy/outlook/attitude.
7. Other (explain) _____

References

Aldwin, C. M. (2007). *Stress, coping, and development: An integrative approach* (2nd ed.). New York: Guilford Press.

Aldwin, C. M., & Levenson, M. R. (2004). Posttraumatic growth: A developmental perspective. *Psychological Inquiry, 15,* 19–21.

Aldwin, C. M., & Levenson, M. R. (2005). Military service and emotional maturation: The Chelsea Pensioners. In K. W. Schaie & G. Elder Jr. (Eds.), *Historical influences on lives and aging* (pp. 255–281). San Diego, CA: Academic Press.

Aldwin, C. M., Levenson, M. R., & Spiro, A., III. (1994). Vulnerability and resilience to combat exposure: Can stress have lifelong effects? *Psychology and Aging, 9,* 33–44.

Aldwin, C. M., Sutton, K., & Lachman, M. (1996). The development of coping resources in adulthood. *Journal of Personality, 64,* 91–113.

Baltes, P. B. (1987). Theoretical propositions of life-span developmental psychology: On the dynamics between growth and decline. *Developmental Psychology, 24,* 611–626

Baltes, P. B., & Staudinger, U. M. (2000). Wisdom: A metaheuristic (pragmatic) to orchestrate mind and virtue toward excellence. *American Psychologist, 55,* 122–136.

Boeninger, D. G., Le, T., & Aldwin, C. M. (2005, March). *Adversarial growth and loss: The roles of stressor type, coping, personality, and cultural values.* Paper presented at the third International Positive Psychology Summit, Washington, DC.

Brandstädter, J. (1999). The self in action and development: Cultural, biosocial, and ontogenetic bases of intentional self-development. In J. Brandstädter & R. M. Lerner (Eds.), *Action and self-development: Theory and research through the life span* (pp. 37–66). Thousand Oaks, CA: Sage.

Buhler, C. M., Massarik, F., & Bugental, J. F. T. (1968). *The course of human life: A study of goals in the humanistic perspective.* New York: Springer Publishing Company.

Burt, M. R., & Katz, B. L. (1987). Dimensions of recovery from rape: Focus on growth outcomes. *Journal of Interpersonal Violence, 2,* 57–82.

Carstensen, L. L., Mikels, J. A., & Mather, M. (2006). Aging and the intersection of cognition, motivation and emotion. In J. Birren & K. W. Schaie (Eds.), *Handbook of the psychology of aging* (6th ed., pp. 343–362). San Diego, CA: Academic Press.

Carver, C. S. (1998). Resilience and thriving: Issues, models, and linkages. *Journal of Social Issues, 54,* 245–266.

Caspi, A., Elder, G. H. J., & Bem, D. J. (1987). Moving against the world: Life-course patterns of explosive children. *Developmental Psychology, 23,* 308–313.

Collins, R. L., Taylor, S. E., & Skokan, L. A. (1990). A better world or a shattered vision? Changes in life perspectives following victimization. *Social cognition, 8,* 263–285.

Curbow, B., Somerfield, M. R., Baker, F., Wingard, J. R., & Legro, M. W. (1993). Personal changes, dispositional optimism, and psychological adjustment to bone marrow transplantation. *Journal of Behavioral Medicine, 16,* 423–443.

Dannefer, D. (1984). Adult development and social theory: A paradigmatic reappraisal. *American Sociological Review, 49,* 100–116.

Davis, C., Nolen-Hoeksema, S., & Larson, J. (1998). Making sense of loss and benefiting from the experience: Two construals of meaning. *Journal of Personality and Social Psychology, 75,* 647–654.

Davis, M. C., Zautra, A. J., Johnson, L. M., Murray, K. E., & Okvat, H. A. (2007). Psychosocial stress, emotion regulation, and resilience among older adults. In C. M. Aldwin, C. L. Park, & A. Spiro III (Eds.), *Handbook of health psychology and aging* (pp. 250–266). New York: Guilford Press.

Douglas-Klotz, N. (2005). *The Sufi book of life: Ninety-nine pathways of the heart for the modern dervish.* London: Penguin Books.

Elder, G. H. J., & Clipp, E. (1989). Combat experience and emotional health: Impairment and resilience in later life. *Journal of Personality, 57,* 311–341.

Elder, G. H. J., & Shanahan, M. J. (2006). The life course and human development. In R. M. Lerner & W. Damon (Eds), *Handbook of child psychology: Vol. 1. Theoretical models of human development* (6th ed., pp. 665–715). Hoboken, NJ: Wiley.

Epstein, S. 1991. The self-concept, the traumatic neurosis, and the structure of personality. In D. J. Ozer, J. M. Healy, & A. J. Stewart (Eds.), *Perspectives in personality* (Vol. 3, pp. 63–98). London: Jessica Kingsley.

Erikson, E. (1950). *Childhood and society.* New York: Norton.

Finkel, N. J., & Jacobsen, C. A. (1977). Significant life experiences in an adult sample. *American Journal of Community Psychology, 5,* 165–175.

Ford, D. H., & Lerner, R. M. (1992). *Developmental systems theory: An integrative approach.* Newbury Park, CA: Sage.

Fowler, J. (1981). *Stages of faith: The psychology of human development and the quest for meaning.* New York: Harper & Row.

Greve, W., Rothermund, K., & Wentura, D. (2005). Introduction. In W. Greve, K. Rothermund, & D. Wentura (Eds.), *The adaptive self: Personal continuity and intentional self-development* (pp. viii–xvi). Cambridge, MA: Hogrefe & Huber.

Hooker, K., & McAdams, D. (2003). Personality reconsidered: A new agenda for aging research. *Journals of Gerontology: Series B. Psychological Sciences & Social Sciences, 58,* 296–304.

Idler, E. (2006). Religion and aging. In R. H. Binstock & L. K. George (Eds.), *Handbook of aging and the social sciences* (6th ed., pp. 277–300). San Diego, CA: Academic Press.

James, W. (1981). *The principles of psychology.* Cambridge, MA: Harvard University Press. (Original work published 1890)

Janoff-Bulman, R. (2004). Posttraumatic growth: Three explanatory models. *Psychological Inquiry, 15,* 30–34.

Jennings, P. A., Aldwin, C. M., Levenson, M. R., Spiro, A., III, & Mroczek, D. (2006). Combat exposure, perceived benefits of military service, and wisdom in later life: Findings from the Normative Aging Study. *Research on Aging, 28,* 115–124.

Kelly, L. (2006). Relationships among pro-active coping, situation-specific stress and coping, and stress-related growth. Unpublished doctoral dissertation, University of California, Davis.

Kohlberg, L. (1984). *Essays on moral development: Vol. 2. The psychology of moral development.* San Francisco: Harper & Row.

Kohlberg, L., & Ryncarz, R. A. (1990). Beyond justice reasoning: Moral development and consideration of a seventh stage. In C. Alexander & E. Langer (Eds.), *Beyond formal operations: Alternative endpoints in human development* (pp. 191–207). New York: Oxford University Press.

Krause, N. (2006). Religion and health in late life. In J. E. Birren & K. W. Schaie (Eds.), *Handbook of the psychology of aging* (pp. 499–518). San Diego, CA: Academic Press.

Kurtz, M. E., Wyatt, G., & Kurtz, J. C. (1995). Psychological and sexual well-being, philosophical/spiritual views, and health habits of long-term cancer survivors. *Health Care for Women International, 16,* 253–262.

Lachman, M. E. (1986). Locus of control in aging research: A case for multidimensional and domain-specific assessment. *Psychology and Aging, 1,* 34–40.

Laub, J. H., & Sampson, R. J. (2005). Coming of age in wartime: How World War II and the Korean War changed lives. In K. W. Schaie & G. H. Elder Jr. (Eds.), *Historical influences on lives & aging* (pp. 208–228). New York: Springer Publishing Company.

Le, T. N., & Levenson, M. R. (2005). Wisdom: What's love (and culture) got to do with it? *Journal of Research in Personality, 39,* 443–457.

Leak, G. K. (2003). Validation of the faith development scale using longitudinal and cross-sectional designs. *Social Behavior and Personality, 31,* 637–642.

Lerner, R. M. (2002). *Concepts and theories of human development.* Mahwah, NJ: Erlbaum.

Lerner, R. M., Theokas, C., & Jelicic, H. (2005). Youth as active agents in their own positive development: A developmental systems perspective. In W. Greve, K. Rothermund, & D. Wentura (Eds.), *The adaptive self: Personal continuity and intentional self-development* (pp. 31–47). Cambridge, MA: Hogrefe & Huber.

Levenson, M. R., Aldwin, C. M., & Cupertino, A. P. (2001). Transcending the self: Towards a liberative model of adult development. In A. L. Neri (Ed.), *Maturidade e Velhice: Um enfoque multi-disciplinar* (pp. 99–116). Sao Paulo, Brazil: Papirus.

Levenson, M. R., & Crumpler, C. A. (1996). Three models of adult psychological development. *Human Development, 39,* 135–194.

Levenson, M. R., Jennings, P. A., Aldwin, C. M., & Shiraishi, R. W. (2005). Self-transcendence, conceptualization and measurement. *International Journal of Aging & Human Development, 60,* 127–143.

Lieberman, M. A. (1992). Limitations of psychological stress model: Studies of widowhood. In M. L. Wykle, E. Kahan, & J. Kowal (Eds.), *Stress and health among the elderly* (pp. 133–150). New York: Springer Publishing Company.

Linley, P. A., & Joseph, S. (2004). Positive change following trauma and adversity: A review. *Journal of Traumatic Stress, 17,* 11–21.

Maercker, A., & Herrle, J. (2003). Long-term effects of the Dresden bombing: Relationships to control beliefs, religious belief, and personal growth. *Journal of Traumatic Stress, 16,* 579–587.

Manne, S., Ostroff, J., Winkel, G., Goldstein, L., Fox, K., & Grana, G. (2004). Posttraumatic growth after breast cancer: Patient, partner, and couple perspectives. *Psychosomatic Medicine, 66,* 442–454.

McAdams, D. P., & Bowman, P. J. (2001). Narrating life's turning points: Redemption and contamination. In D. P. McAdams, R. Josselson, & A. Lieblich (Eds.), *Turns in the road: Narrative studies of lives in transition* (pp. 3–34). Washington, DC: American Psychological Association.

McCrae, R. R., Costa, P. T., Jr., Pedroso de Lima, M., Simoes, A., Ostendorf, F., Angleitner, A., et al. (1999). Age differences in personality across the adult life span: Parallels in five cultures. *Developmental Psychology, 35,* 466–477.

McCullough, M. E., Enders, C. K., Brion, S. L., & Jain, A. R. (2005). The varieties of religious development in adulthood: A longitudinal investigation of religion and rational choice. *Journal of Personality and Social Psychology, 89,* 78–89.

McKee, P., & Barber, C. (1999). "On defining wisdom." *International Journal of Aging and Human Development, 49,* 149–164.

Moos, R. H., & Schaefer, J. A. (1984). The crisis of physical illness. In R. Moos (Ed.), *Coping with physical illness* (pp. 3–26). New York: Plenum Press.

Neugarten, B. L. (1969). Continuities and discontinuities of psychological issues into adult life. *Human Development, 12,* 121–130.

Park, C. L., Mills-Baxter, M. A., & Fenster, J. R. (2005). Posttraumatic growth from life's most traumatic event: Influences on elders' current coping and adjustment. *Traumatology, 11,* 297–306.

Parker, R. A., & Aldwin, C. M. (1995). Desiring careers but loving families: Period, cohort, and gender effects in career and family orientations. In G. P. Keita & J. J. Hurrell (Eds.), *Job stress in a changing workforce: Investigating gender, diversity, and family issues* (pp. 23–38). Washington, DC: American Psychological Association.

Parker, R., & Aldwin, C. M. (1997). Do aspects of gender identity change from early to middle adulthood? Disentangling age, cohort, and period effects. In M. Lachman & J. James (Eds.), *Multiple paths of midlife development* (pp. 67–107). Chicago: University of Chicago Press.

Polatinsky, S., & Esprey, Y. (2003). An assessment of gender differences in the perception of benefit resulting from the loss of a child. *Journal of Traumatic Stress, 13,* 709–718.

Powell, S., Rosner, R., Butollo, W., Tedeschi, R. G., & Calhoun, L. G. (2003). Posttraumatic growth after the war: A study with former refugees and displaced people in Sarajevo. *Journal of Clinical Psychology, 59,* 71–83.

Ryff, C. D. (1989). Happiness is everything, or is it? Explorations on the meaning of psychological well-being. *Journal of Personality and Social Psychology, 57,* 1069–1081.

Salmon, P., Manzi, F., & Valori, R. M. (1996). Measuring the meaning of life for patients with incurable cancer: The Life Evaluation Questionnaire (LEQ). *European Journal of Cancer: Part A, 32,* 755–760.

Schwarzwaelder, S. (2004). *The role of loss in the development of wisdom.* Unpublished master's thesis, University of Heidelberg, Heidelberg, Germany.

Schwarzwaelder, S., Shiraishi, R. W., Levenson, M. R., & Aldwin, C. M. (2004, August). *Wisdom: A higher order construct.* Paper presented at the Annual Meeting of the American Psychological Association, Honolulu, HI.

Sears, S. R., Stanton, A. L., & Danoff-Burg, S. (2003). The Yellow Brick Road and the Emerald City: Benefit finding, positive reappraisal, and posttraumatic growth in women with early stage breast cancer. *Health Psychology, 22,* 487–497.

Settersten, R. A., Jr. (2005). Social policy and the transition to adulthood: Toward stronger institutions and individual capacities. In R. A. J. Settersten, F. F. J. Furstenberg, & R. G. Rumbaut (Eds.), *On the frontier of adulthood: Theory, research, and public policy* (pp. 534–560). Chicago: University of Chicago Press.

Settersten, R. A., Jr. (2006). Aging and the life course. In R. H. Binstock & L. K. George (Eds.), *Handbook of aging and the social sciences* (6th ed., pp. 3–19). San Diego, CA: Academic Press.

Shaw, A., Joseph, S., & Linley, P. A. (2005). Religion, spirituality, and posttraumatic growth: A systematic review. *Mental Health, Religion & Culture, 8,* 1–11.

Skaff, M. (2007). Control and aging. In C. M. Aldwin, C. L. Park, & A. Spiro III (Eds.), *Handbook of health psychology and aging* (pp. 186–209). New York: Guilford Press.

Stanton, A. L., Bower, J. E., & Low, C. A. (2006). Posttraumatic growth after cancer. In L. G. Calhoun & R. G. Tedeschi (Eds.), *Handbook of posttraumatic growth: Research and practice* (pp. 138–175). Mahwah, NJ: Erlbaum.

Tedeschi, R. G., & Calhoun, L. G. (2004). Posttraumatic growth: Conceptual foundations and empirical evidences. *Psychological Inquiry, 15,* 1–18.

Tornstam, L. (1994). Gerotranscendence: A theoretical and empirical exploration. In L. E. Thomas & S. A. Eisenhandler (Eds.), *Aging and the religious dimension* (pp. 203–225). London: Auburn House.

Twenge, J. M. (2000). The age of anxiety? Birth cohort change in anxiety and neuroticism, 1952–1993. *Journal of Personality and Social Psychology, 79,* 1007–1021.

Vaillant, G. E. (2002). *Aging well: Surprising guideposts to a happier life from the landmark Harvard study of adult development.* New York: HarperCollins.

Werner, E. E., & Smith, R. S. (2001). *Journeys from childhood to midlife: Risk, resilience, and recovery.* Ithaca, NY: Cornell University Press.

Wethington, E., Kessler, R. C., & Pixley, J. E. (2004). Turning points in adulthood. In O. G. Brim, C. D. Ryff, & R. C. Kessler (Eds.), *How healthy are we? A national study of well-being at midlife* (pp. 586–613). Chicago: University of Chicago Press.

Wink, P., & Dillon, M. (2002). Spiritual development across the adult life course: Findings from a longitudinal study. *Journal of Adult Development, 9,* 79–94.

Part III

Factors That Influence Positive Life Change

6

Lessons Learned About Benefit Finding Among Individuals With Cancer or HIV/AIDS

Suzanne C. Lechner and Kathryn E. Weaver

HIV/AIDS and cancer are two diseases that strike fear into the hearts of most individuals. On being told that one has cancer or has been infected with HIV, a sense of panic sets in. Many individuals report that they do not recall much of the conversation with their physician after hearing this news. During our clinical work with people with HIV and cancer over the past 10 years, we have observed that receiving a diagnosis of HIV or cancer is often a "seismic event" (Tedeschi & Calhoun, 2004). This "earth-shattering news" causes a cascade of emotions and cognitions. In the ensuing days, weeks, and months, patients speak of the hardships and struggles that result from the illness and its treatment. Concurrently, however, many patients experience positive life changes, often referred to as benefit finding and positive growth (BFG).

Patient self-reports suggest that BFG may be manifested in different ways. For example, many patients have told us that they feel closer to their friends and family members and appreciate the love and support they receive. Others report finding a new clarity about relationships, such as knowing who their "true" friends are. Some patients emphasize a newfound sense of self-confidence or awareness of their strengths (e.g., "I never thought I could get through this. If I can get through this, I can get through anything"). This often translates into a desire to help other people through the journey of diagnosis, treatment, and rebuilding. We have also observed other patients who seem to find a new path for their life, by either changing their priorities or making lifestyle changes to bring their daily activities into accord with their life goals. For example, one woman with HIV asserted, "HIV saved my life." Following an initial period of denial and despair, she felt that her diagnosis was a wake-up call to stop using drugs and living on the street. She was able to use this motivation to complete drug rehabilitation, pass her General Education Development (i.e., GED) exam, regain custody of her children, and work as a peer counselor for other women who are HIV-positive. These clinical examples illustrate how patients view growth in the midst of the illness experience.

In this chapter, we examine some of the lessons that researchers have learned from empirical studies of BFG in persons with HIV and cancer, with the goal of informing clinical work with these populations. HIV and cancer are clearly life-limiting diseases, but advances in medical treatment have resulted in longer survival rates. For many individuals with HIV and cancer, this translates into living with a chronic disease for years following the initial diagnosis. Although mortality concerns are common, death is not imminent for most people diagnosed with HIV/AIDS or cancer; rather, they must learn to deal with complex and confusing medical regimens that they may need to follow for an extended period. In addition, persons with cancer or HIV/AIDS may face challenges associated with life disruption due to symptoms (e.g., fatigue, loss of appetite), side effects of treatment (e.g., nausea, changes in physical appearance), and frequent medical appointments. Often, social support networks are disrupted because of stigma and social discomfort. Despite their similarities, there are differences between the illnesses, particularly in social responses to individuals with HIV compared with those with cancer. HIV is an infectious disease, and people who are HIV-positive may face more negative responses from others because of fear, lack of knowledge concerning transmission, and greater perceived personal accountability. In addition, marginalized groups such as gay men, intravenous drug users, and people belonging to an ethnic minority have been disproportionately burdened by HIV/AIDS, thereby increasing the stigma. In contrast, persons with cancer are typically viewed with greater empathy and concern (Fife, 2005); fears regarding transmission of cancer are far less typical.

Lesson 1: Benefit Finding or Growth in Cancer Is Similar to Benefit Finding or Growth in HIV/AIDS

As evidenced by qualitative reports and quantitative research literature, people with HIV/AIDS report similar types of BFG as compared with individuals with cancer. Spontaneously, individuals with these medical illnesses report finding benefits in similar domains. The few studies that compare individuals with cancer and HIV/AIDS suggest that BFG can be conceptualized in the same way across illnesses.

Numerous qualitative and quantitative studies support our clinical observations of BFG in people with cancer or HIV/AIDS. Regardless of the method of assessment (e.g., spontaneous reports, direct questioning regarding BFG, structured questionnaires), studies reveal that the majority of people with these illnesses report some type of growth or benefits from their illness (e.g., see Fromm, Andrykowski, & Hunt, 1996; Sears, Stanton, & Danoff-Burg, 2003; Siegel & Schrimshaw, 2000). Qualitative studies reveal that individuals with cancer or HIV/AIDS report similar domains of BFG, including enhanced relationships with others, deeper spiritual or religious faith, greater appreciation for life, and changes in life priorities or goals (e.g., see Barroso, 1996; Brashers et al., 1999; Coward, 1994; Coward & Lewis, 1993; Dunn et al., 2006; Foley et al., 2006; Fromm et al., 1996; Plattner & Meiring, 2006; Schwartzberg, 1993; Siegel & Schrimshaw, 2000; Viney, Crooks, Walker, & Henry, 1991). Persons with cancer or HIV/AIDS may also report making positive changes relating to their physical health, including increasing physical activity, making dietary changes, improving adherence to medical screening or treatment, or reducing negative health behaviors, such as smoking or using drugs and alcohol (e.g., see Fromm et al., 1996; Siegel & Schrimshaw, 2000; Updegraff, Taylor, Kemeny, & Wyatt, 2002).

Although few studies have directly compared the two disease groups using the same measures, it appears that several categories of BFG are relevant for both patient populations (e.g., see Lechner, Carver, Antoni, Weaver, & Phillips, 2006; Milam, 2004; Sears et al., 2003). One of the few studies to directly compare these groups of patients (Fife, 2005) found that individuals with HIV/AIDS report less positive meaning (as assessed by questions concerning personal identity, relationships with others, and possibilities for the future) with regard to their illness compared with individuals with cancer. Similarly, Weaver (2006) suggested that BFG, as measured by the Benefit-Finding Scale (Antoni et al., 2001), could be conceptualized in the same multidimensional manner across people with breast cancer, prostate cancer, and HIV/AIDS. Patients may demonstrate differences in the levels of BFG they report, but the content of scale items appear to be appropriate for both patient groups; the theoretically derived construct can be conceptualized in the same way. Taken together, the various lines of research suggest that perceptions of BFG may be similar whether the patient has cancer or HIV/AIDS.

BFG shows equally high prevalence rates among persons with HIV and cancer. Between 59% and 83% of participants who were HIV-positive endorsed BFG (Milam, 2004; Schwartzberg, 1994; Siegel & Schrimshaw, 2000), and similar rates have been reported in the cancer literature (Cella & Tross, 1986; Taylor, 1983; Wasserman, Thompson, Wilimas, & Fairclough, 1987). These studies also indicate that BFG may occur relatively early in the disease trajectory in both populations. The evidence of the stability of BFG is more limited. In one of the few longitudinal studies of BFG, Courtenay, Merriam, Reeves, and Baumgartner (2000) observed that reports of BFG at the time of diagnosis with HIV were maintained over 2 years. Stability over time in other sociodemographic and disease groups needs to be investigated further.

Lesson 2: Sociodemographic Variables Are Not Consistently Related to Benefit Finding and Growth From Cancer or HIV/AIDS

The research literature has attempted to identify sociodemographic predictors of BFG in both cancer and HIV populations without much success in finding consistent relationships. We posit that inconsistencies are the result of methodological differences in the assessment of BFG, sample characteristics, or complex interactions between sociodemographic variables.

It would be highly efficient if a clinician could identify an individual who is most likely to report BFG simply by knowing that person's sociodemographic characteristics. However, the current state of the literature provides little guidance in this realm. The results of studies examining characteristics such as gender, age, race/ethnicity, and socioeconomic status (SES) are inconsistent at best, and confusing and counterintuitive at worst. Some studies rely on small samples, and no studies report findings of BFG in population-based studies.

Gender

Are there gender-based characteristics that could predispose one toward greater BFG? In healthy undergraduate samples, women reported greater BFG than did men (Park, Cohen, & Murch, 1996; Tedeschi & Calhoun, 1996). Findings are replicated in some samples of individuals with mixed cancers (e.g., see Bellizzi, 2004; Foley et al., 2006) and HIV/AIDS (e.g., see Milam, 2004; Weaver, 2006). Yet other studies find no gender differences in BFG in samples of patients with gastric cancer (Schulz & Mohamed, 2004), mixed cancers (Lechner, Zakowski, et al., 2003), or those undergoing bone marrow transplant (Andrykowski, Brady, & Hunt, 1993; Fromm et al., 1996). Although some have suggested that women may experience greater positive changes from difficult life experiences through greater use of social support, emotional expression, and spiritual coping strategies (Park et al., 1996; Tedeschi & Calhoun, 1996), the inconsistencies between published studies suggest more complexity regarding the role of gender in BFG.

Age

Developmental stage or age at the time of diagnosis may be a particularly promising predictor of BFG for clinicians to consider. Theoretically, older individuals may view illness as an expected aspect of aging or may find the experience less traumatic because of previous medical illnesses and other challenging life experiences. This might, in turn, lead to the perception of fewer positive changes directly resulting from illness (Foley et al., 2006; see also chap. 5, this volume). At least two studies found that older cancer survivors reported less BFG than did younger survivors (Bellizzi, 2004; Lechner, Zakowski, et al., 2003). Whereas some studies observed a similar negative relationship between age and BFG in women with breast cancer (Bellizzi & Blank, 2006; Bower et al., 2005; Widows, Jacobsen, Booth-Jones, & Fields, 2005), others found no relationship (Cordova, Cunningham, Carlson, & Andrykowski, 2001; Sears et al., 2003; Tomich & Helgeson, 2004). Results relating age and BFG in people with HIV/AIDS are similarly mixed, with some studies finding increasing age related to less BFG (Milam, 2004) and others finding no relationship (Siegel, Schrimshaw, & Pretter, 2005; Weaver, 2006).

Why these discrepancies? First, none of these studies sought to determine the impact of age on subsequent BFG. These results are simply correlations that were noted in the reports. Because the researchers were not looking for the causal mechanisms for an age–BFG relationship, they did not have data to address this topic. Cancer is also typically a disease that occurs more frequently in older people (age is the number one risk factor for cancer), yielding samples of older adults for cancer studies. HIV does not discriminate on the basis of age, but many HIV studies have younger participants, on average, than do cancer studies. Thus, many samples may not include a wide range of ages. If there is little variability in age, statistical analyses may not detect significant associations with BFG. This lack of range in age is also problematic when trying to compare studies. Aging, and its associated wisdom, maturity, and life stage changes should be a potentially rich area of study with regard to positive life changes following illness (see chap. 5, this volume).

Socioeconomic Status

SES is often measured by a combination of educational attainment and current income. Individuals with lower income and less education might perceive the experience of receiving a diagnosis of a medical illness to be more stressful or threatening because of barriers associated with access to health care, limited health knowledge, and greater financial concerns. Individuals who find their medical illness more threatening because of limited resources might struggle more and therefore perceive more benefits (Cordova et al., 2001; Lechner, Zakowski, et al., 2003). Individuals with low SES may also have experienced more traumatic or stressful events in their lifetimes and therefore may have more practice in searching for and/or finding benefits from negative experiences, resulting in greater reported BFG following medical illness (Tomich & Helgeson, 2004). Accordingly, several researchers have observed significant negative relationships between BFG and income and education in individuals with cancer (e.g., see Carver & Antoni, 2004; Tomich & Helgeson, 2004; Urcuyo, Boyers, Carver, & Antoni, 2005; Widows et al., 2005). Other studies have found no relationship between indicators of SES and BFG in people with cancer or HIV/AIDS (Fromm et al., 1996; Lechner, Zakowski, et al., 2003; Milam, 2004; Siegel et al., 2005), or have found positive relationships between SES and BFG (Sears et al., 2003; Updegraff et al., 2002). A full range of SES levels is necessary to conclusively evaluate SES as a predictor of BFG; however, because of patient characteristics, it can be challenging to recruit individuals from all economic strata, particularly in studies of women who are HIV-positive.

Marital Status

Marital or relationship status might be expected to be related to BFG through its impact on social networks and support, yet many studies have reported no relationship between marital or relationship status and BFG in people with cancer (e.g., see Fromm et al., 1996; Lechner, Zakowski, et al., 2003) and HIV/AIDS (Weaver, 2006). It is possible that marital status is related only to certain dimensions of BFG, particularly those involving social or family relationships (e.g., see Bellizzi & Blank, 2006; Weaver, 2006). This may explain the lack of findings in studies that used overall BFG scores.

The relationship between marital or partner status and BFG may also differ between cancer and HIV/AIDS. Because HIV/AIDS is a sexually transmitted disease, concerns about infecting a partner (if the couple is serodiscordant), disclosure of sexual preference or serostatus, or guilt (if one partner transmitted the virus to the other) would be expected to deleteriously affect the relationship. This may influence BFG, especially in the domain of intimate relationships. For example, if an HIV diagnosis results in the breakup of a relationship, or decreased sexual intimacy, positive changes in the area of intimate relationships are unlikely to be reported. Demonstrating possible differences between

HIV/AIDS and cancer, Weaver (2006) found that being married or in an equivalent relationship was a significant predictor of improved family relations in
individuals with breast cancer and prostate cancer but was unrelated to all
dimensions of BFG in women with HIV/AIDS and men who are HIV-positive
and who have sex with men.

Ethnicity

Many studies have found that members of racial and ethnic minority groups report
greater BFG than non-Hispanic white individuals (Bower et al., 2005; Milam, 2004;
Siegel et al., 2005; Urcuyo et al., 2005; Weaver, 2006). However, a few studies
have shown that individuals from ethnic minorities report less BFG (Updegraff
et al., 2002) or that ethnicity was unrelated to BFG (Sears et al., 2003). Drawing
conclusions about whether BFG is related to race and ethnicity is difficult
because most studies were not designed to directly compare different racial or
ethnic groups. Few studies include balanced numbers of Hispanic, African-
American, and non-Hispanic white individuals, thereby affecting the validity of
statistical analyses. In addition, because members of ethnic minority communi-
ties have a lower SES than the general population, it may be difficult to disentangle the effects of SES and ethnicity. Furthermore, the ethnic and cultural
differences that have been observed may be due to variations in spirituality, coping strategies, social support, health beliefs, or discrimination. For example,
Urcuyo et al. (2005) found that one reason why some minority women with
breast cancer reported higher levels of BFG was their greater use of religious
coping strategies.

    In sum, the inconsistencies in the reported relationships between socio-
demographic variables and BFG may be due to several factors, including differing methods of assessing BFG (e.g., interview vs. questionnaire; single vs.
multiple items) and sample composition (e.g., education, ethnicity, disease site,
time since diagnosis). Much of the reviewed data appear to come from studies
whose primary aim was other than elucidating the relations between sociodemographic variables and BFG. Thus, the assessment of sociodemographic
characteristics may be limited, and information on potential mechanisms by
which constructs such as ethnicity, developmental stage, and SES influence
BFG is limited. It is likely that several sociodemographic characteristics may
interact to influence BFG in complex ways. This complexity is demonstrated by
results showing that one characteristic influences the effect of another. For
example, Weaver (2006) found that SES was related to BFG in men with
prostate cancer or HIV/AIDS but not in women with breast cancer or
HIV/AIDS. This result suggests that the relationship between SES and BFG
may be different for men and women. In addition, sociodemographic variables
may be related to certain dimensions of BFG but not to others. For example,
Bellizzi and Blank (2006) found that marital status was a significant predictor
of BFG in the domains of relationships with others and new possibilities in life
but not appreciation for life on the Posttraumatic Growth Inventory (PTGI;
Tedeschi & Calhoun, 1996). Clearly, these relationships need to be studied in
much greater depth before they can be used as clinical predictors of BFG.

Lesson 3: Psychological Characteristics Are Associated With Benefit Finding and Growth in Cancer and HIV

In accordance with BFG theories, psychosocial variables such as optimism, coping, and emotional expressiveness are related to the development and maintenance of BFG.

As reports of BFG became more common in the literature, scholars began to try to understand how BFG develops, and the psychosocial factors that might be associated with its development. As outlined in chapter 1 of this volume, many theories have arisen to explain the phenomenon of BFG. All of these theories identify the role of dispositional traits, coping styles, social support, and the capacity to regulate emotions as key variables in facilitating or hindering BFG. For example, according to Tedeschi and Calhoun's (2004) model, interpersonal and intrapersonal variables can influence the initiation of a search for meaning in an event such as being diagnosed with cancer or HIV. Highly optimistic persons might be more likely to find benefits in cancer because they already have a tendency to view challenging situations as conquerable and expect that things will work out for them. Conversely, individuals who frequently cope with adversity by using denial or disengaging from the situation may find fewer benefits because they do not allow themselves to work through many of the thoughts and emotions that are associated with being diagnosed with a life-threatening illness.

It is important to note that coping and optimism may facilitate development of BFG in a reciprocal fashion. When people acknowledge or recognize areas of BFG, they may also observe that they are coping well or feeling more optimistic, thereby strengthening these psychological characteristics. In turn, this new-found confidence could augment BFG over time. In a hypothetical example, a young woman has been diagnosed with breast cancer. Although she is feeling distressed, she comes to realize that she is more capable of handling adversity than she believed. This recognition enhances her confidence in her ability to manage a new stressful situation related to treatment, such as an unexpected hospitalization. When she handles the situation well, she feels even more self-confident and perhaps even dares to try out new adaptive coping strategies. In this way, her belief in her ability to overcome adversity (i.e., optimism) is strengthened with each new experience, and thus BFG grows over time.

Research studies using both cross-sectional and longitudinal designs have shed light on the relationships between BFG and key psychosocial variables. Evidence suggests that each of these variables may exert reciprocal influences on one another as well as BFG, but, for the sake of simplicity, we consider each of them separately. In this chapter, we summarize some findings related to dispositional optimism, coping, and emotional processing. Although these variables have received the most attention in the empirical and theory-based literature, a wide range of predictor variables has been examined (see Stanton, Bower, & Low, 2006).

Dispositional Optimism

Dispositional optimism is a personality trait that reflects an individual's expectancies of positive or negative outcomes (Scheier & Carver, 1985). In cross-sectional studies, researchers have observed a strong correlation between optimism and BFG in a sample of patients with mixed cancers (Lechner, 2000) and individuals with HIV/AIDS (Milam, 2004; Updegraff et al., 2002). However, there are inconsistencies in the breast cancer literature. In a sample of survivors of breast cancer who were 1 to 4 years postdiagnosis, there was no relationship between optimism and subscales of the PTGI relating to changed relationships, new possibilities, or appreciation for life posttreatment (Bellizzi & Blank, 2006).

Cross-sectional studies can yield only a limited amount of information about variables that may change over time. Therefore, it is important to examine BFG as it relates to other variables over time using longitudinal designs. Longitudinal studies indicate that the relationship between optimism and reports of BFG may change over the course of the illness. In one longitudinal study of women with breast cancer, Sears et al. (2003) found a positive relationship between baseline optimism and baseline BFG but no relationship between baseline optimism and BFG scores 12 months later. Among women with early-stage breast cancer entering a stress management intervention trial, optimism and BFG were not significantly correlated at baseline or posttreatment; however, changes in these two variables were moderately related over time (Antoni et al., 2001; Carver & Antoni, 2004). Thus, the relationship between optimism and BFG over time may be quite complex, and research is being conducted to understand how these variables relate to one another in a dynamic way.

Coping

As noted in chapter 1, BFG is sometimes described as a coping strategy. In this section, we discuss the relationship between BFG and traditionally measured coping strategies. The results presented here do not answer the question of whether BFG is a coping strategy per se but show important relationships between BFG and coping that may validate some of the pathways thought to be involved in the development of BFG (e.g., see chap. 12, this volume).

Use of approach-oriented or active coping strategies has been identified as a critical component in the development of BFG (Tedeschi & Calhoun, 1996). Most studies that have investigated the relationship between BFG and coping have been derived from Lazarus and Folkman's (1984) model, which posits that coping is a response that is initiated when a stressor is appraised as exceeding the individual's ability to meet the demands of a situation. The Ways of Coping Scale (Folkman & Lazarus, 1988) and the COPE (Carver, Scheier, & Weintraub, 1989) are examples of measures that assess various domains of this construct.

In general, studies seem to find that approach-oriented or active coping strategies are associated with greater BFG. In a sample of individuals who were HIV-positive, Siegel et al. (2005) observed a moderate association between the use of positive reappraisal coping and BFG. Similarly, positive reappraisal coping was positively associated with BFG 12 months later in women with breast cancer who had completed primary medical treatment (Sears et al., 2003). Active coping was related to higher levels of BFG in a sample of older men with prostate cancer (Kinsinger et al., 2006) and in a sample of women who had completed breast cancer treatment 1 to 4 years prior to study enrollment (Bellizzi & Blank, 2006). In another study, women who had early-stage breast cancer were recruited to participate in a randomized intervention trial and were followed over the course of a year. Hierarchical multiple regression analyses revealed that during the early period of dealing with the diagnosis of and treatment for breast cancer, BFG was associated with greater positive reframing, more religious coping, greater self-distraction, higher emotional processing, less substance use, and less need to seek social support. However, by the middle of treatment (i.e., 3 months after surgery), active coping and religious coping were important positive correlates of BFG. After treatment completion (i.e., after 6 months), greater BFG was related to higher levels of active coping, emotional processing, seeking social support, and religious coping, and to lower levels of acceptance coping. One year postsurgery, greater BFG was associated with higher levels of positive reframing and planning coping strategies (Lechner, Antoni, & Carver, 2003). The research team postulated that because different coping strategies are more or less adaptive at different points in an illness, certain forms of coping may also be more or less related to a person's ability to derive positive sequelae at different points in the illness trajectory (Lechner & Antoni, 2004). These findings highlight the potentially dynamic nature of the relationship between coping and BFG.

Emotional Processing

Any discussion of life-threatening illness would be incomplete without mentioning the role of emotional processing. For many persons who have been diagnosed with cancer or HIV/AIDS, there are social taboos against expressing hopelessness, helplessness, fear, or depression. As a result, patients may feel isolated because they do not have outlets to share these feelings. This may hinder their opportunities for emotional processing and may particularly affect the type of processing that occurs when one shares his or her feelings with other people. Antoni et al. (2001) found that those women who reported that they engaged in higher levels of emotional processing also reported greater BFG at the initial assessment, at the posttreatment assessment, at 3 months postintervention, and at 9 months postintervention (rs ranging from .23 to .32). However, in examining whether emotional processing could prospectively predict growth, results showed that emotional processing at earlier time points did not predict subsequent BFG scores. Thus, we can conclude only that emotional processing at a given time point was associated with BFG at the same time point, but that earlier emotional processing was not related to BFG at later assessment points.

Lesson 4: Social Environment Is Related to Benefit Finding and Growth, but the Mechanism Is Unclear

A person's social environment can have a powerful impact on the identification of benefits or growth. The presence of supportive others may promote self-disclosure, which provides opportunities for expression of feelings and the development of new life narratives.

Research has consistently shown that having supportive others to rely on may be especially important for individuals diagnosed with cancer and HIV/AIDS. Patients encounter numerous stressors and challenges on a daily basis as well as broad existential issues. We have theorized that individuals who are able to share their experience with concerned others, and who perceive adequate instrumental and informational support, should be more likely to successfully find positive attributes of their illness (Lechner, 2000; Schaefer & Moos, 2001; Tedeschi & Calhoun, 1996; see also chap. 8, this volume). However, the few empirical studies that have investigated the relationship between social support and BFG among people with cancer and people who are HIV-positive have been inconsistent. This topic is covered more broadly in chapter 8 of this volume, but we comment on a few studies here.

Some studies of persons with HIV/AIDS or cancer failed to find a relationship between aspects of social support and BFG (e.g., see Sears et al., 2003; Updegraff et al., 2002; Weiss, 2004), whereas others found that perceptions of support were related to greater BFG (e.g., see Siegel et al., 2005). Fife (1995), for example, observed a strong relationship between BFG and social support from family, friends, and health care professionals in a sample of 422 patients with a variety of stages and types of cancer. In one notable study of women with breast cancer, Cordova et al. (2001) found that general social support satisfaction was not related to finding benefit in cancer. However, talking about cancer with other people was related to greater BFG. Cancer-specific discussions may serve several functions, and it is unclear which process might account for these findings. On the one hand, the action could be labeled as a coping strategy whereby an individual deals with a stressor by actively problem solving in the presence of another person. On the other hand, perhaps the social process of reflecting or validating emotions provides opportunities for greater self-insight. To talk about cancer, one must also have supportive persons available and willing to listen. Thus, a number of different processes could be occurring to facilitate BFG in this scenario.

Collectively, these findings generate interesting theoretical possibilities. Perhaps the act of talking about cancer topics with other people promotes greater BFG, but general satisfaction with social support may not be an important predictor of growth. We suggest that these findings indicate a need for greater specificity in the questions that researchers ask about the relationships between social support and BFG, as well as the domains and dimensions of social support that are being measured.

Whether or not an individual is married or in a partnered relationship does not seem to be a stable predictor of BFG in individuals with HIV and cancer, as discussed earlier; however, the quality of relationships may play an important role in whether the person who is diagnosed with the illness experiences positive life changes. More specifically, simply being married or in a partnered relationship might not promote BFG, but being in an emotionally expressive, loving, and caring partnered relationship may facilitate the process of growth. Again, the lack of consistent associations highlights the need for greater specificity in examining the social variables that may be related to BFG in cancer and HIV.

It is notable that studies have shown that positive life changes from medical illness may not be limited to the person with the illness. Watching a partner grow and find benefits in illness can spread between partners, resulting in a shared sense of meaning making, possibly culminating in BFG (Manne et al., 2004; Thornton & Perez, 2006; Weiss, 2004). In one of the first longitudinal studies examining this process, Manne et al. (2004) found that BFG increased over an 18-month period in male partners of women with breast cancer. Moreover, when examining dyadic BFG in the form of growth within a unit as a couple, there was a significant correlation between patient BFG and partner BFG over time. These findings highlight the importance of understanding the process of finding benefits within the context of social relationships.

There is a small but growing literature on BFG in caregivers of persons with HIV/AIDS and cancer (e.g., see Kim, Schulz, & Carver, 2007). However, caution must be taken in comparing these two bodies of literature directly. In the cancer literature, the caregivers are more commonly spouses or romantic partners. Typically, studies in the HIV/AIDS area have focused primarily on bereaved caregivers. This leads to natural questions about whether the BFG resulted from bereavement experiences or from the experience of caring for an ill romantic partner as in the cancer studies (e.g., see Cadell, 2001, 2003; Clipp, Adinolfi, Forrest, & Bennett, 1995; McCausland & Pakenham, 2003).

Lesson 5: Treatment Factors and Illness Prognoses Provide a Context for Benefit Finding and Growth

Diagnostic and treatment variables may have important effects on BFG in individuals with medical illnesses. Disease severity provides some information about probability of recovery and survival and thus is directly linked to perceptions of threat. Treatment-related variables may be linked to differences in the perceived stressfulness of the illness because of differences in side effects and impact on functioning. As the process of BFG is thought to unfold over time, time since diagnosis may be an important variable to consider.

Diagnostic and treatment variables appear to affect BFG in individuals with medical illnesses. One important contextual variable to consider is disease severity, typically conceptualized in cancer as the American Joint Committee on Cancer (i.e., AJCC) stage of disease, and in HIV using detectable viral load, disease symptoms, or AIDS diagnosis. Disease severity provides some information about probability of recovery and/or survival and thus is directly linked to perceptions of medical threat. Patients with cancer may perceive greater disease threat when their prognosis is communicated in direct or subtle ways by medical staff or when they have to undergo extensive and painful treatments. However, they are not always correct in detecting their levels of threat or in knowing their stage of disease (Vothang, Lechner, Tocco, & Glück, 2006). Patients with HIV experience a growing number of symptoms as their disease worsens, and thus they may be better informed about their levels of threat than are cancer patients, although this has not been tested empirically. Several studies have supported the link between greater perceived threat with greater BFG in medical patients (e.g., see Bellizzi & Blank, 2006; Cordova et al., 2001; Lechner & Yanez, 2006). In contrast, other research has shown no relationship between disease severity and BFG in individuals with HIV/AIDS (e.g., see

Mellors, Riley, & Erlen, 1997; Milam, 2004; Siegel et al., 2005) or cancer (e.g., see Andrykowski et al., 1993; Manne et al., 2004; Thornton & Perez, 2006; Weaver, 2006).

One potential explanation for this discrepancy is that threat and BFG may not track together in a one-to-one relationship. Consistent with this hypothesis, in a study of cancer patients (Lechner, Zakowski, et al., 2003), we observed that patients with medium levels of disease severity reported greater BFG than those with low severity and those with very high disease severity. We suggest that when disease threat is low, people do not need to engage in the cognitive processes leading to BFG. Because the event is not seismic enough (e.g., see Tedeschi & Calhoun, 2004), individuals can get through it with a minimum amount of struggle. However, if severe disease results in great threat to life or serious distress, an individual's ability to tolerate threatening emotions and cognitions may be overwhelmed. When an individual's ability to cope is significantly compromised, searching for meaning is unlikely, as is ultimately finding benefits (Lechner, Zakowski, et al., 2003). Thus, a little threat is necessary to provide a context for BFG, but too much threat may overwhelm coping resources and undermine BFG.

In addition, the relationship between various indicators of disease severity and BFG may be moderated by patients' knowledge and understanding of their prognosis. For example, Vothang et al. (2006) found that 43% of patients incorrectly reported the stage of their cancer. Incomplete understanding of disease severity may lead individuals to either overestimate or underestimate threat, possibly obscuring relationships between objective medical indicators and BFG.

As BFG is conceptualized as a dynamic process, time since diagnosis may be an important variable to consider when examining BFG in medical patients. Results from cross-sectional studies of individuals with cancer, typically 1 to 5 years postdiagnosis, are mixed, with some studies suggesting that BFG is significantly related to time since diagnosis (Sears et al., 2003) and others finding no relationship (e.g., see Bellizzi & Blank, 2006; Cordova et al., 2001; Lechner, Zakowski, et al., 2003). Results from studies of adults who are HIV-positive do not typically support a relationship between time since diagnosis and BFG (e.g., see Milam, 2004; Siegel et al., 2005); however, both of these studies included individuals who were, on average, 6 to 7 years postdiagnosis. It is possible that there are critical periods during which changes in BFG occur that are related to disease processes. For example, BFG could increase in the time immediately following diagnosis and then remain relatively stable if a person's health status is also relatively stable. In one of the few longitudinal studies examining the period immediately after diagnosis, Manne et al. (2004) observed progressive increases in BFG in both patients with breast cancer and their partners between the time shortly after surgery and the first 18 months thereafter. Disease recurrence or progression (e.g., discovery of metastatic disease in cancer patients, diagnosis with an AIDS-defining symptom) might lead to further changes in BFG. Longitudinal studies of medical patients beginning soon after diagnosis will be necessary to identify critical periods during which changes in BFG occur.

Finally, whether individuals are actively receiving treatment, and what type of treatment they receive, may be important factors in the development and maintenance of BFG. Treatment-related side effects may affect physical functioning and/or perceptions of threat, thereby influencing BFG as described earlier. Although most studies have exclusively examined either cancer patients currently receiving treatment or those finished with treatment, one study including both populations found that overall BFG did not differ between cancer patients who were receiving active treatment and those whose treatment was complete (Lechner, Zakowski, et al., 2003). In women with breast cancer, having received chemotherapy predicted greater BFG (Bower et al., 2005; Weaver, 2006). Yet, studies have not typically observed relationships between type of cancer surgery and BFG in women with breast cancer and men with prostate cancer (e.g., see Bellizzi & Blank, 2006; Weaver, 2006; Weiss, 2004). It is possible that some treatments and their side effects are more salient to cancer patients (e.g., chemotherapy-related hair loss) than others. Similarly, Milam (2004) observed no relationship between current use of antiretroviral medications and BFG in people with HIV/AIDS. Future research will need to clarify how medical treatments for cancer and HIV are related to BFG and the role of mediating mechanisms such as perceptions of threat, illness-related stress, and treatment side effects.

One exciting aspect of BFG clinical research is that there are so many unanswered questions to address in future work. Possible questions stemming from the lessons identified in this chapter are listed in Exhibit 6.1.

Clinical Implications

The lessons identified in this chapter may have clinical implications for clinicians working with persons with HIV/AIDS or cancer. First, we have evidence that BFG is similar in these populations. The majority of persons with HIV and cancer report some sort of positive changes resulting from their illness. The types of positive changes reported are similar between the groups, although we recognize that some aspects of BFG may be more important to different populations at different points in the illness trajectory. This suggests that BFG can be approached in a similar clinical manner across groups of people. Second, it may be difficult to predict from sociodemographic characteristics who is likely to find benefits; psychological characteristics may provide better information. Assessments of psychological strengths such as optimism, coping strategies, and emotional processing may provide clinicians with clues about their clients' readiness for and/or likelihood of engaging in the cognitive processing associated with BFG. Next, clinicians should consider a client's social network (including the client–therapist relationship) when addressing BFG in therapy. Therapy may provide some clients with unique opportunities to express their emotions in a supportive environment, thereby facilitating BFG. Finally, it is important for clinicians to recognize that treatment and medical prognostic factors provide a context for BFG. Assessment of treatment-related stressors and a client's expectations for the future may guide BFG work in therapy.

Clinicians can address BFG in individual sessions by asking clients, in a gentle and encouraging manner, to consider how their lives have changed as a result of their medical illness. Ideally, patients will initiate the idea of positive changes

Exhibit 6.1.   Future Directions and Unanswered Questions About Benefit Finding and Growth (BFG) Following Cancer and HIV

The Nature of BFG

---

1. How does BFG develop after a seismic life event? What processes or premorbid characteristics are truly necessary for BFG?
2. The qualities of BFG may be similar across different medical illnesses, but is BFG stemming from medical illness different from BFG from other types of trauma?
3. Is BFG that results from a single traumatic event (e.g., rape) different from an ongoing long-term stressor such as daily HAART therapy?
4. Does BFG that results from different types of ongoing traumas differ on the basis of the type of hardship? Is living through a Category 5 hurricane likely to produce qualitatively or quantitatively different BFG compared with daily HAART, weekly chemotherapy, daily radiation and/or follow-up check-ups every 6 months?
5. Health behavior changes appear to be an important aspect of response to HIV/AIDS, cancer, and other illnesses. What are some of the reasons why health behaviors are not typically identified as aspects of BFG in qualitative reports of other types of stressors and traumas?
6. How do the types of losses associated with different illnesses (e.g., threat to life, loss of femininity or masculinity, inability to do one's job or carry out social roles, isolation from friends and family, loss of dignity, loss of physical abilities, disfigurement) affect BFG?

The Trajectory of BFG

---

1. Is there a critical period for the initial development of BFG? Does this period vary by the type and nature of the traumatic event (e.g., single event vs. ongoing stressor)?
2. What is the long-term trajectory of BFG? Is growth stable over time?

Predictors of BFG

---

1. What role does medical uncertainty regarding prognosis play?
2. What role does fear of death play?
3. What is the role of specific cognitive processes such as intentionally searching for or reminding oneself about positive change?

Outcomes of BFG

---

1. How may BFG affect disease outcomes and mortality? Does it affect disease outcomes and mortality (e.g., see Bower, Kemeny, Taylor, & Fahey, 1998; Moskowitz, 2003)?
2. Some have suggested that BFG is unrelated to outcomes because BFG can co-occur with distress, intrusive thoughts, and other traditional outcome variables. Is there support for the idea that these constructs are not mutually exclusive?

Note.   HAART = highly active antiretroviral therapy.

themselves, but we have also successfully broached the topic by mentioning, without violating confidentiality, the experience of other clients who have experienced BFG. If timed correctly, most clients will receive this intervention well and will be grateful for the opportunity to discuss both positive and negative life changes resulting from cancer and HIV. At this point, it is too early to suggest specific interventions to enhance BFG or to know whether encouraging

BFG would be beneficial for all clients. Instead, we advocate being aware of the process of BFG and providing a supportive forum for the discussion of positive changes resulting from medical illness. Chapter 12 of this volume presents a useful framework for conducting therapy with survivors that the authors call "expert companionship." Other work involving meaning-making interventions may also be useful in this context (Lee, Cohen, Edgar, Laizner, & Gagnon, 2006).

It is important for clinicians to be sensitive to the timing of BFG discussions. Suggesting that there are positive aspects to a life challenge that a person continues to experience as profoundly distressing may be upsetting to the client and could even lead to a rupture in the therapeutic alliance. Our clinical experiences with HIV and cancer patients warrant this cautionary clinical vignette. A young man, whom we will call Adam, is an active and insightful member of a support group for people who are HIV-positive. He contracted HIV through unprotected sex and feels a great deal of responsibility for his illness. He has changed some health behaviors: He has stopped smoking, eats healthier foods, and exercises more frequently. Adam is feeling a great deal of distress over his new medication regimen and the implications of HIV on his sex life, and he voices fears and concerns about disease course, mortality, and other existential issues. In group sessions, the novice therapist suggests that perhaps Adam might want to view HIV as an opportunity for growth and positive change. If the therapist suggests that there may be positive sequelae to HIV before Adam is ready to process that idea, Adam may feel misunderstood and abandoned, and may become defensive. This scenario could happen in one-to-one treatment, but is probably more prevalent in group work when a therapist needs to consider the needs of many people who are at different stages of processing their illness.

It is certainly challenging to address BFG in a sensitive manner during group-based interventions. An intervention that addresses positive reframing and growth needs to be delivered at the right time, which clinical experience suggests will differ for every client. We also lack empirical guidance on the most opportune time to intervene. Thus, if the therapist in a group setting proposes such ideas, group members may feel alienated. There is also the danger that clients may also experience high levels of peer pressure from group members, who are further along on the BFG trajectory, to endorse positive changes before they are ready, or to minimize the distress they are experiencing. However, if clients are at similar stages of BFG, group discussion of positive changes may be profoundly moving and helpful to them. It is often much easier for a group member to hear these ideas and thoughts from another group member than from the therapist. Although some colleagues disagree with this point, we feel that it is premature to develop group-based interventions to specifically augment BFG. As discussed in this chapter, many questions have yet to be answered about BFG in persons with cancer and HIV/AIDS. We recommend that more prospective research needs to be conducted to determine the optimal time to deliver such interventions before these group-based interventions are developed.

In summary, inquiry into BFG in persons with medical illnesses has flourished in recent years. This is an exciting time to study the sequelae of medical illness, as we gain more knowledge regarding how people adjust to challenging life experiences. The inconsistencies that have been highlighted in this chapter can be the impetus for enhanced attention to the complexities of people's reactions to illness. Clinicians have the privilege of joining patients along the journey toward well-being and contentment. BFG is only one aspect of positive adaptation to illness, and we are encouraged by the attention that has been paid to this phenomenon.

References

Andrykowski, M. A., Brady, M. J., & Hunt, J. W. (1993). Positive psychosocial adjustment in potential bone marrow transplant recipients: Cancer as a psychosocial transition. *Psycho-Oncology, 2,* 261–276.

Antoni, M. H., Lehman, J. M., Kilbourn, K. M., Boyers, A. E., Culver, J. L., Alferi, S. M., et al. (2001). Cognitive-behavioral stress management intervention decreases the prevalence of depression and enhances benefit finding among women under treatment for early-stage breast cancer. *Health Psychology, 20,* 20–32.

Barroso, J. (1996). Focusing on living: Attitudinal approaches of long-term survivors of AIDS. *Issues in Mental Health Nursing, 17,* 395–407.

Bellizzi, K. M. (2004). Expressions of generativity and posttraumatic growth in adult cancer survivors. *International Journal of Aging and Human Development, 58,* 267–287.

Bellizzi, K. M., & Blank, T. O. (2006). Predicting posttraumatic growth in breast cancer survivors. *Health Psychology, 25,* 47–56.

Bower, J. E., Kemeny, M. E., Taylor, S. E., & Fahey, J. L. (1998). Cognitive processing, discovery of meaning, CD4 decline, and AIDS-related mortality among bereaved HIV-seropositive men. *Journal of Consulting and Clinical Psychology, 66,* 979–986.

Bower, J. E., Meyerowitz, B. E., Desmond, K. A., Bernaards, C. A., Rowland, J. H., & Ganz, P. A. (2005). Perceptions of positive meaning and vulnerability following breast cancer: Predictors and outcomes among long-term breast cancer survivors. *Annals of Behavioral Medicine, 29,* 236–245.

Brashers, D. E., Neidig, J. L., Cardillo, L. W., Dobbs, L. K., Russell, J. A., & Haas, S. M. (1999). "In an important way, I did die": Uncertainty and revival in persons living with HIV or AIDS. *AIDS Care, 11,* 201–219.

Cadell, S. (2001). Post-traumatic growth in HIV/AIDS caregivers in Quebec. *Canadian Social Work, 3,* 86–94.

Cadell, S. (2003). Trauma and growth in Canadian carers. *AIDS Care, 15,* 639–648.

Carver, C. S., & Antoni, M. H. (2004). Finding benefit in breast cancer during the year after diagnosis predicts better adjustment 5 to 8 years after diagnosis. *Health Psychology, 23,* 595–598.

Carver, C. S., Scheier, M. F., & Weintraub, J. K. (1989). Assessing coping strategies: A theoretically based approach. *Journal of Personality and Social Psychology, 56,* 267–283.

Cella, D. F., & Tross, S. (1986). Psychological adjustment to survival from Hodgkin's disease. *Journal of Consulting and Clinical Psychology, 54,* 616–622.

Clipp, E. C., Adinolfi, A. J., Forrest, L., & Bennett, C. L. (1995). Informal caregivers of persons with AIDS. *Journal of Palliative Care, 11*(2), 10–18.

Cordova, M. J., Cunningham, L. L. C., Carlson, C. R., & Andrykowski, M. A. (2001). Posttraumatic growth following breast cancer: A controlled comparison study. *Health Psychology, 20,* 176–185.

Courtenay, B. C., Merriam, S., Reeves, P., & Baumgartner, L. (2000). Perspective transformation over time: A 2-year follow-up study of HIV-positive adults. *Adult Education Quarterly, 50,* 102–119.

Coward, D. D. (1994). Meaning and purpose in the lives of persons with AIDS. *Public Health Nursing, 11,* 331–336.

Coward, D. D., & Lewis, F. M. (1993). The lived experience of self-transcendence in gay men with AIDS. *Oncology Nursing Forum, 20,* 1363–1368.

Dunn, J., Lynch, B., Rinaldis, M., Pakenham, K., McPherson, L., Owen, N., et al. (2006). Dimensions of quality of life and psychosocial variables most salient to colorectal cancer patients. *Psycho-Oncology, 15,* 20–30.

Fife, B. L. (1995). The measurement of meaning in illness. *Social Science & Medicine, 40*, 1021–1028.

Fife, B. L. (2005). The role of constructed meaning in adaptation to the onset of life-threatening illness. *Social Science & Medicine, 61*, 2132–2143.

Foley, K. L., Farmer, D. F., Petronis, V. M., Smith, R. G., McGraw, S., Smith, K., et al. (2006). A qualitative exploration of the cancer experience among long-term survivors: Comparisons by cancer type, ethnicity, gender, and age. *Psycho-Oncology, 15*, 248–258.

Folkman, S., & Lazarus, R. S. (1988). The relationship between coping and emotion: Implications for theory and research. *Social Science & Medicine, 26*, 309–317.

Fromm, K., Andrykowski, M. A., & Hunt, J. (1996). Positive and negative psychosocial sequelae of bone marrow transplantation: Implications for quality of life assessment. *Journal of Behavioral Medicine, 19*, 221–240.

Kim, Y., Schulz, R., & Carver, C. S. (2007). Benefit finding in the cancer caregiving experience. *Psychosomatic Medicine, 69*, 283–291.

Kinsinger, D. P., Penedo, F. J., Antoni, M. H., Dahn, J. R., Lechner, S., & Schneiderman, N. (2006). Psychosocial and sociodemographic correlates of benefit-finding in men treated for localized prostate cancer. *Psycho-Oncology, 15*, 954–961.

Lazarus, R. S., & Folkman, S. (1984). *Stress, appraisal, and coping.* New York: Springer Publishing Company.

Lechner, S. C. (2000). *Found meaning in individuals with cancer.* Unpublished doctoral dissertation, Finch University of Health Sciences/The Chicago Medical School, Chicago.

Lechner, S. C., & Antoni, M. H. (2004). Posttraumatic growth and group-based interventions for persons dealing with cancer: What have we learned so far? *Psychological Inquiry, 15*, 35–41.

Lechner, S. C., Antoni, M. H., & Carver, C. S. (2003). Associations between benefit-finding and coping with breast cancer over a one-year period [Abstract]. *Annals of Behavioral Medicine, 25*, S053.

Lechner, S. C., Carver, C. S., Antoni, M. H., Weaver, K., & Phillips, K. (2006). Curvilinear associations between benefit finding and adjustment to breast cancer. *Journal of Consulting and Clinical Psychology, 74*, 828–840.

Lechner, S. C., & Yanez, B. (2006). *Perceived threat mediates the relationship between cancer severity and benefit finding.* Manuscript submitted for publication.

Lechner, S. C., Zakowski, S. G., Antoni, M. H., Greenhawt, M., Block, K., & Block, P. (2003). Do sociodemographic and disease-related variables influence benefit finding in cancer patients? *Psycho-Oncology, 12*, 491–499.

Lee, V., Cohen, S. R., Edgar, L., Laizner, A. M., & Gagnon, A. (2006). Meaning-making intervention during breast or colorectal cancer treatment improves self-esteem, optimism, and self-efficacy. *Social Science & Medicine, 62*, 3133–3145.

Manne, S., Ostroff, J., Winkel, G., Goldstein, L., Fox, K., & Grana, G. (2004). Posttraumatic growth after breast cancer: Patient, partner, and couple perspectives. *Psychosomatic Medicine, 66*, 442–454.

McCausland, J., & Pakenham, K. I. (2003). Investigation of the benefits of HIV/AIDS caregiving and relations among caregiving adjustment, benefit finding, and stress and coping variables. *AIDS Care, 15*, 853–869.

Mellors, M. P., Riley, T. A., & Erlen, J. A. (1997). HIV, self-transcendence, and quality of life. *Journal of the Association of Nurses in AIDS Care, 8*, 59–69.

Milam, J. E. (2004). Posttraumatic growth among HIV/AIDS patients. *Journal of Applied Social Psychology, 34*, 2353–2376.

Moskowitz, J. T. (2003). Positive affect predicts lower risk of AIDS mortality. *Psychosomatic Medicine, 65*, 620–626.

Park, C. L., Cohen, L. H., & Murch, R. L. (1996). Assessment and prediction of stress-related growth. *Journal of Personality, 64*, 71–105.

Plattner, I. E., & Meiring, N. (2006). Living with HIV: The psychological relevance of meaning making. *AIDS Care, 18*, 241–245.

Schaefer, J. A., & Moos, R. H. (2001). Bereavement experiences and personal growth. In M. S. Stroebe, R. O. Hansson, W. Stroebe, & H. Schut (Eds.), *Handbook of bereavement research: Consequences, coping, and care* (pp. 145–167). Washington, DC: American Psychological Association.

Scheier, M. F., & Carver, C. S. (1985). Optimism, coping, and health: Assessment and implications of generalized outcome expectancies. *Health Psychology, 4*, 219–247.

Schulz, U., & Mohamed, N. E. (2004). Turning the tide: Benefit finding after cancer surgery. *Social Science & Medicine, 59,* 653–662.

Schwartzberg, S. S. (1993). Struggling for meaning: How HIV-positive gay men make sense of aids. *Professional Psychology, Research and Practice, 24,* 483–490.

Schwartzberg, S. S. (1994). Vitality and growth in HIV-infected gay men. *Social Science & Medicine, 38,* 593–602.

Sears, S. R., Stanton, A. L., & Danoff-Burg, S. (2003). The Yellow Brick Road and the Emerald City: Benefit finding, positive reappraisal coping and posttraumatic growth in women with early-stage breast cancer. *Health Psychology, 22,* 487–497.

Siegel, K., & Schrimshaw, E. W. (2000). Perceiving benefits in adversity: Stress-related growth in women living with HIV/AIDS. *Social Science & Medicine, 51,* 1543–1554.

Siegel, K., Schrimshaw, E. W., & Pretter, S. (2005). Stress-related growth among women living with HIV/AIDS: Examination of an explanatory model. *Journal of Behavioral Medicine, 28,* 403–414.

Stanton, A. L., Bower, J. E., & Low, C. A. (2006). Posttraumatic growth after cancer. In L. G. Calhoun & R. G. Tedeschi (Eds.), *Handbook of posttraumatic growth: Research and practice* (pp. 138–175). Mahwah, NJ: Erlbaum.

Taylor, S. E. (1983). Adjustment to threatening events: A theory of cognitive adaptation. *American Psychologist, 38,* 1161–1173.

Tedeschi, R. G., & Calhoun, L. G. (1996). The Posttraumatic Growth Inventory: Measuring the positive legacy of trauma. *Journal of Traumatic Stress, 9,* 455–471.

Tedeschi, R. G., & Calhoun, L. G. (2004). Posttraumatic growth: Conceptual foundations and empirical evidence. *Psychological Inquiry, 15,* 1–18.

Thornton, A. A., & Perez, M. A. (2006). Posttraumatic growth in prostate cancer survivors and their partners. *Psycho-Oncology, 15,* 285–296.

Tomich, P. L., & Helgeson, V. S. (2004). Is finding something good in the bad always good? Benefit finding among women with breast cancer. *Health Psychology, 23,* 16–23.

Updegraff, J. A., Taylor, S. E., Kemeny, M. E., & Wyatt, G. E. (2002). Positive and negative effects of HIV infection in women with low socioeconomic resources. *Personality and Social Psychology Bulletin, 28,* 382–394.

Urcuyo, K. R., Boyers, A. E., Carver, C. S., & Antoni, M. H. (2005). Finding benefit in breast cancer: Relations with personality, coping, and concurrent well-being. *Psychology and Health, 20,* 175–192.

Viney, L. L., Crooks, L., Walker, B. M., & Henry, R. (1991). Psychological frailness and strength in an AIDS-affected community: A study of seropositive gay men and voluntary caregivers. *American Journal of Community Psychology, 19,* 279–287.

Vothang, T., Lechner, S., Tocco, J., & Glück, M. (2006, March). *Beware of self-report medical data: Lessons learned at a cancer center.* Poster session presented at the annual meeting of the Society of Behavioral Medicine, San Francisco.

Wasserman, A. L., Thompson, E. I., Wilimas, J. A., & Fairclough, D. L. (1987). The psychological status of survivors of childhood/adolescent Hodgkin's disease. *American Journal of Diseases of Children, 141,* 626–631.

Weaver, K. E. (2006). *Assessing positive growth from the experience of chronic illness: A measurement model of benefit-finding in breast cancer, prostate cancer, and HIV/AIDS.* Unpublished doctoral dissertation, University of Miami, Coral Gables, FL.

Weiss, T. (2004). Correlates of posttraumatic growth in married breast cancer survivors. *Journal of Social and Clinical Psychology, 23,* 733–746.

Widows, M. R., Jacobsen, P. B., Booth-Jones, M., & Fields, K. K. (2005). Predictors of posttraumatic growth following bone marrow transplantation for cancer. *Health Psychology, 24,* 266–273.

7

Illness Perceptions and Benefit Finding Among Individuals With Breast Cancer, Acoustic Neuroma, or Heart Disease

Keith J. Petrie and Arden Corter

One important factor that seems to influence the types of positive effects reported from illness is the way patients view the demands of their illness (Affleck & Tennen, 1996; Petrie, Buick, Weinman, & Booth, 1999). This chapter highlights the important role played by patients' perceptions of illness in affecting positive changes following the diagnosis of a major illness. Much of this work draws from self-regulation theory, developed by Howard Leventhal and others (Leventhal et al., 1997; Leventhal, Nerenz, & Steele, 1984), which highlights the important role of patients' understanding and conceptualization of their illness in directing personal coping with health threats. The theory starts with the premise that individuals are active problem solvers who make sense of a threat to their health, such as symptoms or an illness, by developing their own cognitive representations of the health threat, which in turn determine coping responses.

Leventhal's (Leventhal et al., 1984, 1997) self-regulation theory is dynamic, proposing that changes in patients' perceptions of their illness result in shifts in emotional response and coping strategies. When faced with the diagnosis of an illness, patients build models of the illness on the basis of their own knowledge and what they may have been told by health professionals, as well as their own personal experience of others with the illness, such as family or friends. As patients develop more knowledge and experience with the illness, their representations often change and lead to different patterns of coping (Petrie, Broadbent, & Meechan, 2003).

Following the diagnosis of a chronic illness, issues of loss of functioning and uncertainties about the future often dominate patients' thoughts as they try to work out how the nature of the illness will impact their life and future plans. Evidence from a growing number of studies shows that the way patients conceptualize the threat of the illness has a profound impact on illness-related and emotional coping strategies as well as eventual adjustment (Fortune, Richards, Griffiths, & Main, 2002; Petrie, Weinman, Sharpe, & Buckley, 1996; Scharloo et al., 1998). There is also some evidence that perceptions of illness may also influence the acquisition of benefits from the illness (Petrie et al., 1999).

In this chapter, we first examine how the acquisition of benefit finding varies across different illness groups: breast cancer, acoustic neuroma, and heart disease. Then we present background information on illness perceptions, including the five main components of illness perceptions. We then discuss the use of patient drawings as one possible way to assess illness perceptions. Next, we discuss the possible link between illness perceptions and benefit finding. Finally, we look at further applications of this work within the health psychology area.

Benefit Finding in Different Illness Groups

In our research, we have examined the nature of benefit finding in patients diagnosed with breast cancer or a heart attack as well as patients who have had surgery to remove an acoustic neuroma tumor near the brain. In this section, we examine more closely the types of benefits reported by breast cancer and acoustic neuroma patients driven by the demands brought on by the disease and specific treatment.

Breast cancer is an illness viewed with fear and dread by all women (see chaps. 1 and 3, this volume). The diagnosis of breast cancer causes patients to deal with the physical effects of the removal of the cancer—usually by surgery and radiation or chemotherapy—as well as confronting the possibility that the cancer will recur and ultimately cause an early death (Buick, 1997). It is not surprising that given the psychological issues that provide the backdrop to this illness, finding increased value in close relationships, changing personal priorities, and reporting a greater appreciation of life feature prominently in the types of benefits that women with breast cancer report.

In a study of women with breast cancer, Petrie et al. (1999) found that an improvement in the quality of personal relationships was reported by 33% of participants. This is illustrated by a quotation from one woman: "My husband and I have been closer than we have been for years with more communication" (p. 541). A greater appreciation of life was reported by 27% of women. A patient commented,

> One can't help feeling that perhaps life is going to be shorter than anticipated—so the most must be made of every minute! I love the time spent with friends and family—every moment seems precious—so I am determined to keep on enjoying and appreciating all life has to offer. (p. 541)

A benefit that is closely related to a greater appreciation of life is a change in personal priorities, which was found in 20% of patients with breast cancer. This is illustrated by a quotation from one woman: "It made you stop and examine your life and where it is heading. Changing priorities—look at what and who is really important. Realise how easy it is to lose life. Do what *you* want to do" (p. 541).

One can see from the types of benefits and from the quotations, that the perceived demands of the illness cause a realignment of life priorities so that important relationships and valued activities become more significant as patients confront the fact that their future is uncertain. The benefits patients report following their illness reflect this change in the alignment of priorities.

A similar process is seen in patients who have had surgery for acoustic neuroma. An acoustic neuroma is a benign tumor that grows along the vestibulo-cochlear nerve and can extend from the internal auditory canal into the brain cavity. The tumor is commonly removed surgically. In most cases the long-term prognosis is excellent, but surgery can leave patients with hearing loss, disequilibrium, facial weakness, and other functional deficits. The dramatic nature of the brain surgery treatment required for removal of the tumor creates a pattern of perceived benefits similar to women diagnosed with breast cancer. In a sample of 119 acoustic neuroma patients, the most frequently reported positive aspect was a greater appreciation of life (33%), followed by improved interpersonal relationships (30%). Feeling fortunate to be alive, perhaps driven by the seriousness of the treatment, was also mentioned by 12% of patients. Patients who following the surgery were left with facial disfigurement were less likely to mention benefits (Browne, Distel, Morton, & Petrie, in press).

For many patients who experience a heart attack, the diagnosis of heart disease is a surprise, as they may have been unaware of the disease process that is likely to have been operating for many years. For some patients, surviving the drama of a heart attack is seen as being given another chance at life and is viewed as a positive opportunity to change long-standing unhealthy behaviors. As a man in one of the studies wrote, "I now eat healthier food. I get regular exercise. I now realize that no one can go through life thinking they will do what they like and their body will take care of itself" (Petrie et al., 1999, p. 540).

How Patients Perceive Illness

The diagnosis of an illness normally starts with noticing physical symptoms. The type of symptom and whether it appears suddenly or causes pain and disruption to an individual's normal activity are all factors that cause individuals to seek medical care (Petrie & Pennebaker, 2004). Howard Leventhal has highlighted the symmetry between symptoms and illness labels (Leventhal et al., 1997). When individuals are experiencing symptoms, there is pressure to find an illness label to explain their sickness. Similarly, receiving a diagnosis of a particular illness often leads the patient to search for symptoms that are consistent with that particular disease label. This process occurs even if the illness is asymptomatic (e.g., hypertension) and may result in the patient misattributing a number of symptoms to their illness, perhaps using them as indicators of their need for medication or other treatment (Baumann & Leventhal, 1985).

Often the knowledge or information patients use to build mental representations of their illness is built on rudimentary or incorrect concepts about their body or health. We have found that the public lacks basic knowledge about where major body organs such as the heart and kidney are located in the body. Weinman, Yusuf, Berks, Rayner, and Petrie (2008) recently found that less than 50% of a general population sample could identify the correct location of their heart, lungs, stomach, or kidney. Furthermore, patients with specific organ-related pathology, such as heart disease or kidney failure, were generally no better than members of the public at locating these organs. In clinical situations, such as in doctors' offices or hospital wards, patients' basic inaccuracies and misperceptions about symptoms and illness are often not picked up by medical staff because patients are rarely asked about their views of their illness.

Over the past 10 years, considerable work has focused on the components that make up patients' illness perceptions, and on developing ways to assess illness beliefs. Through this work it has become clear that patients with similar illnesses often have very different perceptions of the illness and that these differences are related to differences in the ways patients manage and cope emotionally with their condition. Although patients may see the same illness differently, the structure of perceptions seems to be consistent between patients, with most studies finding that patients organize their beliefs about their illness around five interrelated components (see Hagger & Orbell, 2003, for a review).

The first of these components is *identity,* incorporating the illness label and the symptoms that patients associate with their condition. It is important to note that the symptoms that patients associate with their illness do not always coincide with the medical view of the illness and typically contain a wider range of symptoms. Many illness labels, such as cancer, have a strong and immediate emotional response. Symptoms are often used by patients as a way of determining the seriousness of their illness (Petrie & Pennebaker, 2004). Both the number of symptoms and patients' emotional response to the illness label are likely to be associated with later benefit finding.

Patients usually develop *causal beliefs* about their illness, particularly following diagnosis. Causal beliefs have important relationships in some illnesses to the types of treatment patients use to manage their condition, adherence to treatment, and emotional reactions to illness. They also may be associated with patients' ability to derive benefits from their illness. Patients who believe their illness has been caused by poor health habits such as poor diet or smoking are more likely to change these behaviors, whereas patients who see their illness as caused by stress are more likely to attempt to reduce their stress by making changes such as giving up or changing their job (Weinman, Petrie, Sharpe, & Walker, 2000). In many illnesses, patients may blame themselves for their condition, which can increase their level of negative emotional response to the illness (Malcarne, Compas, Epping-Jordan, & Howell, 1995). Patients who have had a heart attack and who change their lifestyle in response to their belief that the illness was caused by faulty health habits often report this as an important positive outcome from their illness.

Patients also normally develop *timeline beliefs* about their condition (Nerenz & Leventhal, 1983). These beliefs usually vary from acute or time-limited to chronic. Occasionally, patients may believe that their condition is cyclical and only use medication when they believe they are currently suffering from their illness. This often happens with "symptomless" conditions such as hypertension, when patients may believe their blood pressure is elevated only when they have been under stress and only take medication at these times (Baumann & Leventhal, 1985).

Patients' ideas about the timeline of their illness tend to be related to *personal and treatment control beliefs.* Patients often develop ideas about how susceptible their illness is to being controlled by their own actions. In some illnesses, such as heart disease, patients often develop strong beliefs that they can manage their illness by changing their health behavior, for example, by improving their diet or stopping smoking. Patients also develop beliefs about how effectively their treatment will control their illness (Horne & Weinman, 1999). High levels of personal and treatment control tend to be related to shorter time-line beliefs, lower identity, and lower emotional reactions to illness (Weinman, Petrie, Moss-Morris, & Horne, 1996).

The final major illness perception component is *consequence beliefs*. This component centers on the perceived consequences of the illness in terms of the effect it will have on patients' work, finances, family, and lifestyle. Soon after being diagnosed with an illness, patients make judgments about how the illness will affect their life on the basis of their knowledge of the illness and its perceived severity. However, patients' views of the severity of their illness often have a low level of concordance with objective clinical markers of illness severity (Broadbent, Petrie, Ellis, et al., 2006). Similarly, patients' personal views of their illness can vary markedly from clinicians' views of the same illness.

Assessing Patients' Views of Their Illness

Although early studies highlighted the importance of illness perceptions in understanding patients' response to illness, it was not until recently that scales have been available to directly measure patients' views of their illness. Previously, illness perceptions were extracted using semistructured interviews with patients. This technique produced variable responses from patients and lacked psychometric validity. Just over 10 years ago, the Illness Perception Questionnaire was developed as a self-report measure for patients (Weinman et al., 1996). The scale provided a method for assessing the major components of illness perceptions and can be tailored to specific illnesses or medical conditions. A later revised version of the scale extended the original scale by adding more items and subscales (Moss-Morris, Weinman, Petrie, Horne, Cameron, & Buick, 2002). A short version of the scale (see Figure 7.1) was published for use in both clinical and research situations when patients are very ill or when there is limited time available for assessment (Broadbent, Petrie, Main, & Weinman, 2006).

A recent innovative assessment procedure for accessing illness perceptions is the use of patient drawings. Patient drawings provide a rich source of data for understanding patients' response to illness. Examples of drawings from patients who have chronic headaches, patients with heart failure, and patients who have experienced a heart attack are shown in Figure 7.2. In a study of patients who had experienced a myocardial infarction, Broadbent, Petrie, Ellis, Ying, and Gamble (2004) found that the size of damage drawn by patients on their heart was associated with a slower return to work and less positive perceptions of their condition 3 months later. Furthermore, drawings were a better predictor of these outcomes than biological measures of damage to the heart following their heart attack. Patients' drawings also provide a more dynamic view of how they perceive their illness as changing over time. Broadbent, Ellis, Gamble, and Petrie (2006) found that by asking patients to draw their hearts again 3 months after their heart attack, a decrease in the size of the heart

For the following questions, please circle the number that best corresponds to your views:

How much does your illness affect your life?

0   1   2   3   4   5   6   7   8   9   10

No effect
at all

Severely
affects my life

How long do you think your illness will continue?

0   1   2   3   4   5   6   7   8   9   10

A very
short time

Forever

How much control do you feel you have over your illness?

0   1   2   3   4   5   6   7   8   9   10

Absolutely
no control

Extreme amount
of control

How much do you think your treatment can help your illness?

0   1   2   3   4   5   6   7   8   9   10

Not at all

Extremely
helpful

Figure 7.1. Examples of items from the Brief Illness Perception Questionnaire. From "The Brief Illness Perception Questionnaire (BIPQ)," by E. Broadbent, K. J. Petrie, J. Main, and J. Weinman, 2006, *Journal of Psychosomatic Research, 60,* p. 637. Copyright 2006 by Elsevier Limited. Reprinted with permission.

patients drew was an indicator of better recovery in terms of increased lower heart-focused anxiety, complaints of ill health, and use of health care.

Drawing tasks could be readily adapted to look at positive effects of illness if valid methods for assessing drawings are developed. In fact, in the studies highlighted here, patients have spontaneously produced drawings that encompass positive aspects of their illness. As an example, Figure 7.3 shows that a patient conceptualized his heart before the heart attack as being surrounded by worry and concern. Represented inside the heart are various topics of concern including money, the family court, truth and lies, as well as his own health.

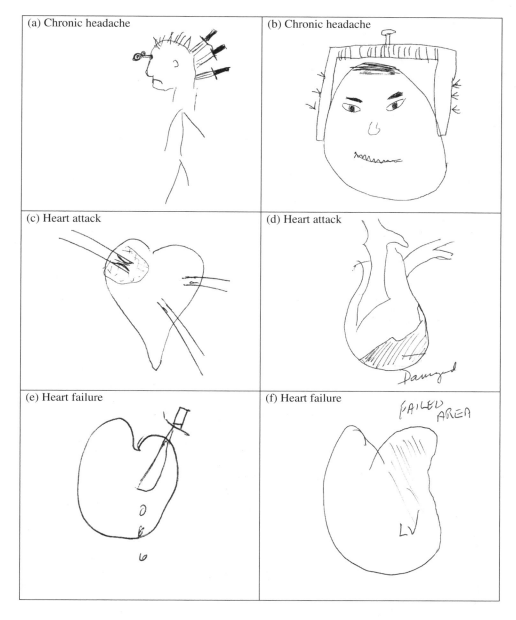

Figure 7.2. Examples of patients' drawings of their illness. Parts (a) and (b) depict chronic headaches; (c) and (d), heart attack; (e) and (f), heart failure.

At the center of the heart, the patient has drawn an area that represents his family. The patient's drawing of his heart following his heart attack shows a changed picture with the outside of the heart now filled with hope and faith. Health now takes a more prominent position in the drawing and the shape of how the family has been represented has been reconfigured. Although the focus

Picture of my heart before my heart attack   Picture of my heart after my heart attack

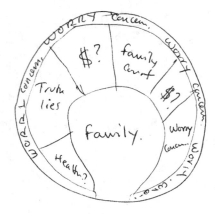
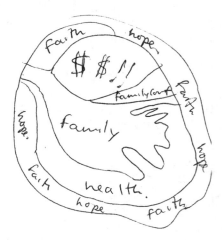

Figure 7.3. A heart attack patient's pictorial representation of life changes following his heart attack represented as areas on his heart.

of some of his worries and concerns is still present in the form of the family court and money, the size of these sections now represent smaller components of the heart.

In a second example, we specifically asked patients who had experienced heart failure to "Draw a picture of how you feel your heart failure is affecting you" and to "Please use some words to describe your drawing." Most drawings and descriptions capture patients' frustrations with the physical limitations caused by living with their heart failure. An example of this is provided in Figure 7.4, in which a 28-year-old male patient drew a broken-down car and accompanied the drawing with the following description: "Sorry. Broken down car—it needs to be fixed." However, a few of the sample of 60 patients drew or described positive aspects of living with their condition. One 64-year-old man wrote, "I have re-evaluated my life. I have changed my diet. I look at food labels intensely now. My concept of eternity has changed somewhat. I realise I am frail." A 66-year-old woman drew the picture in Figure 7.5, wherein she stated that because of her illness she had "lots of time to lie down and watch TV."

As shown in these examples, patients' drawings offer a valuable way of understanding their view of their illness and a quick way of capturing the meaning of the illness in their lives. Drawings as a means of assessment have had limited development in the health field. However, they have been used to measure children's health knowledge (Bendelow, Williams, & Oakley, 1996) and to improve communication between children and their doctors (Quinn, 1988). In adults, drawings have been used to assess illness suffering (Buchi et al., 2002) but have not been used specifically to evaluate benefit finding. The potential

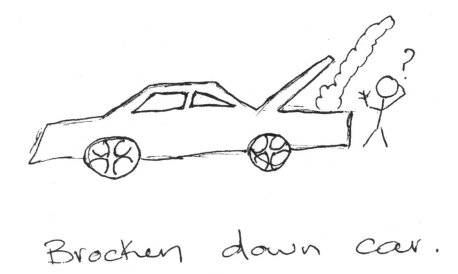

Figure 7.4.   Patient's drawing of his heart failure as a broken-down car.

exists to use this rich data source if methods are developed to construct useful and reliable metrics to analyze drawings.

Illness Perceptions and Benefit Finding

This chapter has highlighted the important role that illness perceptions play in patients' reports of positive effects from their illness. Although there has been only limited work in this area to date, the data indicate that patients' beliefs

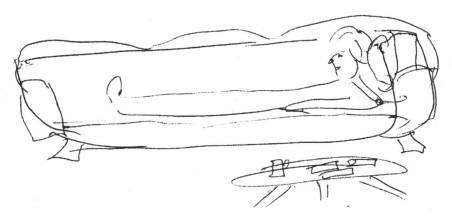

Figure 7.5.   Patient describing the benefits of her heart failure as having more leisure time.

about the consequences of their illness, and their initial level of emotional response to the diagnosis, are factors that predict later benefit finding. A recent meta-analysis of cross-sectional studies in the area has found that perceptions of the severity of an illness or traumatic event are related to benefit finding (Helgeson, Reynolds, & Tomich, 2006). A further review of both cross-sectional and longitudinal studies of patients with cancer showed that indicators of illness threat were among the most consistent predictors of benefit finding (Stanton, Bower, & Low, 2006).

Consistent with these findings, a prospective study found that patients' illness beliefs measured at the beginning of the study predicted adversarial growth 4 to 6 months following medical treatment for psoriasis. Specifically, it was found that stronger beliefs in the chronicity or likelihood of recurrence, stronger beliefs in the emotional causes of the condition, and stronger beliefs in the severity of the consequences of the condition were predictive of growth (Fortune et al., 2002).

These findings suggest that a certain threshold of concern about the illness and its impact may need to be reached before positive effects of the illness are seen. It seems that the illness must be perceived as threatening or stressful enough to challenge one's assumptions about the self and the world for positive changes to be apparent (Parkes, 1971). St Jean, Broadbent, Ellis, Gamble, and Petrie (2008) found support for this hypothesis in a recent study examining how illness perceptions measured following hospitalization for a heart attack predicted later benefit finding in a sample of 78 patients and 37 spouses. While patients were in the hospital, they completed the Brief Illness Perception Questionnaire exhibited in Figure 7.1. Patients and spouses were contacted between 12 and 18 months following their heart attack and asked to rate the effect of the heart attack on their lives using a scale from −5 (very negative) to +5 (very positive). They were also asked about any positive effects that had occurred in their life as a result of their own or their partner's heart attack. As can be seen from Figure 7.6, both patients and spouses were consistent in the way they viewed the impact of the heart attack on their life: Approximately 60% viewed it positively and 16% negatively, with the remainder seeing it as having a neutral impact.

We next examined how illness beliefs, demographics, and various objective measures of illness severity predicted the reporting of positive effects from the illness. We found no relationship between demographic factors and positive effects or between the biological markers of the severity of the heart attack and the reported benefits from the illness. Although causal beliefs about the heart attack were not related to benefits, patients' perceptions of the consequences of the illness were related to later reports of benefits. Those patients who were concerned after their admission to hospital that their heart attack would have more serious consequences that were more serious were more likely to report benefits from their illness 12 to 18 months later. The pattern was slightly different for spouses: Spouses who had higher identity beliefs (i.e., they believed that their partner's illness caused lots of symptoms and had high levels of concern about the illness) were more likely to report later positive benefits.

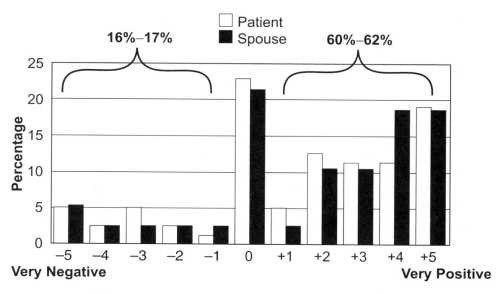

Figure 7.6. Ratings by patients and their spouses of the overall effect of heart attack on their lives according to their responses to the Brief Illness Perception Questionnaire (Broadbent, Petrie, Main, & Weinman, 2006).

Future Directions

Very little research has yet explored the relationship between the various illness perception components and benefit finding. The research discussed in this chapter suggests that, along with the patient's initial emotional response to the illness, the consequences component is likely to show the most consistent relationship with later benefit finding. Both of these components encompass the perceived disruption and threat that the illness presents to the patient's life and social world. The data suggest that the perceived disruption in these areas needs to be substantial before benefits from the illness are recognized.

It is interesting to speculate on some of the clinical implications of changing patients' perceptions of illness and the impact of this on later benefit finding. Recent work has found that stress management programs have improved adjustment and increased benefit finding in women following treatment for breast cancer (Antoni et al., 2006; see also chap. 11, this volume). Interventions to change illness perceptions are only a recent development in health psychology but have been shown to change patients' perceptions to a more positive view of their illness and to result in a faster functional recovery (Petrie, Cameron, Ellis, Buick, & Weinman, 2002). If more negative perceptions of illness are associated with later benefit finding, it may be that interventions designed to change illness perceptions will reduce benefit finding in certain illnesses.

One recent interesting application of illness perception assessment has been the use of patient drawings to examine patients' perceptions of illness. Drawings offer a rich source of data for understanding the patient's viewpoint and the impact of events such as illness. Although drawings have not yet been specifically used to look at positive effects of illness, the evidence we have collected from other studies shows that there is potential to examine how drawings relate to other measures of benefit finding (e.g., see Antoni et al., 2001; Tedeschi & Calhoun, 1996). Drawings may offer a means of accessing aspects of the patient's experience that are not readily captured by existing measures.

The way patients develop ideas and beliefs about their illness, and the effect of these psychological processes on later adjustment is a fascinating and useful area of research for health psychology. It puts the patient at the center of the research and offers researchers the potential to develop specific cognitive interventions that can have a major impact on the lives of patients and their families. The application of illness perceptions to benefit finding has only recently been the focus of research attention but it promises to provide important insights into understanding how patients cope with illness.

References

Affleck, G., & Tennen, H. (1996). Construing benefits from adversity: Adaptational significance and dispositional underpinnings. *Journal of Personality, 64,* 899–922.

Antoni, M. H., Lechner, S. C., Kazi, A., Wimberly, S. R., Sifre, T., Urcuyo, K. R., et al. (2006). How stress management improves quality of life after treatment for breast cancer. *Journal of Consulting and Clinical Psychology, 74,* 1143–1152.

Antoni, M. H., Lehman, J. M., Kilbourn, K. M., Boyers, A. E., Culver, J. L., & Alferi, S. M., et al. (2001). Cognitive–behavioral stress management intervention decreases the prevalence of depression and enhances benefit finding among women under treatment for early-stage breast cancer. *Health Psychology, 20,* 20–32.

Baumann, L. J., & Leventhal, H. (1985). "I can tell when my blood pressure is up, can't I?" *Health Psychology, 4,* 203–218.

Bendelow, G., Williams, S. J., & Oakley, A. (1996). It makes you bald: Children's knowledge and beliefs about health and cancer prevention. *Health Education, 3,* 12–19.

Broadbent, E., Ellis, C. J., Gamble, G., & Petrie, K. J. (2006) Changes in patient drawings of the heart identify slow recovery following myocardial infarction. *Psychosomatic Medicine, 68,* 910–913.

Broadbent, E., Petrie, K. J., Ellis, C. J., Anderson, J., Gamble, G., Anderson, D., & Benjamin, W. (2006). Acute myocardial infarction patients have an inaccurate understanding of their risk of a future cardiac event. *Internal Medicine Journal, 36,* 643–647.

Broadbent, E., Petrie, K. J., Ellis, C. J., Ying, J., & Gamble, G. (2004). A picture of health—myocardial infarction patients' drawings of their hearts and subsequent disability: A longitudinal study. *Journal of Psychosomatic Research, 57,* 583–587.

Broadbent, E., Petrie, K. J., Main, J., & Weinman, J. (2006). The Brief Illness Perception Questionnaire (BIPQ). *Journal of Psychosomatic Research, 60,* 631–637.

Browne, S., Distel, E., Morton, R. P., & Petrie, K. J. (in press). Patients' quality of life, reported difficulties and benefits following surgery for acoustic neuroma. *Journal of Otolaryngology.*

Buchi, S., Buddeberg, C., Klaghofer, R., Russi, E. W., Brandli, O., Schlosser, C., et al. (2002). Preliminary validation of PRISM (Pictorial Representation of Illness and Self Measure)—A brief method to assess suffering. *Psychotherapy & Psychosomatics, 40,* 314–320.

Buick, D. L. (1997) Illness representations and breast cancer: Coping with radiation and chemotherapy. In K. J. Petrie & J. Weinman (Eds.), *Perceptions of health and illness* (pp. 379–410). Amsterdam: Harwood Academic.

Fortune, D. G., Richards, H. L., Griffiths, C. E. M., & Main, C. J. (2002). Psychological stress, distress and disability in patients with psoriasis: Consensus and variation in the contribution of illness perceptions, coping and alexithymia. *British Journal of Clinical Psychology, 41,* 157–174.

Hagger, M., & Orbell, S. (2003). A meta-analytic review of the common-sense model of illness representations. *Psychology and Health, 18,* 141–184.

Helgeson, V. S., Reynolds, K. A., & Tomich, P. L. (2006). A meta-analytic review of benefit finding and growth. *Journal of Consulting and Clinical Psychology, 74,* 797–816.

Horne, R., & Weinman, J. (1999). Patients' beliefs about prescribed medicines and their role in adherence to treatment in chronic physical illness. *Journal of Psychosomatic Research, 47,* 555–567.

Leventhal, H., Benyamini, Y., Brownlee, S., Diefenbach, M., Leventhal, E. A., Patrick-Miller, L., & Robitaille, C. (1997). Illness representations: Theoretical foundations. In K. J. Petrie & J. Weinman (Eds.), *Perceptions of health and illness* (pp. 19–46). Amsterdam: Harwood Academic.

Leventhal, H., Nerenz, D. R., & Steele, D. J. (1984). Illness representations and coping with health threats. In A. Baum & J. Singer (Eds.), *A handbook of psychology and health* (Vol. 4, pp. 219–252). Hillsdale, NJ: Erlbaum.

Malcarne, V. L., Compas, B. E., Epping-Jordan, J. E., & Howell, D. C. (1995). Cognitive factors in adjustment to cancer: Attributions of self-blame and perceptions of control. *Journal of Behavioral Medicine, 18,* 401–417.

Moss-Morris, R., Weinman, J., Petrie, K. J., Horne, R., Cameron, L. D., & Buick, D. (2002). The Revised Illness Perception Questionnaire (IPQ-R). *Psychology and Health, 17,* 1–16.

Nerenz, D. R., & Leventhal, H. (1983). Self-regulation theory in chronic illness. In T. G. Burish & L. A. Bradley (Eds.), *Coping with chronic disease: Research and applications* (pp. 13–38). New York: Academic Press.

Parkes, C. L. (1971). Psycho-social transitions: A field for study. *Social Science & Medicine, 5,* 101–115.

Petrie, K. J., Broadbent, E., & Meechan, G. (2003). Self-regulatory interventions for improving the management of chronic illness. In L. D. Cameron & H. Leventhal (Eds.), *The self-regulation of health and illness behaviour* (pp. 247–277). London: Routledge.

Petrie, K. J., Buick, D. L., Weinman, J., & Booth, R. J. (1999). Positive effects of illness reported by myocardial infarction and breast cancer patients. *Journal of Psychosomatic Research, 47,* 537–543.

Petrie, K. J., Cameron, L. D., Ellis, C. J., Buick, D., & Weinman, J. (2002). Changing illness perceptions following myocardial infarction: An early intervention randomized controlled trial. *Psychosomatic Medicine, 64,* 580–586.

Petrie, K. J., & Pennebaker, J. W. (2004). Health-related cognitions. In S. Sutton, A. Baum, & M. Johnston (Eds.), *The Sage handbook of health psychology* (pp. 127–142). New York: Sage.

Petrie, K. J., Weinman, J., Sharpe, N., & Buckley, J. (1996). Role of patients' view of their illness in predicting return to work and functioning after myocardial infarction: Longitudinal study. *British Medical Journal, 312,* 1191–1194.

Quinn, C. M. (1988). Children's asthma: New approaches, new understandings. *Annals of Allergy, 60,* 283–292.

Scharloo, M., Kaptein, A. A., Weinman, J., Hazes, J. M., Willems, L. N. A., Bergman, W., & Rooijmans, H. G. (1998). Illness perceptions, coping and functioning in patients with rheumatoid arthritis, chronic obstructive pulmonary disease and psoriasis: A 1-year follow-up. *British Journal of Dermatology, 142,* 899–907.

St Jean, K., Broadbent, E., Ellis, C., Gamble, G., & Petrie, K. J. (2008). *The relationship between illness perceptions and later benefit finding in patients and their spouses following myocardial infarction.* Manuscript submitted for publication.

Stanton, A. L., Bower, J. E., & Low, C. A. (2006). Posttraumatic growth after cancer. In L. G. Calhoun & R. G. Tedeschi (Eds.), *Handbook of posttraumatic growth: Research and practice* (pp. 138–175). Mahwah, NJ: Erlbaum.

Tedeschi, R. G., & Calhoun, L. G. (1996). The Posttraumatic Growth Inventory: Measuring the positive legacy of trauma. *Journal of Traumatic Stress, 9,* 455–471.

Weinman, J., Petrie, K. J., Moss-Morris, R., & Horne, R. (1996). The Illness Perception Questionnaire: A new method for assessing illness perceptions. *Psychology and Health, 11,* 431–446.

Weinman, J., Petrie, K. J., Sharpe, N., & Walker, S. (2000). Causal attributions in patients and spouses following a heart attack and subsequent lifestyle changes. *British Journal of Health Psychology, 5,* 263–273.

Weinman, J., Yusuf, G., Berks, R., Rayner, S., & Petrie, K. J. (2008). *Do patients know the location of key body organs?* Manuscript submitted for publication.

8

Positive Life Change and the Social Context of Illness: An Expanded Social-Cognitive Processing Model

Stephen J. Lepore and William D. Kernan

This chapter identifies and discusses the processes through which interpersonal relationships may contribute to positive experiences, benefit finding, and personal growth in the aftermath of a serious illness such as cancer. In particular, we examine the interplay between social and cognitive factors in producing positive outcomes in illness. By doing so, we aim to contribute to theory in this area and inform social interventions designed to facilitate adjustment to cancer. To address our aims, we review social factors that have been implicated in adjustment to cancer, and we emphasize positive outcomes (e.g., benefit finding, personal growth). We then review two cognitive models that emphasize the role of social relationships in achieving positive life outcomes. Both models claim that the social environment can indirectly help achieve positive life outcomes by influencing cognitive adaptation processes. We expand on these models by adding the idea that the social environment can *directly* help achieve positive life outcomes in ways that are not mediated through cognitive adaptation processes, such as buffering stress, providing diversion from one's worries, and reinforcing a sense of belonging and self-worth. We conclude by discussing clinical implications and areas for future research.

Positive Life Outcomes in the Context of Cancer

There is great variability in the quality and intensity of individuals' psychological responses to cancer. Negative reactions run the gamut from disbelief to self-blame to helplessness and social alienation. People often feel anxious and depressed about cancer, especially around the time of diagnosis. These negative reactions are not surprising given the life threat, disability, disfigurement, pain, and uncertainty that can accompany cancer and its treatments. What may be somewhat surprising, however, is the emerging evidence that patients also experience personal growth and positive life changes in the aftermath of cancer (Stanton, Bower, & Low, 2006). Thus, like other life stressors, cancer

We, the chapter authors, thank Tracey Revenson for her helpful comments on an earlier draft of this chapter.

can signal a period of psychosocial transition, with the potential for both positive and negative changes (Cordova & Andrykowski, 2003).

Cancer survivors report various positive outcomes. They include a more positive outlook on life, adoption of a healthier lifestyle, a greater appreciation of life, increased spirituality, and an enhanced ability to relate to others (Antoni et al., 2001; Bower et al., 2005; Cordova, Cunningham, Carlson, & Andrykowski, 2001). A frequently reported outcome is a positive change in social relationships (Petrie, Buick, Weinman, & Booth, 1999; Sears, Stanton, & Danoff-Burg, 2003). People with cancer have reported improved marital and family relations, an increased awareness of their importance to others, and a greater compassion for others (Cordova et al., 2001; Fromm, Andrykowski, & Hunt, 1996; Gritz, Wellisch, Siau, & Wang, 1990; Northouse, Laten, & Reddy, 1995; Sears et al., 2003).

Cognitive Models of Positive Life Outcomes

The predominant theoretical models of how people adjust to illness, including cancer, emphasize cognitive adaptation processes. Few theoretical models specifically emphasize positive life changes associated with illness. However, two prominent cognitive theories of adjustment to life stressors address positive life changes and even acknowledge social factors that might influence cognitive processes of adaptation.

Cognitive Adaptation Theory

One highly influential model is Taylor's (1983) cognitive adaptation theory (CAT), which emphasizes the role of constructive meaning making and self-enhancement processes in adjustment to serious illness or stressful life events (see also Updegraff & Taylor, 2000). According to CAT, serious illnesses evoke a search for meaning in the experience, elicit attempts to regain mastery over the illness in particular and over one's life more generally, and encourage efforts to restore self-esteem through self-enhancing evaluations. The search for meaning is driven by the individual's need to understand why the illness occurred and its full implications. Efforts to regain a sense of mastery are often cognitive, including adopting a positive attitude in the belief that such a stance will somehow ward off future harm.

An important feature of CAT is that the cognitions related to finding meaning, regaining mastery, and enhancing self-concept are constructions, or *positive illusions*. Taylor (e.g., see Taylor & Brown, 1988) has championed the notion that positive illusions are beneficial to mental health. For example, persons with cancer may believe that they can control the disease through prayer. Whether this is true or not, the illusion of control may help to reduce fear. Increasingly, investigators are providing data on the potentially adaptive role of various kinds of cognitive distortions, such as denial, self-enhancement, and dissociation from stressful events (see Bonanno, 2004). There is even some evidence that these cognitive distortions may be related to the social environment.

For example, in one study, individuals near the World Trade Center during the terrorist attacks in 2001 who had higher levels of trait self-enhancement reported better social relationships and emotional outcomes (Bonanno, Rennicke, & Dekel, 2005). Thus, self-enhancement processes may increase individuals' positive perceptions of the quality of their social relationships.

Self-enhancement can also be achieved through social comparison processes. Taylor observed that in a sample of women who had been diagnosed with breast cancer, virtually all women managed to find a comparison target who appeared to be doing worse. These downward social comparisons are cognitive processes that can buoy self-esteem in the face of threats (Taylor & Lobel, 1989). The act of making social comparisons also has the potential to produce perceived benefits in illness. For example, individuals who learn through social comparisons about someone who is more isolated than they are might feel better about the quality of their relationships and view this insight as a benefit of their illness experience.

Posttraumatic Growth Theory

Another influential model is the posttraumatic growth theory (PTGT) by Tedeschi and Calhoun (2004). PTGT focuses on adaptation to severe stressors, including serious illness, and includes positive (i.e., growth) outcomes. PTGT includes elements of CAT and other cognitive processing theories. For instance, the model starts with the assumption that major stressors challenge or shatter individuals' worldviews and self-views because there is a discrepancy between the information inherent in the stressor, on the one hand, and people's expectations and beliefs about the world, on the other hand. Because it is distressing, this discrepancy, or psychological discord, leads people to exert cognitive coping efforts to resolve it.

According to PTGT, it is necessary to experience distress to experience growth, particularly if the distress results from efforts to assimilate or accommodate novel stress-related information into preexisting mental models. Tartaro et al. (2005) reported findings consistent with this theory in a longitudinal study of women treated for breast cancer. Compared with women who did not report finding any benefits in their experience of breast cancer, those who did report benefits had higher distress before diagnosis and a significant decline subsequently (see also Tomich & Helgeson, 2004). However, as Tedeschi and Calhoun (2004) noted, findings from the broader literature have been mixed (see also Lepore & Revenson, 2006; chap. 10, this volume).

The model proposed by Tedeschi and Calhoun (2004; see also Calhoun & Tedeschi, 2006) further suggests that various personal traits and social factors may produce positive outcomes or what they call "posttraumatic growth" in the aftermath of severe stressors. In terms of social factors, Tedeschi and Calhoun suggested that the social environment can facilitate psychological growth by providing new perspectives and schemas related to growth, and by giving empathic responses to disclosures about stressors. For example, a friend may help a person with cancer to see how strong he or she has been in coping with the illness. Empathic responses from others also can stimulate people to see the importance and benefits that they had hitherto not noticed in their social relationships. Thus, social relations can create a sense of both agency and relatedness where there might previously have been none.

Summary of Cognitive Theories of Positive Outcomes in Illness

Both CAT and PTGT are rooted in theories of stress and trauma that emphasize cognitive adaptation processes. Both models emphasize a need to restore or maintain positive mental models of the world, the self, and the self–world relation following highly stressful events, including the onset or progression of a serious illness. In addition, both models describe various ways, including some social processes, through which individuals assimilate or accommodate stress-related information to restore or create positive mental models. For instance, people may (a) engage in downward social comparison processes that can make their situation seem better, (b) interpret social interactions and outcomes of situations in ways that bolster self-image, (c) search for ways to make sense or meaning of a stressful situation to restore a sense of order and coherence, (d) reinterpret or reframe stress-related information to assimilate it into preexisting mental models, and (e) interpret outcomes of situations in ways that enhance feelings of self-efficacy or control. Although both CAT and PTGT note that the social environment can influence cognitive adaptation processes and, as a result, lead to personal growth and benefit finding, to date, these models have not produced much evidence for these processes or discussed the multitude of pathways through which the social environment can influence cognitive adaptation and positive outcomes.

Social Influences on Positive Life Outcomes in Illness

In this section, we further discuss some of the important independent and moderating effects of the social context of stressors, especially the emotionally important social context consisting of close friends and family members. We concur with Tedeschi and Calhoun's (2004; see also Calhoun & Tedeschi, 2006) suggestion that the social environment may influence cognitive processes of adaptation related to benefit finding and personal growth. We would add, however, that the social environment also may have direct positive influences that are not mediated through cognitive adaptation processes. In this section, we discuss both the direct and the indirect cognitively mediated pathways through which social relationships might influence positive outcomes in patients with cancer.

In the context of illness, the presence of supportive others and the absence of critical and unsupportive others can exert powerful and independent influences on patients' adjustment. Significant others often influence individuals' thinking about their situation, especially if individuals choose to disclose or socially process their thoughts and feelings. For example, if others are validating, they can reinforce a thought or feeling, and if they are confrontational, they might broaden and change a thought or feeling (Lepore, Fernandez-Berrocal, Ragan, & Ramos, 2004). The mere act of trying to put thoughts and feelings into words can shape and change them. After intense emotional experiences, either positive or negative, people often wish to share these experiences with others, so the social environment plays an important role in adaptation to stressors.

Direct Influences of the Social Environment on Positive Outcomes

People who are integrated in a social network, have diverse social roles, and perceive that they have adequate social support are generally healthier and live longer than people who have a relatively low level of social integration and social support (Uchino, 2004). Social integration and support also are associated with positive emotional states and well-being (e.g., see Chesney, Chambers, Taylor, Johnson, & Folkman, 2003). There has been extensive research and theorizing on the direct benefits of social relationships with regard to mental and physical health outcomes. In contrast, little research or theorizing is available on the direct benefits of social relationships with regard to positive life changes, such as personal growth and perceived benefits in the context of illness. The dominant theories in this area have been social control theory (Lewis, Butterfield, Darbes, & Johnston-Brooks, 2004) and social support theory (Uchino, 2004).

According to social control theory, people who have a higher level of social integration are more likely to have role obligations and relationships with others that infuse their life with purpose and meaning (Lewis et al., 2004). Because of significant social bonds with others, individuals are motivated to stay healthy and be able to fulfill social obligations. For example, a woman who has dependent children may avoid risky health behaviors and engage in health-promoting behaviors so that she can provide the resources necessary to maintain her children's health and well-being. Social control theory also maintains that people with higher social integration are more likely to be prompted by others to engage in health-promoting behaviors and to avoid health-compromising behaviors. Theoretically, social control is linked to improved physical health outcomes but, paradoxically, also to poorer mental health outcomes. To imagine how this might happen, consider a scenario in which a woman is trying to get her husband to follow a doctor's orders about losing weight; she does so by frequently reminding him not to eat the fatty and sugary foods he normally enjoys. The husband might lose the weight but feel needled and deprived in the process. It is easy to imagine both positive and negative outcomes in this situation because the husband might simultaneously resent his wife's admonitions but appreciate her concern and the resulting weight loss.

According to social support theory, people who have relatively high social integration have more positive outcomes because members of their social network help to mitigate stressors, perhaps by providing informational, material, instrumental, or emotional support (Wills & Filer, 2001). Alternatively, being integrated in a social network may prevent a number of stressors from occurring and give individuals a sense of well-being simply by being connected with others. Some scholars have suggested that the need to belong is a fundamental human motivation (Baumeister & Leary, 1995), possibly derived through selective processes of evolution that favored the survival of people who could successfully form social relations. Thus, individuals who feel a sense of belonging may have less negative affect (e.g., fear, anger) and more positive affect (e.g., happiness, calmness). Positive emotional states also may arise naturally out of the pleasant exchanges and activities that occur between companions (Rook, 1987).

A half-dozen published studies of the aftermath of cancer have examined the association between indicators of social support (e.g., received support, support seeking, support satisfaction) and measures of benefit finding or personal growth. In a study of people with cancers of the gastrointestinal system, a greater level of received social support was associated with greater benefit finding (Schulz & Mohamed, 2004). In studies of survivors of prostate cancer, greater perceived emotional and tangible social support was associated with greater benefit finding (Kinsinger et al., 2006) and men who tended to cope by using emotional support tended to report a high level of posttraumatic growth (Thornton & Perez, 2006). In a study by Weiss (2004), survivors of breast cancer who reported greater social support from their husbands tended to report more posttraumatic growth, although there was no association between a global measure of satisfaction with social support and posttraumatic growth. In another study of survivors of breast cancer (Cordova et al., 2001), women who reported talking about their cancer with others had greater posttraumatic growth, although, again, there was no association between a global measure of satisfaction with social support and posttraumatic growth. Finally, Widows, Jacobsen, Booth-Jones, and Fields (2005) found no association between posttraumatic growth and a composite measure of perceived tangible, belonging, and appraisal support among people undergoing bone marrow transplant.

In summary, on the basis of social control and social support theory, one would expect that the social context of illness could reduce negative emotional outcomes and increase positive emotional outcomes through various mechanisms, including buffering stress, providing diversion from one's worries, and reinforcing a sense of belonging and self-worth (i.e., being needed by others). Furthermore, when people are feeling sick and needy, the kindness of others may become especially salient. In the absence of a specific need to tap one's social resources, these resources may, to a degree, be taken for granted. Recent studies suggest a correlation between social support and positive outcomes such as personal growth and perceived benefits. Whether these benefits are direct or mediated through cognitive processes is not yet clear. Indeed, as discussed in the next section, evidence is emerging that the social context of illness can alter cognitive processes of adaptation, which in turn can generate a range of positive outcomes, including positive emotional states, benefit finding, and feelings of personal growth.

Indirect Influences of the Social Environment on Positive Outcomes

Close interpersonal relationships could influence cognitive adaptation processes by either supporting or challenging the positive mental models people are trying to maintain or recreate in the context of illness. For example, when individuals are seriously ill, the kindly and supportive acts of loved ones can help them to maintain or reestablish positive views of the world and self. In contrast, when loved ones violate expectations for support or, worse yet, act in a hostile or insensitive manner, their behaviors can undermine a patient's ability to maintain or establish positive beliefs at a time when these beliefs may be under siege.

In previous work (for reviews, see Lepore, 2001; Lepore & Revenson, 2007), we have used a social-cognitive processing (SCP) model to understand adjustment to cancer, but we have not emphasized positive outcomes or discussed how those outcomes might be generated. The SCP model shares many of the elements of cognitive processing theories described earlier. It assumes that cognitive integration of the challenging aspects of cancer, including diagnosis, treatment, pain, and implications for the future, could occur through mental processes of assimilation, reappraising events to fit preconceptions, or accommodation, changing mental models to fit information inherent in a traumatic event (see chap. 1, this volume). Through assimilation and accommodation processes, people can interpret their illness in personally meaningful terms, integrate threatening and confusing aspects of the disease into a coherent conceptual framework, and achieve intellectual or emotional resolution. In addition, as suggested by cognitive processing theories, particularly Taylor's CAT, these processes of assimilation and accommodation should be biased toward constructing positive interpretations of the situation and future outcomes. The SCP model extends the basic cognitive models by considering the role of the social context in shaping these cognitive adaptations to illness.

According to SCP theory (Lepore, 2001), there are various pathways through which the social environment can influence cognitive adaptations to stressors including cancer and other serious illnesses. For example, the social environment can help to shape worldviews, such as expectancies about future outcomes related to health. Social networks are most receptive to patients who are optimistic about their condition and thus may reinforce optimism and possibly even discourage pessimism. In an interesting demonstration of this effect, Silver, Wortman, and Crofton (1990) manipulated the self-presentation of a person with Hodgkin's disease and examined how people reacted to different self-presentations. There were four experimental conditions: positive coping (i.e., patient conveys no negative affect, is coping well), poor coping (i.e., patient conveys negative affect, is not coping well), no information about coping, and balanced coping (i.e., patient discloses some distress along with optimistic statements and information that coping efforts are being exerted). Research participants indicated that they would be most comfortable with, and preferred interacting with, the patients with Hodgkin's disease who presented themselves as balanced copers who were struggling with their condition but had an optimistic outlook. Poor copers were the least attractive to the research participants. Similarly, in a longitudinal survey study, Lepore and Ituarte (1999) found that among women treated for breast or colon cancer, greater optimism about recovery was associated with fewer negative reactions from others when patients talked about their cancer. In response to social demands, people with cancer may feel a need to identify and express to others some reason for expecting positive future outcomes.

Supportive others can also help people to maintain a positive self-concept during a serious illness by validating their experiences and affirming that they are loved and esteemed (Albrecht & Adelman, 1987). Discussing fears and concerns associated with illness also can help people to maintain or reestablish a coherent worldview (Lepore, 2001). Supportive others can suggest new and positive perspectives on a traumatic experience, provide information on how to cope, or encourage individuals to accept their situation (Clark, 1993; Lepore, Silver, Wortman, & Wayment, 1996). By helping individuals to make sense of illness, accept the illness and its implications, and establish a positive self-view and a positive worldview, positive social relations can reduce the need for ongoing cognitive processing (e.g., ruminating, searching for meaning; see Lepore, Ragan, & Jones, 2000). As noted earlier, relationships can help to build positive self-views and positive worldviews in part by bolstering a person's sense of agency and relatedness.

SCP theory distinguishes positive, supportive social ties from constraining (i.e., critical and otherwise unsupportive) social ties. In contrast to the benefits of supportive social ties, constraining social ties can impede cognitive processing of adaptation and emotional adjustment. When individuals disclose stressful experiences in a negative, constraining social context, or one in which network members are not fully supportive, it can result in increased psychological distress (for reviews, see Lepore, 1997b, 2001). Lepore et al. have argued that unexpected or negative social responses to disclosures about stressors, including cancer, can impede cognitive processing if disclosers counterrespond to the negative social responses by trying not to think or talk about the stressors (Kliewer, Lepore, Oskin, & Johnson, 1998; Lepore, 1997a; Lepore & Helgeson, 1998; Lepore et al., 1996). Active attempts at inhibiting or suppressing thoughts can have the ironic effect of prolonging them (Wegner, 1994).

Inhibition of talking and thinking about stressors also can interfere with cognitive processing in other ways, including limiting individuals' access to new information and alternative perspectives, which may be critical for cognitive integration of stress-related information. A longitudinal study of men with prostate cancer revealed that men with relatively poor social support were more likely to engage in a prolonged search for meaning and were less likely to resolve cancer-related ruminations or intrusive thoughts (a marker of incomplete cognitive processing) than were their counterparts who had adequate social support (Roberts, Lepore, & Helgeson, 2006). Furthermore, baseline social support was positively associated with mental health at follow-up; this relation was mediated by baseline indicators of cognitive processing, intrusive thoughts, and searching for meaning. These findings suggest that supportive social relations may improve mental health by helping men cognitively process (i.e., make sense of, or stop searching for, meaning in) their cancer experience.

Thus, the social context of illness can influence individuals' ability to gain mental and emotional control. We also would argue that the research literature supports the theory that the social context of illness can influence cognitive adaptation processes related to perceived benefits and personal growth in the aftermath of illness. One of the mechanisms for promoting benefit finding and personal growth is the reaffirmation of self-worth and the belief in the benevolence of the world that can occur when support expectations are fulfilled. Another mechanism is the facilitation of cognitive adaptation processes (i.e., resolving ruminations and the search for meaning) that may help people to establish or maintain positive self-views (e.g., esteem, efficacy) and worldviews (e.g., predictability, benevolence).

In the literature on adjustment to cancer, the evidence linking unsupportive and supportive social environments, respectively, to more or less negative psychological outcomes is robust. For example, evidence from several survey studies with cancer patients confirms that being able to safely confide in significant others about cancer-related thoughts tends to reduce the negative effects of intrusive thoughts on depressive and somatic symptoms (Lepore, 2001; Lepore & Helgeson, 1998; Manne, 1999). Of interest here, as we attempt to extend the SCP model to positive outcomes in illnesses such as cancer, is whether the social context of illness is related to perceived benefits and personal growth through cognitive adaptation processes.

We could find only one study that tested whether cognitive adaptation processes mediate the effects of social support on positive outcomes. Porter et al. (2006) used baseline data from 524 women in an intervention study designed to manage uncertainty in long-term survivors of breast cancer. The study included a measure of satisfaction with social support, cognitive reframing (i.e., the ability to address concerns from a positive point of view), and personal growth. In a structural equation model, cognitive reframing mediated the positive relation between support satisfaction and personal growth. Specifically, a higher level of support satisfaction was associated with more cognitive reframing which, in turn, was associated with a higher level of reported personal growth.

We could not find any published studies examining the association between social constraints and benefit finding or growth in patients with cancer or survivors of cancer. We were able to find one study of women with rheumatoid arthritis that examined social constraints and their relation to a particular form of benefit finding, namely, interpersonal benefits. In that study, Danoff-Burg and Revenson (2005) found that a lower level of perceived social constraints against talking about one's illness was associated with higher levels of interpersonal benefits.

Summary of Social Influences on Positive Outcomes in Illness

The social context of illness can influence positive life outcomes, benefit finding, and personal growth, in direct and indirect ways. Being socially integrated provides people with opportunities for rewarding social exchanges that can provide direct benefits, including increased positive affect and a sense of belonging. In addition, social interdependencies create mutual obligations and provide people with a sense of purpose and meaning. Thus, when members of patients' social networks remind them that they continue to be needed and wanted despite their illness, patients' self-views are directly bolstered, which may help them to see some purpose in life. When network members address patients' emotional and practical needs, they may help patients to maintain a positive self-view and a positive worldview by demonstrating that they are persons worthy of help and that there is good in the world. The kindness of friends, or even strangers, is a counterweight to the sense of worthlessness, isolation, and injustice that may accompany a life-threatening illness such as cancer.

The social context of illness also can influence positive outcomes indirectly through its effects on cognitive adaptation processes. In the process of sharing illness-related experiences with others, people have to articulate a story of their illness. Illness narratives that include some hopeful and optimistic messages are likely to be better received and reinforced by others, whereas pessimistic illness narratives may alienate others. Thus, individuals who are sensitive to maintaining positive social relationships during their illness may collaborate with members of their social network to establish and maintain a positive spin on their illness and the future.

The presence of supportive others and the absence of constraining others also can influence benefit finding and personal growth by influencing assimilation and accommodation processes. For example, supportive others may facilitate assimilation by directing patients' attention to positive information and by helping them to positively reframe their situation. Friends and family members may remind patients that they have improved, despite the persistence of some health problems, or they might point out that some individuals with the same condition are far worse (i.e., downward social comparison). Alternatively, instead of helping patients to assimilate negative information about their health and future, social network members can help them to accommodate the information by changing their beliefs and expectations. For example, members of patients' social networks may help them accept that they cannot control important outcomes, such as health. Indeed, social networks may introduce patients to new beliefs, such as the belief that God controls health outcomes. Through these varied channels, members of patients' social networks may help them to see things in a more positive light and maintain a positive self-view and a positive worldview.

It is important to note that social experiences also can impede normal cognitive adaptation processes that people use to maintain or reestablish positive self-views and positive worldviews. In particular, when people are attempting to reestablish shattered self-views and shattered worldviews, violations of expectations for support can further erode positive beliefs about the self and the world. In the context of cancer, patients may feel that their fundamental sense of safety has been shattered. When patients feel vulnerable and when the people they love are not supportive, essential beliefs about trust in others can be shattered. In such situations, people may feel a tenuous connection with reality as many different basic beliefs are challenged. A violation of support expectations can thus make the patient wonder which of their fundamental beliefs are reliable and which are not.

Clinical Implications

Considering the direct and indirect effects of the social context of illness on positive outcomes, we can enumerate a number of clinical implications. First, people coping with illness may derive great benefits from simply participating in normal social activities and talking about things other than their illness. Family members can be reminded that it is important to maintain some usual social rituals, routines, and expectations in order to help people who are ill to continue to feel needed and valued, and to feel that there is some predictability in their life. In addition, normal companionate and diversionary activities can reinstate a sense of belonging and generate positive feelings in people coping with serious illness. Theoretically, discussions with supportive, noncritical others can also help people who are ill to find meaning or make sense of their illness experience and to accept their illness and stop searching for meaning. They can be helped to reframe or reappraise negative implications and experiences associated with the illness, or to change their beliefs to accommodate the realities of their illness. The primary ways in which others can support patients' cognitive adaptation is through providing opportunities for safe disclosure and offering alternative perspectives.

Several pioneering studies of the aftermath of cancer have examined the effects of social interventions on benefit finding and personal growth. One study was a pilot test of an Internet-based social support group for 32 survivors of breast cancer (Lieberman et al., 2003). Women completed baseline measures, participated in an Internet-based support group for 16 weeks, and completed a follow-up interview. Participants manifested significant declines in depressive symptoms over time, and exhibited a trend that suggested increases on two indicators of growth: new possibilities and spirituality. Interpretations of these findings, however, are hampered by the small sample size and selective attrition, as the authors noted. Another study (Antoni et al., 2001) tested the effects of a 10-week group-based cognitive–behavioral stress management (CBSM) intervention on psychological distress and benefit finding among women treated for early-stage breast cancer. Compared with women in the control group who attended a 1-day stress management seminar, women in the group-based CBSM group evidenced greater gains in benefit finding over time. However, there was no condition-by-time interaction effect on distress measures (see chap. 11, this volume). A third study (Penedo et al., 2006) used a research design similar to the one used by Antoni et al. (2001), except that the population consisted of men treated for localized prostate cancer. Compared with control participants who received a half-day educational seminar, participants who were randomized to receive 10-week group-based CBSM exhibited greater increases in benefit finding and quality of life outcomes. Further, mediation analyses suggested that the effects of group-based CBSM were mediated by increases in stress management skills, including cognitive reframing. One limitation of the CBSM studies is that the control groups were not equated for attention, and the effect sizes were small in magnitude. In general, it is not clear how researchers or clinicians should assess the clinical significance of small effects, or even large effects, on outcomes such as benefit finding and personal growth.

In summary, there is scant evidence of the efficacy of social interventions to improve benefit finding or personal growth, but there is some emerging evidence that these outcomes may be influenced by social interventions, even when the interventions do not effectively reduce distress. There are many questions about how social interventions might influence positive outcomes and whether the effects are clinically meaningful or long-lasting. Thus, the clinical implications of the findings from social experiments are far from clear.

Future Directions

The examination of positive outcomes in illness, including benefit finding and personal growth, has received relatively scant research attention. Because this field is new, there are numerous directions for future research. Among these are (a) examining the relation between specific elements of the social environment and specific positive outcomes in illness, with a focus on intervening cognitive processes; (b) developing and testing controlled social interventions not only to reduce distress but also to increase positive outcomes in people with cancer; and (c) conducting research to more specifically identify the shared and unique pathways through which the social environment can influence positive versus negative outcomes.

As we and other contributors to this volume have noted, cognitive processing theories offer one promising perspective for understanding how people come to identify and construct positive outcomes. However, people are fundamentally social creatures and, as a result, their thoughts, emotions, and actions are all influenced by their social world. By expanding cognitive processing theories to include an interpersonal dimension, we have suggested a more complex model of adaptation to illness. In doing so, we hope to contribute to psychological researchers' understanding of why some people are more successful than others in responding to the cognitive and emotional challenges of serious illnesses, such as cancer. The expanded SCP model of adaptation to illness suggests that the social context of illness can have direct and indirect, cognitively mediated, effects on positive states of mind, benefit finding, and personal growth. Future research is needed to explicate the specific pathways leading to positive and negative outcomes, in addition to identifying efficacious, practical, and acceptable social intervention techniques for facilitating cognitive processes of adaptation to illness.

References

Albrecht, T. L., & Adelman, M. B. (1987). *Communicating social support*. Newbury Park, CA: Sage.

Antoni, M. H., Lehman, J. M., Kilbourn, K. M., Boyers, A. E., Culver, J. L., Alferi, S. M., et al. (2001). Cognitive–behavioral stress management intervention decreases prevalence of depression and enhances benefit finding among women under treatment for early-stage breast cancer. *Health Psychology, 20,* 20–32.

Baumeister, R. F., & Leary, M. R. (1995). The need to belong: Desire for interpersonal attachments as a fundamental human motivation. *Psychological Bulletin, 117,* 497–529.

Bonanno, G. A. (2004). Loss, trauma, and human resilience: Have we underestimated the human capacity to thrive after extremely aversive events? *American Psychologist, 59,* 20–28.

Bonanno, G. A., Rennicke, C., & Dekel, S. (2005). Self-enhancement among high-exposure survivors of the September 11th terrorist attack: Resilience or social maladjustment? *Journal of Personality and Social Psychology, 88,* 984–998.

Bower, J. E., Meyerowitz, B. E., Desmond, K. A., Bernaards, C. A., Rowland, J. H., & Ganz, P. A. (2005). Perceptions of positive meaning and vulnerability following breast cancer: Predictors and outcomes among long-term breast cancer survivors. *Annals of Behavioral Medicine, 29,* 236–245.

Calhoun, L. G., & Tedeschi, R. G. (2006). The foundations of posttraumatic growth: An expanded framework. In L. G. Calhoun & R. G. Tedeschi (Eds.), *Handbook of posttraumatic growth: Research and practice* (pp. 1–23). Mahwah, NJ: Erlbaum.

Chesney, M. A., Chambers, D. B., Taylor, J. M., Johnson, L. M., & Folkman, S. (2003). Coping effectiveness training for men living with HIV: Results from a randomized clinical trial testing a group-based intervention. *Psychosomatic Medicine, 65,* 1038–1046.

Clark, L. F. (1993). Stress and the cognitive-conversational benefits of social interaction. *Journal of Social and Clinical Psychology, 12,* 25–55.

Cordova, M. J., & Andrykowski, M. A. (2003). Responses to cancer diagnosis and treatment: Post-traumatic stress and posttraumatic growth. *Seminar in Clinical Neuropsychiatry, 8,* 286–296.

Cordova, M. J., Cunningham, L. L. C., Carlson, C. R., & Andrykowski, M. A. (2001). Posttraumatic growth following breast cancer: A controlled comparison study. *Health Psychology, 20,* 176–185.

Danoff-Burg, S., & Revenson, T. A. (2005). Benefit finding among patients with rheumatoid arthritis: Positive effects on interpersonal relationships. *Journal of Behavioral Medicine, 28,* 91–103.

Fromm, K., Andrykowski, M. A., & Hunt, J. (1996). Positive and negative psychosocial sequelae of bone marrow transplantation: Implications for quality of life assessment. *Journal of Behavioral Medicine, 19,* 221–240.

Gritz, E. R., Wellisch, D. K., Siau, J., & Wang, H. J. (1990). Long-term effects of testicular cancer on marital relationships. *Psychosomatics, 31,* 301–312.

Kinsinger, D. P., Penedo, F. J., Antoni, M. H., Dahn, J. R., Lechner, S., & Schneiderman, N. (2006). Psychosocial and sociodemographic correlates of benefit finding in men treated for localized prostate cancer. *Psycho-Oncology, 15,* 954–961.

Kliewer, W., Lepore, S. J., Oskin, D., & Johnson, P. D. (1998). The role of social and cognitive processes in children's adjustment to community violence. *Journal of Consulting and Clinical Psychology, 66,* 199–209.

Lepore, S. J. (1997a). Expressive writing moderates the relation between intrusive thoughts and depressive symptoms. *Journal of Personality and Social Psychology, 73,* 1030–1037.

Lepore, S. J. (1997b). Social–environmental influences on the chronic stress process. In B. Gottlieb (Ed.), *Coping with chronic stressors* (pp. 133–160). New York: Plenum Press.

Lepore, S. J. (2001). A social-cognitive processing model of emotional adjustment to cancer. In A. Baum & B. L. Andersen (Eds.), *Psychosocial interventions for cancer* (pp. 99–116). Washington, DC: American Psychological Association.

Lepore, S. J., Fernandez-Berrocal, P., Ragan, J., & Ramos, N. (2004). It's not that bad: Social challenges to emotional disclosure enhance adjustment to stress. *Anxiety, Stress and Coping: An International Journal, 17,* 341–361.

Lepore, S. J., & Helgeson, V. S. (1998). Social constraints, intrusive thoughts, and mental health after prostate cancer. *Journal of Social and Clinical Psychology, 17,* 89–106.

Lepore, S. J., & Ituarte, P. H. G. (1999). Optimism about cancer enhances mood by reducing negative social interactions. *Cancer Research, Therapy and Control, 8,* 165–174.

Lepore, S. J., Ragan, J. D., & Jones, S. (2000). Talking facilitates cognitive–emotional processes of adaptation to an acute stressor. *Journal of Personality and Social Psychology, 78,* 499–508.

Lepore, S. J., & Revenson, T. A. (2006). Resilience and posttraumatic growth: Recovery, resistance, and reconfiguration. In L. G. Calhoun & R. G. Tedeschi (Eds.), *Handbook of posttraumatic growth: Research and practice* (pp. 24–46). Mahwah, NJ: Erlbaum.

Lepore, S. J., & Revenson, T. A. (2007). Social constraints on disclosure and adjustment to cancer. *Social & Personality Psychology Compass: Health, 1,* 313–333.

Lepore, S. J., Silver, R. C., Wortman, C. B., & Wayment, H. A. (1996). Social constraints, intrusive thoughts, and depressive symptoms among bereaved mothers. *Journal of Personality and Social Psychology, 70,* 271–282.

Lewis, M. A., Butterfield, R. M., Darbes, L. A., & Johnston-Brooks, C. (2004). The conceptualization and assessment of health-related social control. *Journal of Social and Personal Relationships, 21,* 669–687.

Lieberman, M. A., Golant, M., Giese-Davis, J., Winzlenberg, A., Benjamin, H., Humphreys, K., et al. (2003). Electronic support groups for breast carcinoma: A clinical trial of effectiveness. *Cancer, 97,* 920–925.

Manne, S. L. (1999). Intrusive thoughts and psychological distress among cancer patients: The role of spouse avoidance and criticism. *Journal of Consulting and Clinical Psychology, 67,* 539–546.

Northouse, L. L., Laten, D., & Reddy, P. (1995). Adjustment of women and their husbands to recurrent breast cancer. *Research in Nursing and Health, 18,* 515–524.

Penedo, F. J., Molton, I., Dahn, J. R., Shen, B. J., Kinsinger, D., Traeger, L., et al. (2006). A randomized clinical trial of group-based cognitive–behavioral stress management in localized prostate cancer: Development of stress management skills improves quality of life and benefit finding. *Annals of Behavioral Medicine, 31,* 261–270.

Petrie, K. J., Buick, D. L., Weinman, J., & Booth, R. J. (1999). Positive effects of illness reported by myocardial infarction and breast cancer patients. *Journal of Psychosomatic Research, 47,* 537–543.

Porter, L. S., Clayton, M. F., Belyea, M., Mishel, M., Gil, K. M., & Germino, B. B. (2006). Predicting negative mood state and personal growth in African American and White long-term breast cancer survivors. *Annals of Behavioral Medicine, 31,* 195–204.

Roberts, K. J., Lepore, S. J., & Helgeson, V. (2006). Social-cognitive correlates of adjustment to prostate cancer. *Psycho-Oncology, 15,* 183–192.

Rook, K. S. (1987). Social support versus companionship: Effects on life stress, loneliness, and evaluations by others. *Journal of Personality and Social Psychology, 52,* 1132–1147.

Schulz, U., & Mohamed, N. E. (2004). Turning the tide: Benefit finding after cancer surgery. *Social Science & Medicine, 59,* 653–662.

Sears, S. R., Stanton, A. L., & Danoff-Burg, S. (2003). The Yellow Brick Road and the Emerald City: Benefit finding, positive reappraisal coping and posttraumatic growth in women with early-stage breast cancer. *Health Psychology, 22,* 487–497.

Silver, R. C., Wortman, C. B., & Crofton, C. (1990). The role of coping in support provision: The self-presentational dilemma of victims of life crises. In B. R. Sarason, I. G. Sarason, & G. R. Pierce (Eds.), *Social support: An interactional view* (pp. 397–426). New York: Wiley.

Stanton, A. L., Bower, J. E., & Low, C. A. (2006). Posttraumatic growth after cancer. In L. G. Calhoun & R. G. Tedeschi (Eds.), *Handbook of posttraumatic growth: Research and practice* (pp. 138–175). Mahwah, NJ: Erlbaum.

Tartaro, J., Roberts, J., Nosarti, C., Crayford, T., Luecken, L., & David, A. (2005). Who benefits? Distress, adjustment and benefit finding among breast cancer survivors. *Journal of Psychosocial Oncology, 23*(2–3), 45–64.

Taylor, S. E. (1983). Adjustment to threatening events: A theory of cognitive adaptation. *American Psychologist, 38,* 1161–1173.

Taylor, S. E., & Brown, J. D. (1988). Illusion and well-being: A social psychological perspective on mental health. *Psychological Bulletin, 103,* 193–210.

Taylor, S. E., & Lobel, M. (1989). Social comparison activity under threat: Downward evaluation and upward contacts. *Psychological Review, 96,* 569–575.

Tedeschi, R. G., & Calhoun, L. G. (2004). Posttraumatic growth: Conceptual foundations and empirical evidence. *Psychological Inquiry, 15,* 1–18.

Thornton, A. A., & Perez, M. A. (2006). Posttraumatic growth in prostate cancer survivors and their partners. *Psycho-Oncology, 15,* 285–296.

Tomich, P. L., & Helgeson, V. S. (2004). Is finding something good in the bad always good? Benefit finding among women with breast cancer. *Health Psychology, 23,* 16–23.

Uchino, B. N. (2004). *Social support and physical health outcomes: Understanding the health consequences of our relationships.* New Haven, CT: Yale University Press.

Updegraff, J. A., & Taylor, S. E. (2000). From vulnerability to growth: Positive and negative effects of stressful life events. In J. E. Harvey & E. D. Miller (Eds.), *Loss and trauma: General and close relationship perspectives* (pp. 3–28). Philadelphia: Brunner-Routledge.

Wegner, D. M. (1994). Ironic processes of mental control. *Psychological Review, 101,* 34–52.

Weiss, T. (2004). Correlates of posttraumatic growth in husbands of breast cancer survivors. *Psycho-Oncology, 13,* 260–268.

Widows, M. R., Jacobsen, P. B., Booth-Jones, M., & Fields, K. K. (2005). Predictors of posttraumatic growth following bone marrow transplantation for cancer. *Health Psychology, 24,* 266–273.

Wills, T. A., & Filer, M. (2001). Social networks and social support. In A. Baum, T. A. Revenson, & J. Singer (Eds.), *Handbook of health psychology* (pp. 209–234). Hillsdale, NJ: Erlbaum.

Part IV

Effects of Positive Life Change

9

Biological Correlates: How Psychological Components of Benefit Finding May Lead to Physiological Benefits

Julienne E. Bower, Elissa Epel, and Judith Tedlie Moskowitz

The majority of studies investigating links between benefit finding and health have focused on mental health, including psychological distress, depression, anxiety, well-being, or quality of life (Helgeson, Reynolds, & Tomich, 2006). However, intriguing preliminary evidence suggests that benefit finding may also have implications for physical health. In this chapter, we examine the association between benefit finding and physical health, focusing on the psychological and physiological mechanisms responsible for this effect. We first review the handful of studies that have specifically examined links between benefit finding, physical health, and physiology. Next, we propose a conceptual model in which we identify the cognitive, affective, motivational, and social components of benefit finding that may translate into physical health outcomes. We then discuss the physiological pathways through which these effects may occur. This chapter is not intended to be a comprehensive review but rather a roadmap that highlights promising links in order to generate directions for future research on benefit finding and health in medical populations.

Benefit Finding, Physical Health, and Physiology

We identified four studies, all of which were conducted with patients with medical illness, that specifically examined the association between benefit finding and objective physiological indicators or physical health measures. Affleck, Tennen, Croog, and Levine (1987) examined perceptions of positive life change among 287 men who had recently experienced their first heart attack. Over 50% of study participants reported benefits, the most common being learning the value of preventative health behaviors (29.6%), changes in mode of life to increase enjoyment (25.1%), and changes in philosophy of life or values (11.8%). Men who perceived benefits were significantly less likely to have a subsequent heart attack and exhibited less morbidity 8 years later. Because of constraints in the study design, the investigators were not able to evaluate possible mechanisms for these effects, such as actual changes in health behavior or physiological parameters. Nonetheless, these results offered the first evidence that benefit finding may have implications for physical health.

Bower, Kemeny, Taylor, and Fahey (1998) assessed perceptions of benefit finding among 40 HIV-positive men who had recently lost a close friend or partner to AIDS. In semistructured interviews, 40% of study participants reported finding some benefit from the bereavement experience, including greater appreciation for loved ones, increased value in and enjoyment of life, and new growth goals. Men who report greater benefit finding showed a significantly less rapid decline in CD4 T cells (a key measure of disease progression) over a 2- to 3-year follow-up, and a lower rate of AIDS-related mortality over a 4- to 9-year follow-up. These effects were not mediated by health status at baseline, health behaviors (e.g., sleep, sexual behavior, drug use), or other potential confounds, including depressed mood.

In a sample of 412 HIV-positive individuals, Milam (2006) evaluated whether reports of HIV-specific benefit finding were associated with changes in two key biological measures of disease progression, CD4 T cell levels, and viral load, over a 16- to 20-month follow-up. Benefit finding was assessed using a modified, shortened version of the Posttraumatic Growth Inventory (PTGI; Tedeschi & Calhoun, 1996). Results showed that benefit finding was associated with positive changes in biological markers among Hispanics and among those who were low in optimism or low in pessimism, but not in the full sample. Effects were independent of potential biobehavioral confounds, including depression, and the use of alcohol and illicit drugs. These findings suggest that the association between benefit finding and physiological outcomes is complex and may vary depending on the characteristics of the patient population.

Antoni et al. (2001) investigated relationships between benefit finding and physiological markers among women with early-stage breast cancer who were enrolled in an intervention trial. Benefit finding was assessed before and after the 10-week intervention using the Benefit-Finding Scale (Tomich & Helgeson, 2004), which assesses potential gains related to cancer, including acceptance, interpersonal growth, and a stronger sense of purpose in life. In analyses of the full patient cohort, results showed a significant increase in benefit finding among women in the intervention group. Increases in benefit finding were correlated with decreases in serum cortisol (Cruess et al., 2000) and with increases in lymphocyte proliferation (McGregor et al., 2004) in subgroup analyses (see chap. 11, this volume).

One additional study examined neural correlates of benefit finding and found that, controlling for positive affect, benefit finding following a motor vehicle accident was correlated with increased relative left frontal activation (Rabe, Zöllner, Maercker, & Karl, 2006). Greater relative left prefrontal activation is also associated with enhancements in certain aspects of immune system function, including a more robust antibody response to vaccination and increased natural killer cell cytotoxicity (Rosenkranz et al., 2003). Thus, benefit finding may be associated with neural processes that favor better immune responses to challenge.

Overall, these results offer preliminary evidence that perceptions of benefit are associated with positive changes in physical health and biological systems relevant to health outcomes, including changes in neural, neuroendocrine, and immune parameters. Positive effects were seen among individuals with cardiovascular disease, HIV/AIDS, and cancer, suggesting that the health consequences of benefit finding may extend across diverse medical conditions (for further review, see chap. 10, this volume). Whether these effects also extend to healthy individuals confronting other, nonmedical stressors has not yet been determined.

How Does Benefit Finding Get Under the Skin to Influence Health?

Despite evidence that benefit finding may have positive effects on physical health, the psychological and physiological mechanisms through which these effects occur have not been identified. Focusing first on psychological mechanisms, we propose that benefit finding may lead to changes in physical health through its effects on five central psychological domains: appraisal, coping processes, interpersonal relationships, priorities and goals, and positive affect.

We identified the first four of these domains by dissecting the construct of benefit finding to identify core components that may be relevant for physical health. Positive changes in interpersonal relationships are among the most widely cited benefits of stressful life events, with many individuals reporting that they feel closer to friends and family members as a result of the stressor. Changes in priorities and goals are also frequently reported, including placing greater importance on relationships and personal growth goals, as well as striving for a deeper sense of meaning or purpose in life. Positive changes in coping are often described as part of a greater feeling of self-reliance; in particular, individuals commonly report feeling stronger and more willing and able to deal proactively with life's difficulties. Although changes in appraisals are rarely labeled as such in the benefit finding literature, there is evidence that individuals report being better able to put things in perspective and not worry about minor concerns.

Changes in these areas are of interest because they map onto constructs that are associated with health outcomes in the broader health psychology literature. In particular, there is evidence that social support is associated with positive health outcomes, as are approach-oriented coping processes, personal coping resources (e.g., self-esteem, mastery, self-efficacy), challenge (vs. threat) appraisals, and, to a lesser degree, pursuit of intrinsic life goals, such as relationships. This literature is reviewed briefly in this chapter, focusing on the links between each of these constructs and disease onset, progression, and mortality, as well as physiological measures relevant for health.

The fifth domain of interest in our model is positive affect. There is compelling evidence from both cross-sectional and longitudinal research that benefit finding is associated with increases in positive affect and other aspects of positive well-being (e.g., see Bower et al., 2005). Indeed, a recent meta-analysis identified positive affect as one of the most consistent and strongest correlates of benefit finding (Helgeson et al., 2006; see also Stanton, Bower, & Low, 2006). A growing body of research has also demonstrated an association between positive affect and physical health outcomes (Pressman & Cohen, 2005). Thus, positive affect may be a factor in mediating the effects of benefit finding on physical health.

As shown in Figure 9.1, we propose that improvements in these five domains of functioning positively affect physiology, particularly how people respond to ongoing or future stressors. Positive changes in these areas will lead to what we label *enhanced allostasis*, or homeostatic responses to stress that minimize wear and tear on the body and/or promote restorative physiological "housekeeping" activities. Enhanced allostasis in turn can lead to improved physical health outcomes.

Appraisal and Health

Appraisals, the value and meaning we assign to stimuli, are the first step in stress perception. Appraisals are the filters determining our evaluations of life events—whether we see stressors optimistically, thus minimizing perceived threat, or whether we have heightened sensitivity to threat information. Here we focus on challenge versus threat appraisals (Lazarus & Folkman, 1984; Tomaka, Blascovich, Kibler, & Ernst, 1997). Challenge appraisals are made when one perceives that demands do not outweigh resources, but rather that one has the ability to cope successfully and may even have an opportunity for growth or gain. In contrast, threat perceptions are made when one perceives that demands outweigh resources and that one's physical or emotional well-being is threatened. We speculate that benefit finding may bias one against threat appraisals and toward challenge appraisals, putting daily stressors in perspec-

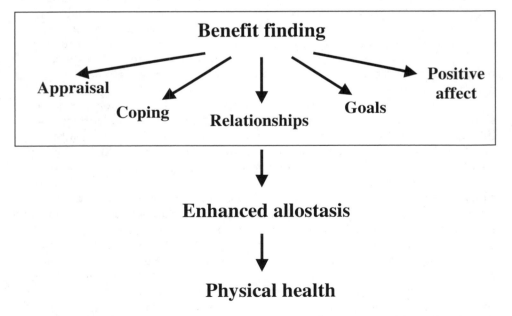

Figure 9.1. Conceptual model identifying psychological and physiological pathways linking benefit finding and physical health.

tive. Challenge versus threat appraisals have been examined primarily in studies evaluating acute physiological responses to experimental stimuli (i.e., *reactivity*), and are discussed in the section on physiological mediators.

Coping and Health

Theoretical models of positive life change posit that coping is an important predictor of benefit finding (e.g., see Tedeschi & Calhoun, 1996), and empirical studies have generally supported this hypothesis (Linley & Joseph, 2004; Stanton et al., 2006). Our model suggests that benefit finding may also lead to more adaptive forms of coping that, ultimately, have an influence on physical health. We focus here on approach coping, a collection of coping strategies characterized by an emotional, cognitive, or behavioral orientation toward the problem or stressor (vs. avoidance of the problem). These strategies include responses such as problem-focused coping, planning, positive reappraisal, emotional approach, and seeking social support.

The findings on coping and disease severity or progression are generally supportive of a positive association between approach coping and better physical health (Penley, Tomaka, & Wiebe, 2002). For example, approach types of coping are related to better metabolic control among people with diabetes (Kvam & Lyons, 1991), better physical health among women with breast cancer (Stanton et al., 2000), and lower risk of mortality in people with HIV (Lee & Powers, 2002). Approach coping was associated with a more adaptive immune response in a sample of healthy older adults with high levels of perceived stress (Stowell, Kiecolt-Glaser, & Glaser, 2001). In contrast, avoidance types of coping are typically associated with more negative physical health outcomes (Taylor & Stanton, 2007).

To better understand the nature and role of coping as a potential link between psychological growth and physical health, one may need to think beyond the traditional conceptualizations of coping. In particular, future studies would benefit from more careful measurement of meaning-focused coping, which includes strategies such as infusing ordinary events with positive meaning, adaptive goal processes, and benefit-reminding (Folkman & Moskowitz, 2007). These types of coping have primarily been described among individuals undergoing chronic life stressors, but may also emerge in the aftermath of a stressful experience. In addition, the experience of benefit finding may also lead to positive changes in coping resources, including perceptions of mastery and self-esteem (Taylor, 1983). There is suggestive evidence that these constructs are linked to health outcomes and may also influence physiological stress responses (Taylor & Stanton, 2007).

Relationships and Health

Our model posits that benefit finding is associated with improvements in interpersonal relationships, which are known to be important contributors to physical health (House, Landis, & Umberson, 1988). For the purpose of this brief review, we group the related literatures of relationship quality, social support, social integration, and social networks under the umbrella term of social ties (Seeman, 1996), although it should be noted that the pathways through which each of these influences physical health might differ (Cohen, 2004; Uchino, 2006).

The association between social ties and lower risk of mortality has been demonstrated in a number of different samples. For example, Berkman and Syme (1979) demonstrated that, controlling for physical health, socioeconomic status, health behaviors, life satisfaction, and preventive health services, social ties (e.g., marriage, social contacts, church, other group affiliations) were associated with lower mortality. Social ties are also associated with slower progression of HIV (Leserman et al., 1999) and cardiovascular disease (Wang, Mittleman, & Orth-Gomer, 2005), lower likelihood of subsequent cardiac event in patients who have had a myocardial infarction (Case, Moss, Case, McDermott, & Eberly, 1992), and decreased risk of mortality after breast cancer (Kroenke, Kubzansky, Schernhammer, Holmes, & Kawachi, 2006).

Social ties are also linked to changes in physiological systems relevant to health, including the immune system (Uchino, Cacioppo, & Kiecolt-Glaser, 1996), with potential benefits for immune-related medical conditions. For example, social network diversity is associated with decreased susceptibility to the common cold (Cohen, Doyle, Skoner, Rabin, & Gwaltney, 1997). Conversely, loss of social relationships is associated with decrements in immune system function (Irwin, Daniels, & Weiner, 1987), and negative and hostile social interactions have been linked to immune dysregulation (Kiecolt-Glaser et al., 1993).

Priorities, Goals, and Health

Individuals who experience benefit finding frequently report a shift in priorities and goals as well as a deeper sense of purpose or meaning in life. Although these constructs have rarely been examined in relation to physical health, there is preliminary evidence suggesting a link with health-related outcomes.

Goals are classified in many different ways; one categorization relevant for benefit finding is the distinction between intrinsic and extrinsic goals (Kasser & Ryan, 1996). Intrinsic goals are those that more directly satisfy inherent psychological needs such as relatedness, autonomy, and personal growth, and are commonly endorsed following stressful life events. There is evidence that individuals who pursue intrinsic life goals have higher levels of psychological adjustment (e.g., see Kasser & Ryan, 1996). Bower, Kemeny, Taylor, and Fahey (2003) found that, controlling for depressed mood and other potential confounds, importance of intrinsic goals was correlated with higher levels of natural killer cell cytotoxicity (NKCC) in a sample of women at high risk for breast cancer. It is interesting to note that importance of life goals in this study was positively correlated with scores on the PTGI, supporting the possibility that intrinsic goal engagement may be a dimension or an outcome of benefit finding. However, PTGI scores were not directly correlated with NKCC.

Purpose in life has also been linked to changes in immune status. In a sample of older women, higher levels of purpose in life were associated with lower plasma levels of the soluble IL-6 receptor, a marker of inflammation (Friedman, Hayney, Love, Singer, & Ryff, 2007). Inflammatory processes have been linked to a host of age-related health problems; thus, lower levels of this marker may be indicative of better physiological well-being. Purpose in life also predicts lower aortic calcification, indicating decreased cardiovascular disease among healthy older women (Matthews, Owens, Edmundowicz, Lee, & Kuller, 2006).

Positive Affect and Health

Benefit finding may be associated with physical health through its association with positive affect. Increasing evidence indicates that positive affect is uniquely associated with lower risk of morbidity and mortality in a number of healthy and chronically ill samples (Pressman & Cohen, 2005). For example, Ostir, Markides, Black, and Goodwin (2000) related positive affect to greater mobility, better functional status, and lower risk of mortality over a 2-year period in a sample of elderly Mexican Americans. In a sample of men with AIDS, positive affect uniquely predicted lower risk of mortality (Moskowitz, 2003). Positive affect is also significantly associated with lower risk of all-cause mortality in people with diabetes (Moskowitz, Epel, & Acree, 2008).

In both laboratory and naturalistic studies, positive affect is associated with more adaptive immune responses (e.g., see Futterman, Kemeny, Shapiro, & Fahey, 1994; Marsland, Cohen, Rabin, & Manuck, 2006). Higher levels of positive affect are also associated with lower levels of cortisol. For example, Steptoe, Wardle, and Marmot (2005) collected salivary cortisol and happiness ratings at eight points over 2 days in a sample of 116 men and 100 women. Total cortisol was inversely related to average happiness, controlling for age, gender, socioeconomic status, body mass, smoking, and distress levels.

It is plausible that benefit finding leads to a fuller experience of the range and depth of emotions, not simply more positive emotion. Future work exploring the affective mechanisms linking benefit finding to health should go beyond a positive or negative affect dichotomy to examine concepts such as emotional complexity (Kang & Shaver, 2004), emotional granularity (Tugade, Fredrickson, & Barrett, 2004), and the association between positive and negative emotion (Zautra, Potter, & Reich, 1997). In addition, researchers should examine a variety of positive emotional states, including feelings of intimacy, compassion, and gratitude, which may be particularly relevant in the aftermath of trauma.

Other Potential Mediators

Our model focuses on several key psychological mediators that are conceptually similar to reports of benefit finding and have demonstrated health relevance. This is certainly not an exhaustive list, and we anticipate that there may be other constructs that mediate effects on physical health. One potentially important mediator is changes in health behaviors, which are frequently cited as positive life changes among individuals confronting medical illnesses (e.g., see Sears, Stanton, & Danoff-Burg, 2003).

None of the psychological mediators we have proposed capture the enhanced sense of living in the moment reported by many individuals after a stressful event. *Mindfulness* can be defined as receptive attention to, and awareness of, present events and experience, and includes a state of present-oriented consciousness that is consistent with reports of benefit finding, although these tend to focus on greater appreciation or enjoyment of moment-to-moment experiences. Mindfulness is associated with higher levels of positive affect and other dimensions of well-being, including social connectedness and improvements in measures of physical health (Brown, Ryan, & Creswell, 2007). Mindfulness has gained increasing attention in the psychological literature and may also be of interest to scholars of benefit finding.

Physiological Mechanisms Through Which Benefit Finding Can Promote Physical Health

As reviewed earlier, measures of benefit finding and related psychological constructs have been associated with better health outcomes and with salutary markers of neuroendocrine and immune function. What are the physiological mechanisms that mediate the link between benefit finding and health? In this section, we propose two pathways through which benefit finding can promote physiological thriving and thus enhance health: (a) stress-buffering mechanisms, which maintain health in the face of chronic stress, and (b) restorative or health-enhancing mechanisms that actually repair damage and promote improvements in health. We include stress buffering and restorative activities as part of enhanced allostasis. *Allostasis* describes the normal repeated fluctuations that the body's regulatory systems make to maintain stability in the ever-changing environment (McEwen, 1998; Sterling & Eyer, 1988). Enhanced allostasis describes an adaptive pattern of responding to stress, which we suggest is partly a result of benefit finding (Bower, Low, Moskowitz, Sepah, & Epel, 2008) and other forms of psychological thriving (Epel, McEwen, & Ickovics, 1998). Here, we propose that enhanced allostasis can be measured by stress response curves that show a peak response with rapid recovery, rapid habituation upon repeated stress exposure, and strong counter-regulatory anabolic processes, including anabolic hormone production and vagal tone.

Overview of the Stress Response

To fully understand physiological thriving, it is necessary to have a basic understanding of the two primary stress response systems: the hypothalamic–pituitary–adrenal (HPA) axis and the sympatho–adrenal–medullary (SAM) axis. When an actual or symbolic (i.e., psychological) threat is perceived, the limbic HPA axis is activated, leading to the release of corticotropin-releasing hormone from the hypothalamus, which triggers the release of adrenocorticotropic hormone from the pituitary, which in turn releases cortisol from the adrenal gland. Catecholamines (i.e., epinephrine and norepinephrine) are released from the adrenal medulla, and norepinephrine from the sympathetic ganglia, in response to sympathetic nerve activity.

Activation of these systems prepares the organism to respond to potential threat and is adaptive in the face of demanding situations, particularly physical threat requiring energy mobilization. However, inappropriate, excessive, or prolonged activation of the stress response may lead to wear and tear on the body, or *allostatic load* (McEwen, 1998; Seeman, McEwen, Rowe, & Singer, 2001). Indeed, overexposure to stress hormones is a prognostic factor for development of cardiovascular disease (Krantz & Manuck, 1984) and respiratory illnesses (Boyce et al., 1995) and may increase risk for disease progression in HIV/AIDS (Cole, Kemeny, Fahey, Zack, & Naliboff, 2003) and some forms of cancer (Antoni et al., 2006).

Role of Benefit Finding in Stress-Buffering Mechanisms

We speculate that benefit finding may lead to more adaptive physiological stress responses, characterized by two features that minimize exposure to stress hormones: rapid recovery and rapid habituation. We focus on recovery and habituation rather than peak response, because these features more unequivocally reflect a healthier stress response. Recovery has been examined primarily in relation to the SAM axis, whereas habituation has been examined primarily in relation to the HPA axis.

RAPID RECOVERY. There is evidence that some of the psychological domains we have linked with benefit finding are associated with faster stress recovery in the SAM system. In particular, challenge appraisals, characterized by greater effort rather than distress, have been associated with positive patterns of SAM response including quick recovery (Dienstbier, 1989). It is of interest to note that challenge appraisals are also associated with a positive profile of autonomic nervous system (ANS) reactivity characterized by high cardiac output, whereas threat appraisals are associated with a more malignant response characterized by lower cardiac output and greater peripheral vasoconstriction (Tomaka et al., 1997). Positive affect may also facilitate quick SAM recovery. In a classic study, Fredrickson and Levenson (1998) induced negative affect in participants by showing them a film that elicited fear. Participants were then shown one of four films designed to elicit contentment, amusement, sadness, or no affect (i.e., a neutral condition). Measures of cardiovascular reactivity indicated that individuals who were shown the films eliciting contentment or amusement had faster recovery to baseline than those who were shown the sad or neutral films.

Psychological resilience, a construct similar to our conceptualization of benefit finding, is characterized by coping flexibility and ability for one's mood to recover quickly from stress. Tugade and Fredrickson (2004) showed that individuals high on trait resilience make fewer threat appraisals and experience more positive emotion in response to a standardized laboratory stressor. More relevant to enhanced allostasis, these individuals also show more rapid cardiovascular recovery following the stressor, an effect that is mediated by the experience of positive emotion.

HABITUATION TO REPEATED STRESS. Habituation to repeated stress is a unique paradigm that allows us to examine adaptation to stress independent from the novelty of the stressor. A healthy stress profile is thought to be characterized by an initial response to novelty, with rapid habituation by the second or later exposure (Dienstbier, 1989). Although habituation has received significantly less attention than the acute stress response, one study directly tested the association between benefit finding and HPA axis response to repeated stress. Epel et al. (1998) found that healthy women who did not habituate to a repeated laboratory stressor (approximately one third of the sample) had the lowest scores on the PTGI, particularly the subscales Appreciation of Life and Spiritual Growth. In contrast, those in the highest tertile on Spiritual Growth showed a positive reactivity curve to novel stress, and greater habituation by the second stressor. Psychological domains (e.g., self-esteem) related to benefit finding in our theoretical model have also been associated with cortisol habituation (Kirschbaum et al., 1995).

Overview of Restorative Processes

To better understand possible pathways that may link benefit finding to health outcomes we now review physiological processes associated with restorative processes such as anabolic and catabolic balance, and heart rate variability (HRV).

ANABOLIC AND CATABOLIC BALANCE. Anabolic hormones are traditionally defined as those that stimulate protein synthesis, and include the androgens—dehydroepiandrosterone (DHEA) and testosterone in men—and the growth hormone axis—growth hormone and insulin-like growth factor 1. These hormones play important roles in restoring homeostasis and repairing mechanisms after stress. Several other hormones can be considered anabolic and may be important in health, such as oxytocin, which decreases blood pressure and suppresses the HPA axis response to social stress in some cases (e.g., see Heinrichs, Baumgartner, Kirschbaum, & Ehlert, 2003; Parker, Buckmaster, Schatzberg, & Lyons, 2005), and neuropeptide Y, an anabolic effector peptide that acts as an anxiolytic.

These anabolic hormones are stress-responsive and typically increase with acute stress, but serve as antistress hormones in that they either directly inhibit the HPA axis or have the opposite effect on target tissues. Although most stress research has focused on overactivation of catabolic hormones such as cortisol, it is now increasingly recognized that catabolic hormones do not act in a vacuum but rather interact with anabolic hormones; the ratio of anabolic to catabolic activity may be a more sensitive index of catabolic stress arousal than either parameter alone. Chronic stress appears to accelerate the age-related shift in the neuroendocrine balance between anabolic and catabolic hormones. In turn, this imbalance is linked to age-related health conditions such as increased adiposity and decreased bone density (Epel, Burke, & Wolkowitz, 2007). Thus, enhanced allostasis may be characterized by strong anabolic activity at rest and in response to stress, which tends to protect the body from catabolic stress responses.

HEART RATE VARIABILITY. HRV, the variability in beat-to-beat intervals, is an indicator of the level of parasympathetic activity. As such, it provides a window into the restorative system, reflecting how strong the "brakes" are on the sympathetic nervous system, and the extent to which the body is in *restorative mode.* HRV decreases with acute stress and with age, and predicts cardiovascular (Villareal, Liu, & Massumi, 2002) and overall mortality (Tsuji et al., 1996). The parasympathetic nervous system may also play an important role in controlling inflammation (Tracey, 2002), with potential relevance for a number of age-related diseases.

Role of Benefit Finding in Restorative Processes

Only a handful of studies have examined the association between psychological factors and restorative hormones and processes. There is preliminary evidence that strong positive affect may trigger release of anabolic hormones. For example, testosterone levels can increase acutely in men after a positive event such as a success experience, an imagined success, or even vicarious success, such as watching one's favorite sports team win (Gonzalez-Bono, Salvador, Serrano, & Ricarte, 1999; McCaul, Gladue, & Joppa, 1992). Higher levels of growth hormone have also been related to positive affect (Epel, Adler, Ickovics, McEwen, & Clayton, 2001) and to other benefit-finding constructs, such as active coping (Epel, Adler, Ickovics, & McEwen, 1999). Oxytocin has been linked to socially related positive emotions, including trust and love (Gonzaga, Turner, Keltner, Campos, & Altemus, 2006; Kosfeld, Heinrichs, Zak, Fischbacher, & Fehr, 2005).

DHEA levels have been associated with positive psychological responses to stress. For example, a positive stressor that induced challenge appraisals also increased DHEA reactivity, and strong positive emotions were linked to greater DHEA reactivity during the exposure to the stressor (Mendes, Ayduk, Epel, Akinola, & Gyurak, 2007). This is an example of an anabolic response to stress, a response that should both protect from the catabolic effects of cortisol and promote quicker recovery back to restorative housekeeping duties after the exposure to the stressor.

Finally, whereas low HRV is related to measures of negative psychological functioning, including depression (e.g., see Carney et al., 2001), high HRV has been linked to positive forms of coping. In a sample of recently bereaved adults, individuals with higher resting HRV scored higher on measures of active coping and acceptance and lower on passive coping (O'Connor, Allen, & Kaszniak, 2002). We replicated these findings in a recent study of breast cancer survivors, finding that higher HRV was associated with approach coping, especially spiritual coping (Low, Bower, Epel, & Moskowitz, 2006). High HRV has also been linked to emotion regulation and constructive coping among undergraduates (Fabes & Eisenberg, 1997).

Future Directions

In this chapter, we have presented an integrative model that identifies central psychological and physiological mechanisms through which benefit finding may influence physical health. We propose that benefit finding from adversity, by influencing the psychological processes reviewed here, promotes enhanced allostasis and eventually better health (see Figure 9.1). Enhanced allostasis works by minimizing exposure to catabolic stress hormones through quick recovery and habituation to familiar stressors, and by promoting repair from stress through calibration of arousal at rest and in response to acute stress, toward a profile of greater anabolic than catabolic activity.

Although we have reviewed studies supporting links between each of our proposed mediators and heath outcomes, we recognize that the relevance of this research for the construct of benefit finding has not been determined. Thus, our hypotheses are speculative and designed to stimulate future research. In particular, longitudinal studies that carefully examine both psychological and physiological mediators of benefit finding are required to clarify these relationships. We conclude by highlighting particular areas of uncertainty and discussing potential limiting conditions for the effects of benefit finding on health.

Links Between Benefit Finding, Psychological and Physiological Mediators, and Health

Our model endeavors to integrate the construct of benefit finding with related psychological constructs in an effort to provide theoretical and empirical grounding for links between perceived benefits and health. However, a major question for future research is whether reports of benefit finding actually lead to improvements in these domains. Do individuals who report that they feel stronger and better able to cope with future difficulties, for example, score higher on measures of coping efficacy? Although approach-oriented coping and other constructs in our model have been examined as predictors and correlates of benefit finding (Helgeson et al., 2006; Stanton et al., 2006), we are not aware of any studies that have examined these variables as outcomes of benefit finding.

We have also speculated that enhanced allostasis should mediate between positive life changes and improvements in health. Given that high levels of psychological stress are linked to certain types of disease, and that stress hormones and ANS activity partially mediate these relationships, it is reasonable to speculate that profiles of stress reactivity that minimize exposure to stress mediators and maximize repair from stress should lead to better health. However, there are no studies of which we are aware that have specifically tested whether our proposed measures of enhanced allostasis—rapid recovery from and habituation to stressors, and the balance between anabolic and catabolic hormones—actually predict morbidity or mortality. Moreover, the links between our proposed psychological mediators and enhanced allostasis have not been carefully evaluated.

Affect as a Common Pathway for Benefit-Finding Effects on Health?

It is temping to speculate that increases in positive affect may be a common pathway through which benefit finding and associated changes in coping, relationships, and priorities and goals might influence physical health. Few studies have specifically tested this pathway, and it is an important issue for future research. However, there is evidence that not all of these effects are mediated by positive affect. In research on eudaimonic well-being, for example, purpose in life and personal growth are associated with biological parameters, whereas happiness is not (Ryff, Singer, & Dienberg, 2004). Furthermore, neural changes associated with eudaimonic well-being (Urry et al., 2004) and with benefit finding (Rabe et al., 2006) appear to be independent of positive affect. Moskowitz and Epel (2006) found that positive affect was a moderator, rather than a mediator, of the association between benefit finding and HPA axis activity in maternal caregivers. Although benefit finding was not directly related to diurnal cortisol slope in this sample, the occurrence of daily positive affect with benefit finding predicted a steeper, more adaptive decline in cortisol levels.

What about negative affect? Given the importance of depression and other negative affective states for physical health, it might be argued that decreases in psychological distress are an alternate common pathway linking benefit finding to health outcomes. However, there is inconsistent evidence that benefit finding is associated with changes in global measures of psychological distress, depression, or anxiety (Helgeson et al., 2006), and many studies have found effects of benefit finding, coping, relationships, and goals on health to be independent of depression (Bower et al., 2003). It is possible that other negative affective states will play a more important role in mediating these effects. These states include hopelessness, loneliness, and social threat with associated feelings of shame (Dickerson, Gruenewald, & Kemeny, 2004). These states are relevant to benefit finding to the extent that individuals become more socially integrated and less concerned about social evaluation following a stressful experience.

Boundary Conditions for Benefit Finding—Is it Always Health Enhancing?

Although we have presented a model postulating positive effects of benefit finding on health, we recognize that there are circumstances in which these effects may not occur. There is currently some debate about whether reports of benefit reflect actual change (Park & Helgeson, 2006), and whether benefit finding serves an approach or avoidant function (Stanton & Low, 2004). To the extent that reports of benefit finding are illusory, or represent avoidance or denial, links to our proposed mediators and to physical health are unlikely.

It is also important to note that efforts to sustain perceptions of benefit may be taxing in the context of extreme or chronic stress. This is illustrated in the following quote from a research participant shortly after her diagnosis with metastatic breast cancer: "I learned so much about life and myself from my first diagnosis, but enough already! I don't need this cancer to teach me anything else" (Stanton et al., 2006, p. 158). Indeed, Ryff and Singer (2006) found that reports of personal growth were associated with higher allostatic load in a small sample of women, although personal growth was associated with lower allostatic load for men. They suggested that "women who are striving to realize their talents through continuing growth and are highly engaged in managing complex environments may have higher activation of stress hormones" (p. 551). Further, PTGI scores were related to shorter telomere length, a marker of leukocyte aging, in a sample of healthy maternal caregivers (Wolfson, Moskowitz, & Epel, 2006). It is unclear whether sustaining growth in the context of a chronic caregiving stressor was taxing or whether growth simply reflected past severity and chronicity of stress, which were related to telomere shortening in this sample

(Epel et al., 2004). We speculate that although cross-sectionally, greater benefit finding may at times be linked to greater physiological wear and tear, in the long run, benefit finding should prevent telomere shortening and other aspects of biological aging. Clearly, the psychological and environmental context in which benefit finding occurs requires careful consideration in future research.

References

Affleck, G., Tennen, H., Croog, S., & Levine, S. (1987). Causal attribution, perceived benefits, and morbidity after a heart attack: An 8-year study. *Journal of Consulting and Clinical Psychology, 55,* 29–35.

Antoni, M. H., Lehman, J. M., Kilbourn, K. M., Boyers, A. E., Culver, J. L., Alferi, S. M., et al. (2001). Cognitive–behavioral stress management intervention decreases the prevalence of depression and enhances benefit finding among women under treatment for early-stage breast cancer. *Health Psychology, 20,* 20–32.

Antoni, M. H., Lutgendorf, S. K., Cole, S. W., Dhabhar, F. S., Sephton, S. E., McDonald, P. G., et al. (2006). The influence of bio-behavioural factors on tumour biology: Pathways and mechanisms. *Nature Reviews Cancer, 6,* 240–248.

Berkman, L. F., & Syme, S. L. (1979). Social networks, host resistance, and mortality: A nine-year follow-up study of Alameda County residents. *American Journal of Epidemiology, 109,* 186–204.

Bower, J. E., Kemeny, M. E., Taylor, S. E., & Fahey, J. L. (1998). Cognitive processing, discovery of meaning, CD4 decline, and AIDS-related mortality among bereaved HIV-seropositive men. *Journal of Consulting and Clinical Psychology, 66,* 979–986.

Bower, J. E., Kemeny, M. E., Taylor, S. E., & Fahey, J. L. (2003). Finding positive meaning and its association with natural killer cell cytotoxicity among participants in a bereavement-related disclosure intervention. *Annals of Behavioral Medicine, 25,* 146–155.

Bower, J. E., Low, C. A., Moskowitz, J. T., Sepah, S., & Epel, E. (2008). Benefit finding and physical health: Positive psychological changes and enhanced allostasis. *Social and Personality Psychology Compass, 2,* 223–244.

Bower, J. E., Meyerowitz, B. E., Desmond, K. A., Bernaards, C. A., Rowland, J. H., & Ganz, P. A. (2005). Perceptions of positive meaning and vulnerability following breast cancer: Predictors and outcomes among long-term breast cancer survivors. *Annals of Behavioral Medicine, 29,* 236–245.

Boyce, W. T., Chesney, M., Alkon, A., Tschann, J. M., Adams, S., Chesterman, B., et al. (1995). Psychobiologic reactivity to stress and childhood respiratory illnesses: Results of two prospective studies. *Psychosomatic Medicine, 57,* 411–422.

Brown, K. W., Ryan, R. M., & Creswell, J. D. (2007). Mindfulness: Theoretical foundations and evidence for its salutary effects. *Psychological Inquiry, 18,* 1–27.

Carney, R. M., Blumenthal, J. A., Stein, P. K., Watkins, L., Catellier, D., Berkman, L. F., et al. (2001). Depression, heart rate variability, and acute myocardial infarction. *Circulation, 104,* 2024–2028.

Case, R. B., Moss, A. J., Case, N., McDermott, M., & Eberly, S. (1992). Living alone after myocardial infarction. Impact on prognosis. *Journal of the American Medical Association, 267,* 515–519.

Cohen, S. (2004). Social relationships and health. *American Psychologist, 59,* 676–684.

Cohen, S., Doyle, W. J., Skoner, D. P., Rabin, B. S., & Gwaltney, J. M., Jr. (1997). Social ties and susceptibility to the common cold. *Journal of the American Medical Association, 277,* 1940–1944.

Cole, S. W., Kemeny, M. E., Fahey, J. L., Zack, J. A., & Naliboff, B. D. (2003). Psychological risk factors for HIV pathogenesis: Mediation by the autonomic nervous system. *Biological Psychiatry, 54,* 1444–1456.

Cruess, D. G., Antoni, M. H., McGregor, B. A., Kilbourn, K. M., Boyers, A. E., Alferi, S. M., et al. (2000). Cognitive–behavioral stress management reduces serum cortisol by enhancing benefit finding among women being treated for early stage breast cancer. *Psychosomatic Medicine, 62,* 304–308.

Dickerson, S. S., Gruenewald, T. L., & Kemeny, M. E. (2004). When the social self is threatened: Shame, physiology, and health. *Journal of Personality, 72,* 1191–1216.

Dienstbier, R. A. (1989). Arousal and physiological toughness: Implications for mental and physical health. *Psychological Review, 96,* 84–100.

Epel, E., Adler, N., Ickovics, J., & McEwen, B. (1999). Social status, anabolic activity, and fat distribution. *Annals of the New York Academy of Science, 896,* 424–426.

Epel, E., Adler, N., Ickovics, J., McEwen, B., & Clayton, P. (2001, June). *Stress-induced reductions in nocturnal growth hormone: Preliminary evidence and relations with fat distribution.* Poster session presented at the annual meeting of the Endocrine Society, Denver, CO.

Epel, E., Blackburn, E. H., Lin, J., Dhabhar, F. S., Adler, N. E., Morrow, J. D., & Cawthon, R. M. (2004). Accelerated telomere shortening in response to life stress. *Proceedings of the National Academy of Sciences U.S.A., 101,* 17312–17315.

Epel, E., Burke, H., & Wolkowitz, O. (2007). Psychoneuroendocrinology of aging: Focus on anabolic and catabolic hormones. In C. Aldwin, A. Spiro, & C. Park (Eds.), *Handbook of health psychology of aging* (pp. 119–141). New York: Guilford Press.

Epel, E., McEwen, B., & Ickovics, J. (1998). Embodying psychological thriving: Physical thriving in response to stress. *Journal of Social Issues, 54,* 301–322.

Fabes, R. A., & Eisenberg, N. (1997). Regulatory control and adults' stress-related responses to daily life events. *Journal of Personality and Social Psychology, 73,* 1107–1117.

Folkman, S., & Moskowitz, J. T. (2007). Positive affect and meaning-focused coping during significant psychological stress. In M. Hewstone, H. Schut, J. de Wit, K. Van Den Bos, & M. Stroebe (Eds.), *The scope of social psychology: Theory and applications* (pp. 193–208). London: Taylor & Francis.

Fredrickson, B. L., & Levenson, R. W. (1998). Positive emotions speed recovery from the cardiovascular sequelae of negative emotions. *Cognition and Emotion, 12,* 191–220.

Friedman, E. M., Hayney, M., Love, G. D., Singer, B. H., & Ryff, C. D. (2007). Plasma interleukin-6 and soluble IL-6 receptors are associated with psychological well-being in aging women. *Health Psychology, 26,* 305–313.

Futterman, A. D., Kemeny, M. E., Shapiro, D., & Fahey, J. L. (1994). Immunological and physiological changes associated with induced positive and negative mood. *Psychosomatic Medicine, 56,* 499–511.

Gonzaga, G. C., Turner, R. A., Keltner, D., Campos, B., & Altemus, M. (2006). Romantic love and sexual desire in close relationships. *Emotion, 6,* 163–179.

Gonzalez-Bono, E., Salvador, A., Serrano, M. A., & Ricarte, J. (1999). Testosterone, cortisol, and mood in a sports team competition. *Hormones and Behavior, 35,* 55–62.

Heinrichs, M., Baumgartner, T., Kirschbaum, C., & Ehlert, U. (2003). Social support and oxytocin interact to suppress cortisol and subjective responses to psychosocial stress. *Biological Psychiatry, 54,* 1389–1398.

Helgeson, V. S., Reynolds, K. A., & Tomich, P. L. (2006). A meta-analytic review of benefit finding and growth. *Journal of Consulting and Clinical Psychology, 74,* 797–816.

House, J. S., Landis, K. R., & Umberson, D. (1988, July 29). Social relationships and health. *Science, 241,* 540–545.

Irwin, M., Daniels, M., & Weiner, H. (1987). Immune and neuroendocrine changes during bereavement. *Psychiatric Clinics of North America, 10,* 449–465.

Kang, S. M., & Shaver, P. R. (2004). Individual differences in emotional complexity: Their psychological implications. *Journal of Personality, 72,* 687–726.

Kasser, T., & Ryan, R. M. (1996). Further examining the American Dream: Differential correlates of intrinsic and extrinsic goals. *Personality and Social Psychology Bulletin, 22,* 280–287.

Kiecolt-Glaser, J. K., Malarkey, W. B., Chee, M., Newton, T., Cacioppo, J. T., Mao, H. Y., & Glaser, R. (1993). Negative behavior during marital conflict is associated with immunological downregulation. *Psychosomatic Medicine, 55,* 410–412.

Kirschbaum, C., Prussner, J. C., Stone, A. A., Federenko, I., Gaab, J., Lintz, D., et al. (1995). Persistent high cortisol responses to repeated psychological stress in a subpopulation of healthy men. *Psychosomatic Medicine, 57,* 468–474.

Kosfeld, M., Heinrichs, M., Zak, P. J., Fischbacher, U., & Fehr, E. (2005). Oxytocin increases trust in humans. *Nature, 435,* 673–676.

Krantz, D. S., & Manuck, S. B. (1984). Acute psychophysiologic reactivity and risk of cardiovascular disease: A review and methodologic critique. *Psychological Bulletin, 96,* 435–464.

Kroenke, C. H., Kubzansky, L. D., Schernhammer, E. S., Holmes, M. D., & Kawachi, I. (2006). Social networks, social support, and survival after breast cancer diagnosis. *Journal of Clinical Oncology, 24,* 1105–1111.

Kvam, S. H., & Lyons, J. S. (1991). Assessment of coping strategies, social support, and general health status in individuals with diabetes mellitus. *Psychological Reports, 68,* 623–632.

Lazarus, R. S., & Folkman, S. (1984). *Stress, appraisal and coping.* New York: Springer Publishing Company.

Lee, C., & Powers, J. R. (2002). Number of social roles, health, and well-being in three generations of Australian women. *International Journal of Behavioral Medicine, 9,* 195–215.

Leserman, J., Jackson, E. D., Petitto, J. M., Golden, R. N., Silva, S. G., Perkins, D. O., et al. (1999). Progression to AIDS: The effects of stress, depressive symptoms, and social support. *Psychosomatic Medicine, 61,* 397–406.

Linley, P. A., & Joseph, S. (2004). Positive change following trauma and adversity: A review. *Journal of Traumatic Stress, 17,* 11–21.

Low, C. A., Bower, J. E., Epel, E., & Moskowitz, J. (2006, March). *Coping processes, spiritual well-being, and heart rate variability among breast cancer survivors.* Poster session presented at the annual meeting of the American Psychosomatic Society, Denver, CO.

Marsland, A. L., Cohen, S., Rabin, B. S., & Manuck, S. B. (2006). Trait positive affect and antibody response to hepatitis B vaccination. *Brain Behavior and Immunity, 20,* 261–269.

Matthews, K. A., Owens, J. F., Edmundowicz, D., Lee, L., & Kuller, L. H. (2006). Positive and negative attributes and risk for coronary and aortic calcification in healthy women. *Psychosomatic Medicine, 68,* 355–361.

McCaul, K. D., Gladue, B. A., & Joppa, M. (1992). Winning, losing, mood, and testosterone. *Hormones and Behavior, 26,* 486–504.

McEwen, B. S. (1998). Protective and damaging effects of stress mediators. *New England Journal of Medicine, 338,* 171–179.

McGregor, B. A., Antoni, M. H., Boyers, A., Alferi, S. M., Blomberg, B. B., & Carver, C. S. (2004). Cognitive–behavioral stress management increases BF and immune function among women with early-stage breast cancer. *Journal of Psychosomatic Research, 56,* 1–8.

Mendes, W. B., Ayduk, O., Epel, E. S., Akinola, M., & Gyurak, A. (2007). *When stress is good for you: Neuroendocrine concomitants of physiological thriving.* Unpublished manuscript, Harvard University, Boston, MA.

Milam, J. (2006). Posttraumatic growth and HIV disease progression. *Journal of Consulting and Clinical Psychology, 74,* 817–827.

Moskowitz, J. T. (2003). Positive affect predicts lower risk of AIDS mortality. *Psychosomatic Medicine, 65,* 620–626.

Moskowitz, J. T., & Epel, E. S. (2006). Benefit finding and diurnal cortisol slope in maternal caregivers: A moderating role for positive emotion. *Journal of Positive Psychology, 1,* 83–91.

Moskowitz, J. T., Epel, E. S., & Acree, M. (2008). Positive affect uniquely predicts lower risk of mortality in people with diabetes. *Health Psychology, 27*(Suppl.), 73–82.

O'Connor, M. F., Allen, J. J., & Kaszniak, A. W. (2002). Autonomic and emotion regulation in bereavement and depression. *Journal of Psychosomatic Research, 52,* 183–185.

Ostir, G. V., Markides, K. S., Black, S. A., & Goodwin, J. S. (2000). Emotional well-being predicts subsequent functional independence and survival. *Journal of the American Geriatric Society, 48,* 473–478.

Park, C. L., & Helgeson, V. S. (2006). Introduction to the special section: Growth following highly stressful life events—Current status and future directions. *Journal of Consulting and Clinical Psychology, 74,* 791–796.

Parker, K. J., Buckmaster, C. L., Schatzberg, A. F., & Lyons, D. M. (2005). Intranasal oxytocin administration attenuates the ACTH stress response in monkeys. *Psychoneuroendocrinology, 30,* 924–929.

Penley, J. A., Tomaka, J., & Wiebe, J. S. (2002). The association of coping to physical and psychological health outcomes: A meta-analytic review. *Journal of Behavioral Medicine, 25,* 551–603.

Pressman, S. D., & Cohen, S. (2005). Does positive affect influence health? *Psychological Bulletin, 131,* 925–971.

Rabe, S., Zöllner, T., Maercker, A., & Karl, A. (2006). Neural correlates of posttraumatic growth after severe motor vehicle accidents. *Journal of Consulting and Clinical Psychology, 74,* 880–886.

Rosenkranz, M. A., Jackson, D. C., Dalton, K. M., Dolski, I., Ryff, C. D., Singer, B. H., et al. (2003). Affective style and in vivo immune response: Neurobehavioral mechanisms. *Proceedings of the National Academy of Sciences U.S.A., 100,* 11148–11152.

Ryff, C. D., & Singer, B. (2006). From social structure to biology: Integrative science in pursuit of human health and well-being. In C. Snyder & S. Lopez (Eds.), *Handbook of positive psychology* (pp. 541–555). New York: Oxford University Press.

Ryff, C. D., Singer, B. H., & Dienberg, L. G. (2004). Positive health: Connecting well-being with biology. *Philosophical Transactions of the Royal Society of London: Series B. Biological Sciences, 359,* 1383–1394.

Sears, S. R., Stanton, A. L., & Danoff-Burg, S. (2003). The Yellow Brick Road and the Emerald City: Benefit finding, positive reappraisal coping and posttraumatic growth in women with early-stage breast cancer. *Health Psychology, 22,* 487–497.

Seeman, T. E. (1996). Social ties and health: The benefits of social integration. *Annals of Epidemiology, 6,* 442–451.

Seeman, T. E., McEwen, B. S., Rowe, J. W., & Singer, B. H. (2001). Allostatic load as a marker of cumulative biological risk: MacArthur studies of successful aging. *Proceedings of the National Academy of Sciences U.S.A., 98,* 4770–4775.

Stanton, A. L., Bower, J. E., & Low, C. A. (2006). Posttraumatic growth after cancer. In L. G. Calhoun & R. G. Tedeschi (Eds.), *Handbook of posttraumatic growth: Research and practice* (pp. 138–175). Mahwah, NJ: Erlbaum.

Stanton, A. L., Danoff-Burg, S., Cameron, C. L., Bishop, M., Collins, C. A., Kirk, S. B., et al. (2000). Emotionally expressive coping predicts psychological and physical adjustment to breast cancer. *Journal of Consulting and Clinical Psychology, 68,* 875–882.

Stanton, A. L., & Low, C. A. (2004). Toward understanding PTG: Commentary on Tedeschi and Calhoun. *Psychological Inquiry, 15,* 76–80.

Steptoe, A., Wardle, J., & Marmot, M. (2005). Positive affect and health-related neuroendocrine, cardiovascular, and inflammatory processes. *Proceedings of the National Academy of Sciences U.S.A., 102,* 6508–6512.

Sterling, P., & Eyer, J. (1988). Allostasis: A new paradigm to explain arousal pathology. In S. Fisher & J. Reason (Eds.), *Handbook of life stress: Cognition and health* (pp. 629–649). Hoboken, NJ: Wiley.

Stowell, J. R., Kiecolt-Glaser, J. K., & Glaser, R. (2001). Perceived stress and cellular immunity: When coping counts. *Journal of Behavioral Medicine, 24,* 323–339.

Taylor, S. E. (1983). Adjustment to threatening events: A theory of cognitive adaptation. *American Psychologist, 38,* 1161–1173.

Taylor, S. E., & Stanton, A. L. (2007). Coping resources, coping processes, and mental health. *Annual Review of Clinical Psychology, 3,* 377–401.

Tedeschi, R. G., & Calhoun, L. G. (1996). The Posttraumatic Growth Inventory: Measuring the positive legacy of trauma. *Journal of Traumatic Stress, 9,* 455–471.

Tomaka, J., Blascovich, J., Kibler, J., & Ernst, J. M. (1997). Cognitive and physiological antecedents of threat and challenge appraisal. *Journal of Personality and Social Psychology, 73,* 63–72.

Tomich, P. L., & Helgeson, V. S. (2004). Is finding something good in the bad always good? Benefit finding among women with breast cancer. *Health Psychology, 23,* 16–23.

Tracey, K. J. (2002). The inflammatory reflex. *Nature, 420,* 853–859.

Tsuji, H., Larson, M. G., Venditti, F. J., Jr., Manders, E. S., Evans, J. C., Feldman, C. L., & Levy, D. (1996). Impact of reduced heart rate variability on risk for cardiac events. The Framingham Heart Study. *Circulation, 94,* 2850–2855.

Tugade, M. M., & Fredrickson, B. L. (2004). Resilient individuals use positive emotions to bounce back from negative emotional experiences. *Journal of Personality and Social Psychology, 86,* 320–333.

Tugade, M. M., Fredrickson, B. L., & Barrett, L. F. (2004). Psychological resilience and positive emotional granularity: Examining the benefits of positive emotions on coping and health. *Journal of Personality, 72,* 1161–1190.

Uchino, B. N. (2006). Social support and health: A review of physiological processes potentially underlying links to disease outcomes. *Journal of Behavioral Medicine, 29,* 377–387.

Uchino, B. N., Cacioppo, J. T., & Kiecolt-Glaser, J. K. (1996). The relationship between social support and physiological processes: A review with emphasis on underlying mechanisms and implications for health. *Psychological Bulletin, 119,* 488–531.

Urry, H. L., Nitschke, J. B., Dolski, I., Jackson, D. C., Dalton, K. M., Mueller, C. J., et al. (2004). Making a life worth living: Neural correlates of well-being. *Psychological Sciences, 15,* 367–372.

Villareal, R. P., Liu, B. C., & Massumi, A. (2002). Heart rate variability and cardiovascular mortality. *Current Atherosclerosis Reports, 4,* 120–127.

Wang, H. X., Mittleman, M. A., & Orth-Gomer, K. (2005). Influence of social support on progression of coronary artery disease in women. *Social Science & Medicine, 60,* 599–607.

Wolfson, W., Moskowitz, J., & Epel, E. (2006, March). *Stress, posttraumatic growth, and leukocyte aging.* Paper presented at the annual meeting of the American Psychosomatic Society, Denver, CO.

Zautra, A. J., Potter, P. T., & Reich, J. W. (1997). The independence of affects is context-dependent: An integrative model of the relationship between positive and negative affect. *Annual Review of Gerontology and Geriatrics, 17,* 75–103.

10

Is Benefit Finding Good for Individuals With Chronic Disease?

Sara B. Algoe and Annette L. Stanton

Chronic diseases such as cancer, cardiovascular disease, and arthritic conditions affect approximately 90 million Americans (Centers for Disease Control, 2005). Despite the intuitive appeal of linking the ability to find benefit in the experience of such serious illnesses to enhanced well-being, the question remains: Does the report of benefit translate to improvement in psychological and physical health? Recent evidence suggests a complex story.

In this chapter, we use the term *benefit finding* (BF) to refer to the report of finding good in the bad (see Tennen & Affleck, 2002). The majority of studies on links between BF and adjustment are cross-sectional. Reviews of these studies (e.g., see Helgeson, Reynolds, & Tomich, 2006; Linley & Joseph, 2004; Stanton, Bower, & Low, 2006) are a good source to begin to address the question of whether BF is good for individuals with chronic disease. A review of the relevant cancer literature (Stanton et al., 2006) and a meta-analysis of 87 cross-sectional studies across several stressors (Helgeson et al., 2006) have shown that relations of BF to measures of adjustment are not uniform across outcomes. Moreover, amid numerous nonsignificant findings, significant relationships often are moderated by other variables (e.g., time since trauma). In considering the relation between BF and outcomes, it is important to note that adjustment to chronic disease is multifaceted (Stanton, Revenson, & Tennen, 2007). For example, examination of daily affect for individuals with rheumatoid arthritis (RA) strongly supports the separate evaluation of positive and negative adjustment indices because they are influenced by different underlying processes (e.g., see Zautra, Affleck, Tennen, Reich, & Davis, 2005). To find out whether BF is good for people with chronic disease, it is important to assess whether it is related to both negative (e.g., depressive symptoms) and positive (e.g., well-being) indicators of adjustment. Stanton et al.'s (2006) review suggests that physical health outcomes represent another promising domain of "good" that might come from finding benefit in chronic disease.

A limitation of these studies is that because most are cross-sectional they bring researchers only marginally closer to an answer to our question: Is BF good for people with chronic disease? Does seeing some good in the bad bolster adjustment in the long run? The purpose of this chapter is to review the literature in which BF is measured in people affected by chronic physical disease (i.e., either they or a loved one has the disease) and is examined as a prospective predictor of adjustment. We then offer ideas about how to account for the inconsistent associations between BF and later adjustment, discuss implications for intervention, and suggest directions for future research.

Finding Benefit in Chronic Disease Has Inconsistent Relations With Adaptive Outcomes

In addition to limiting our review to longitudinal, naturalistic studies in which BF was used to predict adaptive outcomes, we restricted the definition of BF to measures in which the participant explicitly listed or rated benefits that were perceived to have happened as a result of the stressor, and we excluded measures in which participants endorsed items about attempts to find benefit. These latter measures (e.g., COPE Positive Reappraisal subscale, Carver, Scheier, & Weintraub, 1989; Ways of Coping Positive Reframing subscale, Folkman & Lazarus, 1985) have sometimes been characterized as BF, but there is debate about whether they measure the same thing (e.g., see Helgeson et al., 2006; Tennen & Affleck, 2002). We searched PsycINFO (http://www.apa.org/psycinfo) and PubMed (http://www.ncbi.nlm.nih.gov/pubmed) for the following terms: *benefit finding, posttraumatic growth, stress-related growth, adversarial growth,* and related phrases. We also reviewed the resulting articles' reference sections as well as recent reviews of the literature. Because a variety of terms have been used to describe the phenomenon of finding benefit in adversity, the resultant articles are likely to compose a representative but not exhaustive sampling of the literature.

Table 10.1 displays methodological features of the studies. The search yielded 16 samples with data involving people who were diagnosed or had a close other diagnosed with chronic disease (i.e., maternal caregivers; Moskowitz & Epel, 2006; Rini et al., 2004); one study included HIV-positive men bereaved over a close friend or partner lost to AIDS (Bower, Kemeny, Taylor, & Fahey, 1998). Three studies were of subsamples of women from a larger study on breast cancer (Antoni et al., 2001; see also chap. 11, this volume), each addressing different outcomes (Cruess et al., 2000; Lechner, Carver, Antoni, Weaver, & Phillips, 2006, Study 2; McGregor et al., 2004). Although one study pertained to an acute illness, we included it because it involved a life-threatening condition (i.e., severe acute respiratory syndrome [SARS]; Cheng, Wong, & Tsang, 2006). BF was indexed by a variety of measures. All studies reported an initial assessment of BF and at least one follow-up assessment of an outcome relevant to mental or physical health. However, although BF can be investigated as an outcome in its own right, examining BF as an outcome was not a goal for this chapter. Follow-up assessments were conducted between 1 day and 8 years after the initial BF measure, with the majority occurring within 1 year. With a few noted exceptions, all prospective analyses statistically controlled for baseline values of the outcome measure.

Participants in the samples were primarily married Caucasian women in their 40s. Sex of the participant often was confounded with disease studied. Eight studies included women with breast cancer or mothers of ill children. Two studies were the only prospective studies on RA, with samples that were

Table 10.1. Longitudinal Studies Predicting Psychological and Physical Health Outcomes From Benefit Finding (BF)

Author(s)	Sample[b]	Timing of baseline	BF measurement[c]	Follow-up	Outcomes
Cancer (from Antoni and Carver research group—breast cancer)					
Carver and Antoni (2004); Lechner (2006), Study 1	96 women, Stage 0, I, or II	3, 6, or 12 months postsurgery	17-item Benefit-Finding Scale (BFS; Tomich & Helgeson, 2004)	4–7 years after T1	Depressive symptoms Distress/negative affect Positive affect Quality of life Social disruption Serum cortisol
Cruess et al. (2000)[a]	34 women, Stage I or II	4–8 weeks post-surgery	Change from T1 to T2 on 17-item BFS	10 weeks after T1	Depressive symptoms Distress/negative affect Social disruption Quality of life
Lechner (2006), Study 2[a]	74 women, Stage 0, I, or II	6 months post-surgery	17-item BFS	5 years postsurgery	
McGregor et al. (2004)[a]	29 women, Stage I or II	T1 = 4–8 weeks postsurgery T2 = 10 weeks after T1	Change from T1 to T2 on 17-item BFS	T3 = 6 months post-surgery	Circulating lympho-cytes (various) Proliferative response to anti-CD3

(continues)

Table 10.1. Longitudinal Studies Predicting Psychological and Physical Health Outcomes From Benefit Finding (BF) (*Continued*)

Author(s)	Sample[b]	Timing of baseline	BF measurement[c]	Follow-up	Outcomes
Cancer (from other research groups)					
Bower et al. (2005)	763 women, Stage I or II breast cancer survivors	1–5 years post-dx (*M* = 3.4 years)	11-item "positive meaning" scale	5–10 years post-dx (*M* = 2.8 years after T1)	Distress/negative affect Positive affect Quality of life
Schwarzer, Luszcynska, Boehmer, Taubert, and Knoll (2006)	117 (73 men) patients with various cancers, Stages I–IV	Week before surgery	7-item "positive changes" scale	T2 = 1 month post-surgery T3 = 12 months postsurgery	Depressive symptoms Health-related worry Health-related quality of life
Sears, Stanton, and Danoff-Burg (2003)	101 women, Stage I or II breast cancer	*M* = 28.5 weeks post-dx	Coded from interview questions (yes/no and total number of benefits found)	T2 = 3 months after T1 T3 = 12 months after T1	Distress/negative affect Positive affect Quality of life Perceived health Cancer-related medical visits
Tomich and Helgeson (2004)	364 women, Stage I, II, or III breast cancer	*M* = 4 months post-dx	20-item BFS (adapted from Behr, Murphy, & Summers, 1991)	T2 = 3 months after T1 T3 = 9 months after T1	Distress/negative affect Positive affect Quality of life
Cardiovascular					
Affleck, Tennen, Croog, and Levine (1987)	205 men after first heart attack	7 weeks after first heart attack	Coded from interview questions (total number of benefits found)	8 years after first heart attack	Heart attack recurrence Morbidity

Caregivers

Study	Sample	Timing	Benefit finding measure	Measurement interval	Outcomes
Moskowitz and Epel (2006)	Maternal caregivers of a chronically ill ($n = 45$) or healthy ($n = 26$) child	(no information)	Posttraumatic Growth Inventory (PTGI) for "most stressful event of their adult lives" (57% reported child-related stressor)	3×/day for 2 days after T1	Distress/negative affect; Positive affect; Salivary cortisol
Rini et al. (2004)	144 mothers of children undergoing hematopoietic stem cell transplantation	In hospital $M = 3.6$ days prior to infusion	2-item scale: looking for and able to find positive things for family from child's illness	6 months after T1	Quality of life

Human Immunodeficiency Virus (HIV)

Study	Sample	Timing	Benefit finding measure	Measurement interval	Outcomes
Bower, Kemeny, Taylor, and Fahey (1998)	40 HIV-positive gay or bisexual men	$M = 8$ months post-bereavement	Coded "discovery of meaning" from interview questions (yes/no)	6-month intervals for 2–3 years	CD4 T lymphocyte levels; AIDS-related mortality
Milam (2006b)	412 (88.1% men) living with HIV	$M = 6.4$ years since initial positive HIV test	PTGI (modified)	16–20 months after T1	Viral load; CD4 count

Rheumatoid Arthritis (RA)

Study	Sample	Timing	Benefit finding measure	Measurement interval	Outcomes
Danoff-Burg and Revenson (2005)	124 (111 women) RA patients	$M = 16$ years post-dx	Coded interpersonal benefits from interview questions (yes/no)	1 year after T1	Distress/negative affect; Functional disability; Pain
Tennen, Affleck, Urrows, Higgins, and Mendola (1992)	54 (41 women) RA patients	9 years post-dx	5-item benefit-appraisal scale	75 daily reports after T1	Positive affect; Activity limitation; Pain

(continues)

Table 10.1. Longitudinal Studies Predicting Psychological and Physical Health Outcomes From Benefit Finding (BF) *(Continued)*

Author(s)	Sample[b]	Timing of baseline	BF measurement[c]	Follow-up	Outcomes
Sudden Acute Respiratory Syndrome (SARS)					
Cheng, Wong, and Tsang (2006)	301 Chinese adults (56% women): 1. Recovered from SARS (23.3%) 2. Family member of recovered (19.6%) 3. No knowledge of affected (57.1%)	1. and 2. 4–5 weeks postdischarge from hospital 3. Same period of time	Coded benefits, costs, or mixed (cost and benefit) from interview questions (i.e., forced choice, then elaborated on each option)	T2 = mailed 4–6 weeks after T1 T3 = 1.5 years after T1	Self-esteem

[a]From Antoni et al., 2001. T1 = Time 1; T2 = Time 2; T3 = Time 3; dx = diagnosis. [b]All Ns are from follow-up analyses, as reported by the researchers, with three exceptions that had two follow-up time points and therefore multiple Ns for these points: Sears et al. (2003), Tomich and Helgeson (2004), Cheng et al. (2006). [c]Researchers who coded benefits from interview questions used an item that asked participants whether they had experienced benefits associated with the disease, and to elaborate if so. Cheng et al. (2006) also asked about costs.

76% and 82% female. The two HIV-positive samples were 100% and 88% male, and a study on BF after myocardial infarction exclusively enrolled men. One study included participants diagnosed with various cancers, and another study included people affected by SARS.

Measures of Negative Psychological Outcomes

A variety of negative outcomes were measured, including depressive symptoms, distress or negative affect (NA), and social disruption. We review the evidence for each and then provide a summary.

DEPRESSIVE SYMPTOMS. Depressive symptoms were measured in three samples using the Center for Epidemiological Studies Depression Scale (CES-D; Radloff, 1977). BF within the year following surgery for breast cancer predicted a decrease in depressive symptoms 4 to 7 years later (Carver & Antoni, 2004), with no curvilinear relation evident (Lechner et al., 2006, Study 1). An increase in BF from 1 month to 1 year following cancer surgery was predictive of fewer depressive symptoms at 1 year (Schwarzer, Luszczynska, Boehmer, Taubert, & Knoll, 2006). In contrast, Lechner et al. (2006, Study 2) found no linear or curvilinear relation between early BF and depressive symptoms 5 years later in breast cancer patients who had undergone a cognitive–behavioral stress management intervention (CBSM; Antoni et al., 2001).

DISTRESS OR NEGATIVE AFFECT. Eight samples reported on distress or negative mood. In three of the samples described earlier, the associations for distress were the same as those for depressive symptoms. The linear effect in the Carver and Antoni (2004) sample was significant, whereas the linear effect in the second sample and curvilinear effects in both samples were nonsignificant (Lechner et al., 2006). An increase in BF was predictive of less health-related worry a year after cancer surgery in Schwarzer et al. (2006).

Tomich and Helgeson (2004) measured NA (Watson, Clark, & Tellegen, 1988) 3 and 9 months after an initial BF measure in women with breast cancer. An interaction model was tested whereby level of BF and stage of disease interact to predict NA, controlling for baseline NA. For women with a poorer prognosis, more BF at baseline predicted more NA at both the 3-month and the 9-month follow-up. It should be noted that this is the only sample of breast cancer patients that included women with poorer-prognosis (i.e., Stage III) cancer.

Four other studies revealed no association between BF and distress or NA. Neither having found benefits in the experience of breast cancer nor the number of benefits found predicted distress 3 or 12 months later (Sears, Stanton, & Danoff-Burg, 2003). In addition, finding interpersonal benefits from having RA did not predict distress 1 year later (Danoff-Burg & Revenson, 2005). Bower et al. (2005) concluded that "positive meaning" 1 to 5 years after a diagnosis of breast cancer did not predict change in NA items from the CES-D 5 to 10 years after diagnosis. Finally, Moskowitz and Epel (2006) measured NA by averaging six assessments across 2 days following mothers' report of BF for the most stressful event of their adult lives. One half of the mothers had a child with chronic illness, and 57% of the sample reported that the most stressful event was related to their child. BF was not associated with NA.

SOCIAL DISRUPTION. Lechner et al. (2006) tested linear and curvilinear models in which BF predicted disease-related disruption of social and recreational activities. In Study 1, BF did not predict social disruption 4 to 7 years later. In Study 2, a curvilinear effect emerged. Women who were low or high in BF had decreased social disruption 5 years later, whereas women with moderate BF had higher social disruption 5 years later. The author suggested that the levels of BF might represent people who are coping with illness in distinct ways; perhaps those who reported low BF were not distressed by their disease and hence not motivated to find benefit, whereas people who reported more BF were distressed initially but used BF to reduce social disruption.

SUMMARY. Amid several nonsignificant effects, four linear effects from two studies (Carver & Antoni, 2004; Schwarzer et al., 2006) suggest that BF predicts decline in depressive symptoms and distress or worry for people with cancer. Two other findings suggest complex associations between BF and negative outcomes. A moderated effect suggests that the relation of BF to adjustment might depend on the severity of one's disease (Tomich & Helgeson, 2004). A curvilinear relation of BF and outcomes was significant for one of three measures (i.e., social disruption, but not depressive symptoms or distress), but for only one of two samples (Lechner et al., 2006, Study 2). This finding suggests a methodological consideration that may affect the interpretation of data in future studies: Samples reporting a broad range of BF and distress may not demonstrate linear effects.

Measures of Positive Psychological Outcomes

Positive aspects of life were measured in the Carver and Antoni (2004) and Lechner et al. (2006) samples using a 10-item rating scale (e.g., challenge in life, spiritual fulfillment; Andrews & Withey, 1976). Curvilinear trends, but no significant relations, were demonstrated for BF. In addition, for women with breast cancer, BF did not predict quality of life at 3- or 12-month follow-up (Sears et al., 2003), or 5 to 10 years after diagnosis (Bower et al., 2005). Tomich and Helgeson (2004) found that women who had a more severe breast cancer diagnosis and high BF at study entry had worse psychological quality of life 3 months, but not 9 months, later.

In contrast, Schwarzer et al. (2006) found that increases in BF predicted increases in health-related quality of life. Cheng et al. (2006) found that people who reported both benefits and costs of an experience with SARS had a greater increase in self-esteem over 1 year than did those who reported only benefits; the benefit-only group had higher self-esteem than those who reported only costs. Rini et al. (2004) assessed BF in mothers of children who were undergoing stem cell transplantation. Psychological quality of life at the 6-month follow-up was not predicted by BF in the days just prior to transplant or by change in BF from study entry to follow-up. However, BF did interact with optimism to predict mental health: For mothers high in optimism prior to transplant, BF predicted better mental health 6 months later, but for mothers low in optimism, BF was a marginally significant predictor of worse mental health at follow-up.

Like distress and NA, positive feelings were assessed with various measures. Although positive affect (PA) was not measured at study entry in Carver and Antoni (2004), initial BF was significantly related to higher later PA. Using the four PA items from the CES-D, Bower et al. (2005) found that initial BF predicted PA between 5 and 10 years following breast cancer surgery. The four other studies that measured PA did not produce significant results. Sears et al. (2003) demonstrated that BF did not predict vigor (Profile of Mood States; McNair, Lorr, & Droppelman, 1971) 3 or 12 months later. Tomich and Helgeson (2004) tested an interaction between disease severity and BF but found no significant interaction on PA. Tennen, Affleck, Urrows, Higgins, and Mendola (1992) asked participants to complete daily reports for 75 days after a measure of BF. BF did not predict average positive mood during this period, nor was daily mood predicted from the interaction between BF and daily pain. Finally, Moskowitz and Epel (2006) found no relations between reports of BF and average PA as assessed six times across 2 days.

In summary, as with negative outcomes, evidence for positive psychological outcomes of BF was inconsistent: Amid several nonsignificant findings, there were a handful of significant associations and one moderated relation of BF to optimism on positive outcomes. However, there were no negative associations between BF and positive psychological functioning.

Physical Health and Markers of Physical Functioning

In addition to the more commonly studied psychological health outcomes described previously, some researchers have assessed changes in physical health. In this section we review the evidence for self-reported and objectively verifiable changes in physical health.

SELF-REPORTED PHYSICAL HEALTH. The first set of perceived health indicators included measures that incorporated multiple components of perceived general health or a one-item global health measure; no indicator of perceived global health was predicted by earlier reports of BF (Bower et al., 2005; Sears et al., 2003; Tomich & Helgeson, 2004). The other measures of perceived health included disease-related composites or specific indices (e.g., pain, activity level). Participants who perceived benefits after a first heart attack had lower cardiac morbidity (e.g., chest pain, difficulty using stairs) 8 years later than those who did not (Affleck, Tennen, Croog, & Levine, 1987). In a group of individuals with RA, Tennen et al. (1992) tested an association of BF with reports of daily pain and also examined whether the person's activity was limited because of pain on a given day. Neither of the direct associations was significant, nor was daily pain predicted by a BF–disease severity interaction. However, BF interacted with pain to predict days of activity limitation, such that people who found more benefit from their pain and had high daily ratings of pain also reported less limited activity because of pain than did people who found less benefit but had high pain.

Finally, Danoff-Burg and Revenson (2005) found that reports of interpersonal benefits mediated an association between social constraints of discussing RA with others and physical functioning: People who thought others were willing to listen to them discuss their RA experience at study entry were more likely to report interpersonal benefits from RA and, in turn, reported better physical functioning the next year. The effect was eliminated if physical functioning at study entry was controlled, which may be due to the stability of this variable over time (Danoff-Burg & Revenson, 2005). Interpersonal BF had no relation to daily pain.

OBJECTIVE MEASURES OF PHYSICAL HEALTH. Researchers have begun to examine relations of BF to objective measures of physical health or markers of healthy functioning (see chap. 9, this volume). Affleck et al. (1987) demonstrated that participants who reported BF as a result of their first heart attack had lower incidence of reinfarction 8 years later than those who did not. Breast cancer patients prospectively recorded medical visits for 3 months following a BF measure in Sears et al. (2003). BF did not predict frequency of cancer-related medical visits at 3 months.

Two groups of researchers used subsamples of CBSM intervention participants from Antoni et al. (2001). Cruess et al. (2000) demonstrated that an increase in BF from preintervention to postintervention was associated with greater reductions in cortisol, a hormone produced in times of stress. Moreover, BF mediated the effect of CBSM on cortisol: Breast cancer patients in the CBSM condition had an increase in BF that in turn predicted reductions in cortisol. McGregor et al. (2004) found that increased BF from pre- to post-CBSM predicted change in lymphocyte proliferation from baseline to 3 months post-CBSM: Participants who found benefit demonstrated better immune function 3 months later.

Two groups of researchers assessed associations between BF and HIV disease progression. In a sample of gay and bisexual men with HIV, Bower et al. (1998) coded "discovery of meaning" in response to the death of a partner or close friend from interviews within a year of bereavement. They measured CD4 T lymphocytes, with low numbers indicating lower immunocompetence. In the 2 to 3 years following bereavement, participants' CD4 levels declined. However, those who found benefit in the loss had a slower rate of CD4 decline than those who did not. Moreover, the rate of AIDS-related mortality was lower for those who found benefit in the loss. The effect of BF on AIDS-related mortality appears to be mediated by the slower rate of CD4 decline for those who found benefit.

Similarly, Milam (2006b) examined CD4 counts and viral load (whereby high numbers indicate risk of disease progression) in people who were HIV-positive. BF at study entry did not directly predict these indicators 16 to 20 months later. However, Milam tested three variables as potential moderators of effects of BF on CD4 counts and viral load: pessimism, optimism, and ethnicity. As predicted, participants who were low in pessimism but high in BF at study entry had lower viral load at follow-up, compared with those low in pessimism and low in BF. In contrast, participants who were low in optimism but high in BF had higher CD4 counts at follow-up, compared with those who were low in optimism and low in BF. These findings were unanticipated; Milam suggested that, for those high in BF, having no future expectancy is better for one's health than being either pessimistic or optimistic about one's future. Finally, approximately 40% of the sample was of Hispanic ethnicity, which moderated the link between BF and CD4 counts. Hispanic participants who had reported high BF had higher CD4 counts than Hispanic participants with low BF; BF did not appear to matter for non-Hispanic participants.

A moderated relation was also obtained in a study of caregivers (Moskowitz & Epel, 2006). BF had no direct effect on neuroendocrine function (i.e., average diurnal cortisol and cortisol slope). However, specific aspects of BF (i.e., personal strength, life appreciation, and spiritual change) interacted with PA to predict cortisol slope, such that greater BF predicted a steeper slope for women who had higher PA during the 2 days of assessment. This effect held when NA was controlled.

Overall Summary

As found in the cross-sectional data, prospective tests of relations between BF and mental health outcomes yield mixed results. A handful of direct associations suggest that BF predicts better psychological adjustment (Bower et al., 2005; Carver & Antoni, 2004; Cheng et al., 2006; Schwarzer et al., 2006), with two complex associations suggesting that BF might contribute to worse adjustment for some people (Lechner et al., 2006, Study 2; Tomich & Helgeson, 2004).

Associations between BF and perceived or objective physical health or physiological markers are somewhat more consistent in suggesting that BF is good for people with chronic disease. However, the associations are not straightforward. The perceived health measures that were significantly predicted by BF were relevant to the disease at hand: daily pain and activity for individuals with RA, and cardiac health in heart attack patients. Effects for the RA samples had nuances: BF interacted with daily pain to predict activity limitation (Tennen et al., 1992) or the benefits were of a specific type (i.e., interpersonal; Danoff-Burg & Revenson, 2005). For objective measures, the results are more straightforward: Across three distinct chronic diseases, BF appears to be good for one's health. Although medical care use for cancer-related morbidities was unrelated to BF (Sears et al., 2003), BF predicted measures of neuroendocrine and immune function that are assumed to reflect better health (see Antoni, Lutgendorf, et al., 2006).

How Can Researchers Understand These Inconsistent Relations?

On the basis of current longitudinal research, we have the most confidence in the evidence showing that BF is good for the physical health or functioning of those with chronic disease. However, it is crucial to note that such evidence has resulted from just six investigations and that unpublished "file drawer" studies containing null effects might exist. The psychological outcomes were more difficult to ascertain. On the basis of our review, we offer three approaches that may help to explain inconsistencies in the evidence.

Back to Basics: Theoretical Rationale

Predicting adjustment from BF in chronic illness is a relatively new line of inquiry, and theories of BF and posttraumatic growth (PTG) provide limited guidance for what to expect as ensuing effects of BF. In fact, the prevailing theory essentially ends with the measurement of PTG or BF as an outcome of a process that is ongoing or has already occurred (Janoff-Bulman, 2004; Tedeschi & Calhoun, 2004). PTG theory allows for numerous hypotheses regarding factors that should contribute to growth (for reviews, see Helgeson et al., 2006; Linley & Joseph, 2004; Stanton et al., 2006), but hypotheses about the effects of growth (other than more growth) will require a theory that is more explicit. Moreover, it is not clear whether reports of BF are simply tapping into the result of a growth process. Many possibilities have been proposed (e.g., see Tennen & Affleck, 2002; Wortman, 2004), which include considering BF as a veridical report of growth, the outcome of a comparison with one's pre-illness self, or the result of a specific coping process, among other possibilities (see chap. 1, this volume). We know that some people find benefits relatively soon after a stressor (e.g., within 8 weeks; Affleck et al., 1987), and Manne et al. (2004) found that BF increased over time for women with breast cancer and their partners. However, what happens next? Certainly, PTG might be an important outcome in its own right, but its place among other indicators of adjustment deserves greater attention.

Despite the uncertainty about processes behind the reporting of BF, we believe it can be conceptualized as a construct in the positive psychological domain, similar to extraversion and positive emotion, among others. Research on PA might provide a good parallel to BF (Stanton & Low, 2004), given that both have opposing psychological systems (i.e., NA and finding detriment, respectively) that may operate alongside the positive. There is evidence from the psychological literature that people who report PA during chronic stress are better off in the long run than those who do not (e.g., see Fredrickson, Tugade, Waugh, & Larkin, 2003, on resilience after 9/11; Moskowitz, 2003, on AIDS-related mortality; Zautra, Johnson, & Davis, 2005, on pain in women with rheumatic disease). This finding is not trivial: It is not because people do not feel bad when they feel good. Rather, positive and negative feelings coexist; when the positive is present, it may serve as a buffer against the downward spiral of negativity that can accompany a chronic stressor (Fredrickson et al., 2003; Moskowitz, 2003). Research on PA may provide a productive theoretical frame from which to work when testing hypotheses about the role of BF in future psychological adjustment.

In addition, the research has demonstrated relatively more consistent findings for relations between BF and physical health than between BF and psychological health. However, there has been no guiding theoretical framework to explain these effects (see chap. 9, this volume). Bower and Segerstrom (2004) suggested that one way to account for links between BF and physiological change might be through evaluating the distinct benefits found. Social support, engagement with intrinsic life goals, PA, and cognitive change—all specific domains of benefit cited by individuals with chronic illness—are each linked to physiological change. Bower and Segerstrom suggested that these positive psychological pathways may influence physiology independent of distress pathways. This view is echoed in a recent review of evidence for the effects of PA on physical health. Pressman and Cohen (2005) presented a theoretical model of the stress-buffering effects of PA on health that might be used to test pathways from BF to health, using PA either as a mediator or as a similar process. They suggested a number of direct pathways by which PA might influence health outcomes. However, they also suggested that PA helps to speed recovery from stress-related activation, through its influence on autonomic nervous system and hypothalamic-pituitary-adrenal axis activation. It also has a positive effect on health practices. Perhaps BF plays a similar role, diminishing activation or motivating positive health behaviors. Indeed, individuals with chronic disease often spontaneously cite attention to health or health behavior change as a positive outcome of their experience with chronic disease (Cheng et al., 2006; Petrie, Buick, Weinman, & Booth, 1999; Sears et al., 2003), a benefit not included in traditional BF categorization schemes (Tedeschi & Calhoun, 1996).

Moderator Hypothesis

Another reason for inconsistent relations between BF and adjustment, particularly given numerous nonsignificant results, may be that important moderating variables exist; whether BF is good for people with chronic disease might depend on other factors. Stanton et al. (2007) recently summarized research from five domains of constructs that influence adjustment to chronic illness: dispositional factors, cognitive appraisals, coping processes, social resources, and macro-level contextual factors (e.g., socioeconomic status). Such constructs provide a good starting point to find theoretically relevant moderators of the BF–adjustment relation.

Two studies produced effects of BF on adjustment that were dependent on dispositional variables, demonstrating the complexity of the associations between BF and adjustment. Similar to a previous finding involving dispositional hope (Stanton, Danoff-Burg, & Huggins, 2002), Rini et al. (2004) demonstrated that BF was moderated by optimism in maternal caregivers, whereby highly optimistic mothers who found benefit reported better mental health 6 months later than those with low optimism and high BF. However, Milam (2006b) found that people with no expectations about the future (i.e., low pessimism or low optimism) who also found benefit in their experience with HIV had better physical health outcomes than those who held optimistic or pessimistic expectations about the future.

Stanton, Danoff-Burg, and Huggins (2002; Stanton & Low, 2004) have suggested that whether BF predicts psychological adjustment may depend on differences in the motivational function of BF for people with different personal attributes. Specifically, perhaps for those who are low in personal resources, BF represents avoidant motivations, whereas for those who are high in personal resources (e.g., hope, optimism), BF represents approach-oriented motives. Findings of Rini et al. (2004) and Stanton, Danoff-Burg, and Huggins (2002) are consistent with this suggestion. In addition, people who reported only benefit from their experience with SARS had higher reports of defensive motivation (i.e., high social desirability) compared with those who had a more balanced assessment of benefits and costs (Cheng et al., 2006). In contrast is Milam's (2006b) evidence for health advantages in individuals who were low in future expectations, including optimism. We believe that these findings highlight the need to consider the disease context. That is, in contrast to early-stage breast cancer, HIV is a disease that will likely lead to an eventual decline in health (Milam, 2006a). In that context, having relatively low expectations about the future but being able to find some positive aspects to one's current experience might bode well for adjustment. Of course, a number of other differences among the studies (e.g., time since diagnosis) may account for these distinct effects of personality.

An example of a macro-level contextual moderator is ethnicity. In Milam's study (2006b), Hispanic participants high in BF had higher CD4 counts than low-BF Hispanic participants. Milam found that this effect was reduced to marginal significance when the two religion-related BF items were removed, suggesting that the finding might be attributed to the higher likelihood among Hispanics of turning to religion. This was one of the only ethnically heterogeneous samples we reviewed, and although others controlled for race/ethnicity (Bower et al., 2005; Tomich & Helgeson, 2004), no other researcher has tested this factor as a moderator in a longitudinal design. Indeed, ethnic minority women with breast cancer (particularly African American and Hispanic women) may be more likely to derive benefits from the experience than Caucasian women (see review in Stanton et al., 2006). The Helgeson et al. (2006) meta-analysis of BF across a variety of stressors demonstrated that the proportion of non-Caucasian participants in the sample moderated cross-sectional associations between BF and adjustment. On the basis of these findings, we encourage researchers to examine ethnic status in future studies, but even more important, to explore pathways through which ethnicity might influence BF-adjustment relations.

Methodological Issues

Finally, our review highlighted a number of methodological issues related to measurement, timing of assessments, and testing hypotheses in context, all of which may influence the associations between BF and adjustment outcomes.

BENEFIT-FINDING MEASURE. What it means to report having found benefits in the midst of chronic disease remains unclear. Helgeson et al. (2006) concluded that researchers found stronger cross-sectional associations between BF and adjustment when they used, instead of researcher-created or interview-based reports, well-established measures of BF, including the Posttraumatic Growth Inventory (PTGI; Tedeschi & Calhoun, 1996) and the Benefit-Finding Scale (BFS; Tomich & Helgeson, 2004, adapted from Behr, Murphy, & Summers, 1991), which were used in seven studies in this review. Stanton et al. (2006) reported that the PTGI is highly correlated with the BFS and discovery of meaning (Bower et al., 2005), suggesting that they are tapping similar constructs. However, given the variety of BF measures across the relatively few studies reviewed, it is not clear whether the inconsistent findings should be attributed to the measure used.

ADJUSTMENT MEASURE. Measures of adjustment in these studies were diverse. If there had been consistent evidence regarding BF-adjustment relations, such variety would be a positive feature of the findings. Given the inconsistencies, this variety makes interpretation difficult. For the purpose of this review, we designated constructs as tapping either negative or positive outcomes. However, many measures contain items that reflect both negative and positive functioning. For example, depressive symptoms assessed by the CES-D are characterized by high negative cognition and affect, and low PA. Bower et al. (2005) found that BF predicted the PA component, but not the NA component, of the CES-D. Moreover, Moskowitz (2003) called PA from the CES-D the "active ingredient" in predicting AIDS-related mortality in a sample of HIV-positive men, after controlling for the other components. Such findings make it difficult to interpret the results of the scale as a whole: Is BF influencing the negative cognitive component, the NA component, or the PA component of the CES-D?

A related measurement issue that may contribute to the apparently inconsistent findings is easily demonstrated with measures of negative feelings. Although most measures covered a range of NA terms, not all of them included the same emotion domains. This is important because specific emotions have distinct antecedents and consequences, essentially serving different functions (e.g., see Keltner & Gross, 1999). Given the inconsistent findings, it would be worthwhile to take a closer look at how these differences might play a role. For instance, the study that demonstrated direct effects of BF on depressive symptoms (Carver & Antoni, 2004) was also one of the only studies to demonstrate links between BF and NA. The NA measure had a range of NA words related to anxiety, anger, and depressive affect (Derogatis, 1975). Were the two findings driven by the depressive affect content in both measures? Danoff-Burg and Revenson's (2005) distress measure excluded the items that overlap with depressive symptoms, whereas Bower et al.'s (2005) measure of NA included the depressive affect items from the CES-D. We do not suggest that these are inappropriate measures of NA, rather, that the variety may contribute to the difficulty of interpretation regarding patterns of associations between BF and affect. We urge researchers to consider the function of emotion in future research.

Research on indicators of positive adjustment as outcomes is insufficient to identify similar measurement issues. However, Pressman and Cohen (2005) were careful to note interpretational concerns with PA constructs in their review of links between PA and health, such as overlap between cognitive and affective components.

Finally, Park (2004) suggested that BF may be better related to outcome measures that are more closely tied to the event; this appeared to be the case in the studies we reviewed. For the most part, the self-report physical health measures were better predicted by BF when the outcomes were specific to the disease (e.g., pain and limited activity for RA patients).

TIMING OF ASSESSMENTS. Despite the limited number of studies producing significant results, our review suggests that timing of the BF measure and the adjustment measure might influence findings. We use the breast cancer studies as examples, although disease context is also relevant to this discussion. The meta-analysis by Helgeson et al. (2006) of cross-sectional findings showed that there were stronger links between BF and adjustment measures when there were 2 or more years since the stressor. However, all but one study of women with breast cancer included in the present review measured BF within a year of diagnosis. The year following a cancer diagnosis is typically the most disruptive (e.g., see Andersen, Anderson, & deProsse, 1989), which suggests that the BF measures for women in the breast cancer samples were taken at a theoretically interesting point: in the midst of their greatest distress and at a time when finding benefit is less likely to be concurrently related to adjustment. Are people who are able to find benefit at this point better off down the road than those who do not conclude that there are benefits until later? Does this effect vary across disease contexts? For example, timing of the BF measure might be the most theoretically interesting, in terms of prediction of adjustment, within the first year for breast cancer patients. However, for someone with RA who deals with regular pain for years, perhaps timing of the BF measure is less important (see chap. 1, this volume, for more discussion of disease contexts).

It is notable that, in the breast cancer samples, the evidence for positive effects from BF came from studies (Bower et al., 2005; Carver & Antoni, 2004) in which the adjustment variable was measured more than 1 year after the BF measure and disease diagnosis. The Tomich and Helgeson (2004) evidence that BF might be bad for some people, however, was found with outcome measures assessed within 9 months of study entry and just more than a year after diagnosis. To the extent that significant disruption of life and worldviews are required to catalyze BF (Janoff-Bulman, 1992; Tedeschi & Calhoun, 2004), measures of BF and adjustment taken in close proximity in the midst of a stressor may not demonstrate positive consequences of BF. It is possible that the positive effects of BF within stressful periods will not be apparent until after sufficient time has passed for the person to come to some resolution of the event.

Implications for Intervention

The purpose of this chapter is not to imply that individuals should necessarily find benefit from their experience with chronic disease. The evidence for the positive effects of BF is inconsistent, and it is not clear what factors were involved in the studies suggesting that BF is beneficial. However, some studies suggest techniques by which BF might contribute to mental and physical health in chronic disease, and these techniques merit consideration.

The CBSM intervention study (Antoni et al., 2001) tested hypotheses about the role of BF in adjustment (Cruess et al., 2000; Lechner et al., 2006, Study 2; McGregor et al., 2004). Although the intervention involved multiple components, making it difficult to isolate mechanisms, it did increase BF in women with breast cancer (Antoni et al., 2001; see also Antoni, Lechner, et al., 2006). Penedo et al. (2006) also found that CBSM increased BF in men with prostate cancer, mediated by the development of stress management skills.

Other work explicitly manipulated participants' consideration of illness-related benefits, again demonstrating relevance to physical health. Stanton, Danoff-Burg, Sworowski, et al. (2002) found that women who were randomly assigned to write about benefits of their breast cancer experience over four sessions reported fewer cancer-related medical visits and physical symptoms 3 months later than did participants in a fact-writing control condition. The BF condition produced slightly weaker results than did a condition in which participants wrote about their deepest thoughts and feelings regarding the cancer experience, suggesting that there may be different mechanisms to consider (Creswell et al., 2007; Low, Stanton, & Danoff-Burg, 2006). A similar BF manipulation in people with RA influenced fatigue and pain, but not psychological adjustment (Danoff-Burg, Agee, Romanoff, Kremer, & Strosberg, 2006). Both trials also found some moderated effects on outcomes. More research is needed to identify the mechanisms underlying effects of BF on outcomes, as well as the moderators of experimentally induced BF effects.

One promising study suggests a link between a gratitude intervention and positive adjustment (Emmons & McCullough, 2001, Study 3). Participants with neuromuscular diseases (NMDs) were randomly assigned to report things they were grateful for on each of 21 days, or to simply fill out the daily questionnaires during this period. After the intervention, the participant's spouse or significant other completed adjustment measures, answering as if he or she were the participant. Observer reports were higher for PA and life satisfaction, but not NA, in the gratitude condition compared with the control participants. Although the intervention did not focus participants on finding benefits specific to NMD, increased appreciation for life is a commonly reported domain of growth (e.g., see Tedeschi & Calhoun, 1996), so the findings are relevant. Observer reports suggest one method by which researchers might verify the effects of BF on adjustment.

Future Directions

The door is open for future research to address the question of whether and how BF is good for individuals with chronic disease. We have already suggested factors that might be considered to account for inconsistencies in current evidence. However, we also offer a number of suggestions for future study design that could clarify the role of BF in contributing to future adjustment and demonstrate the magnitude of the effects for individuals with chronic disease.

Longitudinal and Experimental Studies

It is clear from this chapter that we think the most compelling answers to the question of whether BF is good for individuals with chronic disease will come from studies with longitudinal designs in which adjustment is measured at some point after initial reports of BF. Experimental designs such as the interventions described earlier will also help to reveal the causal role of BF in adjustment and to isolate mechanisms responsible for the effects.

Behavioral Mediators

There are a number of ways in which BF might influence how individuals with chronic disease interact with the world. In turn, these behaviors may help to account for effects of BF on mental and physical health. Improvement of health behaviors is one potential mediator, but there are others. For example, BF (particularly, renewed appreciation for life) might contribute to prosocial behavior (e.g., see Emmons & McCullough, 2001); recent evidence is converging to demonstrate the potential salubrious effects of providing help to others (e.g., see Brown, Nesse, Vinokur, & Smith, 2003). In addition, BF may contribute to the quantity and quality of one's social interactions (e.g., see Danoff-Burg & Revenson, 2005) and social support is linked with health benefits (e.g., see House, Landis, & Umberson, 1988). These behaviors may demonstrate the concrete ways in which BF influences health and well-being, and may help to shift the evidence away from reliance on self-report measures.

Moderating Variables

Our review and others (e.g., see Helgeson et al., 2006; Stanton et al., 2006) have uncovered a number of moderating variables that will be worth consideration in future studies. Of note from the studies reviewed in this chapter are ethnicity (Milam, 2006b), personality factors (Milam, 2006b; Rini et al., 2004), and disease severity (Tomich & Helgeson, 2004). To advance this line of inquiry, we urge researchers to consider why a particular variable should play a moderating role in the effects of BF on adjustment in the context of chronic disease. Doing so will help to form a comprehensive understanding of the conditions under which BF might be good for individuals with chronic disease.

Outcome Measures: Inclusion of Physical Health and Positive Adjustment

Finally, we were surprised by the relative consistency of the findings, albeit from a handful of investigations, suggesting links between BF and physical health or physiological markers that may relate to health outcomes. These outcomes may be a fruitful line of inquiry for researchers who wish to demonstrate the impact of BF on individuals with chronic disease. Equally important will be to examine the mechanisms through which BF affects physical health.

We believe that the message is out about the importance of considering positive as well as negative psychological outcomes in chronic disease (e.g., see Stanton et al., 2007). However, more work is needed. The range of positive outcomes measured is limited, with PA being the primary outcome; it will be important for researchers to consider the ways in which hypotheses may be different for effects of BF on negative and positive indicators of adjustment.

Conclusion

The recent performance of prospective tests of the effects of BF on mental and physical health is a promising step toward determining whether BF is good for individuals with chronic disease. Although there were few reported negative effects of BF for these individuals, the positive effects were not consistent. This line of inquiry appears open to theoretical advancement; the question of whether BF is good for individuals with chronic disease should be modified to ask instead under what conditions BF might be beneficial. We have suggested a number of methodological considerations that might provide insight into this process. Although the variety of disease contexts and measurement approaches makes it difficult to interpret the evidence, it also signals the increasingly broad empirical and theoretical interest in the meaning of positive psychological processes in the midst of distress. We look forward to future empirical tests that will elucidate the role of finding benefit in living well with chronic disease.

References

Affleck, G., Tennen, H., Croog, S., & Levine, S. (1987). Causal attribution, perceived benefits, and morbidity after a heart attack: An 8-year study. *Journal of Consulting and Clinical Psychology, 55,* 29–35.

Andersen, B. L., Anderson, B., & deProsse, C. (1989). Controlled prospective longitudinal study of women with breast cancer: II. Psychological outcomes. *Journal of Consulting and Clinical Psychology, 57,* 692–697.

Andrews, F. M., & Withey, S. B. (1976). *Social indicators of well-being: Americans' perceptions of life quality.* New York: Plenum Press.

Antoni, M. H., Lechner, S. C., Kazi, A., Wimberly, S. R., Sifre, T., Urcuyo, K. R., et al. (2006). How stress management improves quality of life after treatment for breast cancer. *Journal of Consulting and Clinical Psychology, 74,* 1143–1152.

Antoni, M. H., Lehman, J. M., Kilbourn, K. M., Boyers, A. E., Culver, J. L., Alferi, S. M., et al. (2001). Cognitive–behavioral stress management intervention decreases the prevalence of depression and enhances benefit finding among women under treatment for early-stage breast cancer. *Health Psychology, 20,* 20–32.

Antoni, M. H., Lutgendorf, S. K., Cole, S. W., Dhabhar, F. S., Sephton, S. E., McDonald, P. G., et al. (2006). The influence of bio-behavioural factors on tumor biology: Pathways and mechanisms. *Nature Reviews Cancer, 6,* 240–248.

Behr, S. K., Murphy, D. L., & Summers, J. A. (1991). *Kansas Inventory of Parental Perceptions.* Lawrence: University of Kansas.

Bower, J. E., Kemeny, M. E., Taylor, S. E., & Fahey, J. L. (1998). Cognitive processing, discovery of meaning, CD4 decline, and AIDS-related mortality among bereaved HIV-seropositive men. *Journal of Consulting and Clinical Psychology, 66,* 979–986.

Bower, J. E., Meyerowitz, B. E., Desmond, K. A., Bernaards, C. A., Rowland, J. H., & Ganz, P. A. (2005). Perceptions of positive meaning and vulnerability following breast cancer: Predictors and outcomes among long-term breast cancer survivors. *Annals of Behavioral Medicine, 29,* 236–245.

Bower, J. E., & Segerstrom, S. C. (2004). Stress management, finding benefit, and immune function: Positive mechanisms for intervention effects on physiology. *Journal of Psychosomatic Research, 56,* 9–11.

Brown, S. L., Nesse, R. M., Vinokur, A. D., & Smith, D. M. (2003). Providing social support may be more beneficial than receiving it: Results from a prospective study of mortality. *Psychological Science, 14,* 320–327.

Carver, C. S., & Antoni, M. H. (2004). Finding benefit in breast cancer during the year after diagnosis predicts better adjustment 5 to 8 years after diagnosis. *Health Psychology, 23,* 595–598.

Carver, C. S., Scheier, M. F., & Weintraub, J. K. (1989). Assessing coping strategies: A theoretically-based approach. *Journal of Personality and Social Psychology, 56,* 267–283.

Centers for Disease Control and Prevention, National Center for Chronic Disease Prevention and Health Promotion. (2005). *Chronic disease overview.* Retrieved September 5, 2006, from http://www.cdc.gov/nccdphp/overview.htm

Cheng, C., Wong, W., & Tsang, K. W. (2006). Perception of benefits and costs during SARS outbreak: An 18-month prospective study. *Journal of Consulting and Clinical Psychology, 74,* 870–879.

Creswell, J. D., Lam, S., Stanton, A. L., Taylor, S. E., Bower, J. E., & Sherman, D. K. (2007). Does self-affirmation, cognitive processing, or discovery of meaning explain cancer-related health benefits of expressive writing? *Personality and Social Psychology Bulletin, 33,* 238–250.

Cruess, D. G., Antoni, M. H., McGregor, B. A., Kilbourn, K. M., Boyers, A. E., Alferi, S. M., et al. (2000). Cognitive–behavioral stress management reduces serum cortisol by enhancing benefit finding among women being treated for early stage breast cancer. *Psychosomatic Medicine, 62,* 304–308.

Danoff-Burg, S., Agee, J. D., Romanoff, N. R., Kremer, J. M., & Strosberg, J. M. (2006). Benefit finding and expressive writing in adults with lupus or rheumatoid arthritis. *Psychology and Health, 21,* 651–665.

Danoff-Burg, S., & Revenson, T. A. (2005). Benefit-finding among patients with rheumatoid arthritis: Positive effects on interpersonal relationships. *Journal of Behavioral Medicine, 28,* 91–103.

Derogatis, L. R. (1975). *The Affects Balance Scale.* Baltimore: Clinical Psychometric Research.

Emmons, R. A., & McCullough, M. E. (2001). Counting blessings versus burdens: An experimental investigation of gratitude and subjective well-being in daily life. *Journal of Personality and Social Psychology, 84,* 377–389.

Folkman, S., & Lazarus, R. S. (1985). If it changes it must be a process: Study of emotion and coping during three stages of college examination. *Journal of Personality and Social Psychology, 48,* 150–170.

Fredrickson, B. L., Tugade, M. M., Waugh, C. E., & Larkin, G. R. (2003). What good are positive emotions in crises? A prospective study of resilience and emotions following the terrorist attacks on the United States on September 11th, 2001. *Journal of Personality and Social Psychology, 84,* 365–376.

Helgeson, V. S., Reynolds, K. A., & Tomich, P. L. (2006). A meta-analytic review of benefit finding and growth. *Journal of Consulting and Clinical Psychology, 74,* 797–816.

House, J. S., Landis, K. R., & Umberson, D. (1988, July 29). Social relationships and health. *Science, 241,* 540–545.

Janoff-Bulman, R. (1992). *Shattered assumptions: Towards a new psychology of trauma.* New York: Free Press.

Janoff-Bulman, R. (2004). Posttraumatic growth: Three explanatory models. *Psychological Inquiry, 15,* 30–34.

Keltner, D., & Gross, J. J. (1999). Functional accounts of emotions. *Cognition and Emotion, 13,* 467–480.

Lechner, S., Carver, C. S., Antoni, M. H., Weaver, K. E., & Phillips, K. M. (2006). Curvilinear associations between benefit finding and psychosocial adjustment to breast cancer. *Journal of Consulting and Clinical Psychology, 74,* 828–840.

Linley, P. A., & Joseph, S. (2004). Positive change following trauma and adversity: A review. *Journal of Traumatic Stress, 17,* 11–21.

Low, C. A., Stanton, A. L., & Danoff-Burg, S. (2006). Expressive disclosure and benefit finding among breast cancer patients: Mechanisms for positive health effects. *Health Psychology, 25,* 181–189.

Manne, S., Ostroff, J., Winkel, G., Goldstein, L., Fox, K., & Grana, G. (2004). Posttraumatic growth after breast cancer: Patient, partner, and couple perspectives. *Psychosomatic Medicine, 66,* 442–454.

McGregor, B. A., Antoni, M. H., Boyers, A., Alferi, S. M., Blomberg, B. B., & Carver, C. S. (2004). Cognitive–behavioral stress management increases benefit finding and immune function among women with early-stage breast cancer. *Journal of Psychosomatic Research, 56,* 1–8.

McNair, D. M., Lorr, M., & Droppelman, L. F. (1971). *EITS manual for the Profile of Mood States.* San Diego, CA: Educational and Industrial Testing Service.

Milam, J. (2006a). Positive changes attributed to the challenge of HIV/AIDS. In L. G. Calhoun & R. G. Tedeschi (Eds.), *Handbook of posttraumatic growth: Research and practice* (pp. 214–224). Mahwah, NJ: Erlbaum.

Milam, J. (2006b). Posttraumatic growth and HIV disease progression. *Journal of Consulting and Clinical Psychology, 74,* 817–827.

Moskowitz, J. T. (2003). Positive affect predicts lower risk of AIDS mortality. *Psychosomatic Medicine, 65,* 620–626.

Moskowitz, J. T., & Epel, E. S. (2006). Benefit finding and diurnal cortisol slope in maternal caregivers: A moderating role for positive emotion. *Journal of Positive Psychology, 1,* 83–91.

Park, C. L. (2004). The notion of growth following stressful life experiences: Problems and prospects. *Psychological Inquiry, 15,* 69–76.

Penedo, F. J., Molton, I., Dahn, J. R., Shen, B., Kinsinger, D., Traeger, L., et al. (2006). A randomized clinical trial of group-based cognitive–behavioral stress management in localized prostate cancer: Development of stress management skills improves quality of life and benefit finding. *Annals of Behavioral Medicine, 31,* 261–270.

Petrie, K. J., Buick, D. L., Weinman, J., & Booth, R. J. (1999). Positive effects of illness reported by myocardial infarction and breast cancer patients. *Journal of Psychosomatic Research, 47,* 537–543.

Pressman, S. D., & Cohen, S. (2005). Does positive affect influence health? *Psychological Bulletin, 131,* 925–971.

Radloff, L. S. (1977). The CES-D scale: A self-report depression scale for research in the general population. *Applied Psychological Measurement, 1,* 385–401.

Rini, C., Manne, S., DuHamel, K. N., Austin, J., Ostroff, J., Boulad, F., et al. (2004). Mothers' perceptions of benefit following pediatric stem cell transplantation: A longitudinal investigation of the roles of optimism, medical risk, and sociodemographic resources. *Annals of Behavioral Medicine, 28,* 132–141.

Schwarzer, R., Luszczynska, A., Boehmer, S., Taubert, S., & Knoll, N. (2006). Changes in finding benefit after cancer surgery and the prediction of well-being one year later. *Social Science & Medicine, 63,* 1614–1624.

Sears, S. R., Stanton, A. L., & Danoff-Burg, S. (2003). The Yellow Brick Road and the Emerald City: Benefit finding, positive reappraisal coping, and posttraumatic growth in women with early-stage breast cancer. *Health Psychology, 22,* 487–497.

Stanton, A. L., Bower, J. E., & Low, C. A. (2006). Posttraumatic growth after cancer. In L. G. Calhoun & R. G. Tedeschi (Eds.), *Handbook of posttraumatic growth: Research and practice* (pp. 138–175). Mahwah, NJ: Erlbaum.

Stanton, A. L., Danoff-Burg, S., & Huggins, M. E. (2002). The first year after breast cancer diagnosis: Hope and coping strategies as predictors of adjustment. *Psycho-Oncology, 11,* 93–102.

Stanton, A. L., Danoff-Burg, S., Sworowski, L. A., Collins, C. A., Branstetter, A. D., Rodriguez-Hanley, A., et al. (2002). Randomized, controlled trial of written emotional expression and benefit-finding in breast cancer patients. *Journal of Clinical Oncology, 20,* 4160–4168.

Stanton, A. L., & Low, C. A. (2004). Toward understanding posttraumatic growth: Commentary on Tedeschi and Calhoun. *Psychological Inquiry, 15,* 76–80.

Stanton, A. L., Revenson, T. A., & Tennen, H. (2007). Health psychology: Adjustment to chronic disease. *Annual Review of Psychology, 58,* 565–592.

Tedeschi, R. G., & Calhoun, L. G. (1996). The Posttraumatic Growth Inventory: Measuring the positive legacy of trauma. *Journal of Traumatic Stress, 9,* 455–471.

Tedeschi, R. G., & Calhoun, L. G., (2004). Posttraumatic growth: Conceptual foundations and empirical evidence. *Psychological Inquiry, 15,* 1–18.

Tennen, H., & Affleck, G. (2002). Benefit-finding and benefit-reminding. In C. R. Snyder (Ed.), *Handbook of positive psychology* (pp. 584–597). New York: Oxford University Press.

Tennen, H., Affleck, G., Urrows, S., Higgins, P., & Mendola, R. (1992). Perceiving control, construing benefits, and daily processes in rheumatoid arthritis. *Canadian Journal of Behavioral Science, 24,* 186–203.

Tomich, P. L., & Helgeson, V. S. (2004). Is finding something good in the bad always good? Benefit finding among women with breast cancer. *Health Psychology, 23,* 16–23.

Watson, D., Clark, L. A., & Tellegen, A. (1988). Development and validation of brief measures of positive and negative affect: The PANAS scales. *Journal of Personality and Social Psychology, 54,* 1063–1070.

Wortman, C. B. (2004). Posttraumatic growth: Progress and problems. *Psychological Inquiry, 15,* 81–90.

Zautra, A. J., Affleck, G. G., Tennen, H., Reich, J. W., & Davis, M. C. (2005). Dynamic approaches to emotions and stress in everyday life: Bolger and Zuckerman reloaded with positive as well as negative affects. *Journal of Personality, 73,* 1511–1538.

Zautra, A. J., Johnson, L., & Davis, M. C. (2005). Positive affect as a source of resilience for women in chronic pain. Applications of a dynamic affect model. *Journal of Consulting and Clinical Psychology, 73,* 212–220.

Part V

Clinical Applications

11

Enhancing Positive Adaptation: Example Intervention During Treatment for Breast Cancer

*Michael H. Antoni, Charles S. Carver,
and Suzanne C. Lechner*

Few studies have tested whether psychosocial interventions using cognitive behavioral techniques can facilitate benefit finding in persons with major medical diseases. In this chapter, we describe an intervention program that we have observed to modulate benefit finding in women undergoing treatment for early- to mid-stage breast cancer. The program is designed to better understand how women with breast cancer deal with the diagnosis and treatment of this life-threatening disease. It examines what they fear most and how their perceptions about the future (e.g., optimism) and their social resources (e.g., social support) facilitate their adaptation and protect them from extended periods of distress. In essence, we have sought to learn which intra- and interpersonal processes are most central to their ability to adapt successfully to this stressful period, and move on with their lives. These questions are central to the study of growth-related processes, such as benefit finding, in the context of adversity faced by many medical patients. By gaining insight into the nature of these processes, health psychologists can be better positioned to help these individuals to not only move on with their lives but also possibly grow in ways that they might otherwise not have experienced.

This chapter draws from our program of research to tell the story of how we approached the questions germane to many cancer patients: What are their experiences? What changes occur in their lives? Which processes govern this? Which resources matter most? Can patients learn techniques to help themselves optimize this period of their lives and beyond? We begin by reviewing the stressors and major concerns that women experience as they deal with diagnosis, surgery, and adjuvant therapy for breast cancer. These stressors set the stage for the development of benefit finding and other aspects of positive adaptation indexed with psychosocial and physiological indicators. We next review individual differences such as optimism, certain cognitive coping strategies, social support, and anxiety reduction, all of which serve as *resilience factors*—qualities that predict better adaptation and benefit finding during treatment. We then consider the role of stress physiology in adapting to illness. Although the research on stress physiology has not been conducted specifically in the context of cancer, the findings may be relevant to cancer.

Next, we describe a model for intervention that we developed for women with breast cancer, which combines anxiety and tension reduction techniques with emotional processing, giving women the confidence to persist in meeting the challenges of their treatment and life beyond treatment. This group-based cognitive–behavioral intervention is designed to enhance resiliency and to increase the likelihood and duration of positive adaptation in women with breast cancer. The design and results of two trial interventions are described, and then the chapter concludes with lessons learned and a discussion of directions for future research.

Stressors and Concerns That Women Experience While Dealing With Breast Cancer

Each year over 200,000 women are diagnosed with breast cancer in the United States (American Cancer Society, 2003). These individuals suddenly leave a healthy world to become patients and to come to terms with a major life crisis. Many questions immediately arise: How bad is it? What are my options? What will be the side effects of the treatments? Will I ever be the same again, or will I be just a part of the woman I am now? Will my partner still view me as the same woman? Will I live to see my kids grow up? We have gained a good deal of insight into the major concerns that these women harbor as they deal with breast cancer and its treatment (Spencer et al., 1999). We learned that many fear an early death through disease recurrence and also fear that this might mean that they will not be able to see their children grow up. Many fear that adjuvant therapies, such as chemotherapy, will degrade or destroy their bodies such that they will never be quite the same. In the face of such adversity and experiences that are life changing and life threatening, how is it that so many women are able to return to their pre-morbid lives as mothers, wives, and workers? Just how do these women with breast cancer, in particular, adapt to what for many is the most stressful period in their lives? These questions were a major starting point for some of our most exciting research.

Resilience Factors

Our work in the area of breast cancer and adaptation began in the late 1980s, led by Charles Carver. We interviewed women shortly after they received a diagnosis of breast cancer and collected information regarding their outlook on life, the ways in which they coped with their diagnosis and treatment, and their distress levels. After these initial interviews, women underwent surgery and were followed through the subsequent months to track changes in their distress levels. We examined whether optimism, certain coping strategies, and social support predicted better adaptation during treatment. We also reviewed studies on whether anxiety reduction helps people better adapt to stress, and we considered whether these studies could be applied to women with breast cancer.

Optimism

We reasoned that having a positive outlook toward the future might induce women to accept aspects of their condition and be able to reframe the most difficult of those in a positive light (i.e., positive reframing). These coping strategies might facilitate dealing with the demands of surgery and adjuvant therapy. This in turn could lead to better adaptation, as reflected by lower negative affect and fewer social and interpersonal disruptions. People who can be flexible in the ways they interpret stressful circumstances might also be less prone to depressive thoughts and negative mood and might remain engaged in the social and interpersonal activities from which they draw pleasure and fulfillment. Thus, affect regulation and interpersonal engagement were hypothesized to follow from the use of certain coping strategies. We learned that optimism did indeed relate to less distress over the period of adjuvant therapy and the months that followed (Carver et al., 1993). Women with an optimistic life view at the time of treatment for breast cancer were at lower risk for difficulties in adaptation than their more pessimistic counterparts. In fact, this initial optimistic view during the time of treatment predicted better quality of life up to 13 years later (Carver et al., 2005).

During this time, optimism appeared to relate to less use of maladaptive coping, such as denial and behavioral disengagement (i.e., giving up on goal pursuits), while promoting the use of more helpful strategies, such as acceptance and positive reframing (Carver et al., 1993). Less disengagement and greater use of positive reframing prospectively predicted lower levels of negative affect in the months after surgery and adjuvant treatment. Thus, the advantage that optimistic women had over pessimistic women was in part mediated by their coping strategies.

Benefit Finding

Another important change that the women reported during this period was finding benefits in the cancer experience (Urcuyo, Boyers, Carver, & Antoni, 2005). They expressed an enhanced sense of meaning, greater spirituality, and deepened interpersonal relationships. This experience has been referred to as benefit finding (Tomich & Helgesen, 2004). The development of benefit finding in these women appears not to be closely linked to distress levels (see chap. 3, this volume). It is of interest to note that the coping strategies that produced less negative affect in previous studies (e.g., positive reframing; Carver et al., 1993) were also related to greater benefit finding in this study (Urcuyo et al., 2005).

In our research, the emergence of benefit finding during active medical treatment for breast cancer predicted better quality of life and less distress several years after treatment was completed (Carver & Antoni, 2004), although not everyone has found the same effects (e.g., Tomich & Helgeson, 2004). These findings, taken together, suggest that women who maintain a more positive view of the future and perceive benefits in the cancer experience early in their treatment may be better off several years later. The accumulated evidence provides a strong rationale for examining further how such factors promote optimal psychosocial adaptation across the experience of cancer. In addition, it hints at the potential usefulness of psychosocial interventions that address cognitions (i.e., appraisals about ongoing events and future possibilities) and behaviors (i.e., coping strategies that involve active engagement).

Social Support

Social support has been shown to be important as women move through treatment for breast cancer. Greater social support from spouses and female family members predicted less distress during active treatment (Alferi, Carver, Antoni, Weiss, & Duran, 2001). However, there was also evidence that such support eroded over time, with greater distress postsurgery predicting a diminution of social support over the subsequent months. Thus, although social support provided short-term benefits, there may have been some inefficiencies in the ways this support was being delivered and received (see chap. 8, this volume). Prior work with breast cancer patients has revealed that certain persons may be better equipped to offer emotional versus instrumental supports and that inadequately delivered support could do more harm than good (Manne et al., 2004). It is plausible that a network member whose supportive efforts are not working well, or are not received with enthusiasm, may burn out prematurely and withdraw further support, even when the patient still needs it (Bolger, Foster, Vinokur, & Ng, 1996). It is also plausible that supportive persons remain plentiful, but that the recipient does not provide them with a clear signal of the need for support (e.g., because of a lack of assertiveness), resulting in a reduction of the supportive person's offers.

This set of observations suggests a few things about how social support processes might play out in facilitating adaptation during and after medical treatment. First, given that social support from female family members was related to less distress, it was plausible that psychosocial interventions delivered in a group of other women might be a useful and efficient format. Second, because social support processes could erode over time for a variety of reasons it seemed important to teach patients to more efficiently communicate their needs to members of their social networks. We reasoned that this could be done through assertiveness training and anger management. In sum, studies of social support suggest that psychosocial interventions conducted in group environments that teach improved communication skills could facilitate adaptation during breast cancer treatment.

Anxiety Reduction

Another aspect of our developmental work focused on the issue of anxiety reduction. We knew that persons dealing with a new diagnosis of breast cancer manifest anticipatory anxiety as they think about the future of their treatment (e.g., surgery, adjuvant chemotherapy, radiation) and disease course (Spencer et al., 1999). From prior research we had also learned that teaching relaxation techniques could allay anxiety and negative affect in the weeks after receiving a diagnosis of HIV infection (Antoni et al., 1991). We reasoned that women diagnosed with breast cancer and who were beginning treatment could benefit from learning physical means of inducing relaxation to manage anxiety. Whether teaching these women to reduce anxiety would be paralleled by changes in benefit finding was something that we also considered.

Stress Physiology

In considering how to incorporate the resilience factors mentioned earlier into an intervention strategy, we also considered the role of stress physiology in adapting to illness. We hypothesized that difficulties with psychosocial adaptation might parallel disruptions in stress physiology. This view was based on a growing body of work on relations between chronic stress, distress states, and dysregulation in neuroendocrine and immunological systems in the context of cancer (for a review, see Antoni, Lutgendorf, et al., 2006). This suggests the more provocative notion that fostering psychosocial adaptation may induce better physiologic adaptation in ways that might promote better health outcomes in persons treated for cancer. Perhaps skills and resources for adapting psychosocially to the cancer treatment experience coincide with more efficient physiological management of stressful experiences. If so, teaching stress management techniques could offer patients the skills and resources to facilitate optimal psychosocial and physiological adaptation in the midst of medical treatment. This might, in turn, accelerate recovery of premorbid functioning, leaving the women less vulnerable to factors that could promote disease progression over the long term. In terms of benefit finding, we were not aware of any studies showing that increases in benefit finding during psychosocial intervention parallel either psychological or physiological indicators of distress, and so investigated this question as an exploratory hypothesis.

It is interesting and provocative to consider whether psychosocial interventions can have physiological effects in women with breast cancer. Although some research has demonstrated that women with breast cancer who complete group-based expressive supportive therapy survive longer (for a review, see Spiegel, 2002), this finding has yet to be replicated. Nevertheless, if psychosocial interventions can indeed facilitate better health outcomes, it is plausible that they may do so by improving regulation of immunologic and neuroendocrine functioning during and after the stress of cancer treatment (Antoni, Lutgendorf, et al., 2006).

We view physiological adaptation during cancer treatment as a normalization of stress-disrupted neuroendocrine and immunologic functioning. Patients with breast cancer display changes in endocrine and immunologic functioning (Antoni, 2003a; Sephton & Spiegel, 2003). For instance, women with localized disease, as well as those with advanced disease, show elevations in resting cortisol levels (van der Pompe, Antoni, & Heijnen, 1996) and changes in cortisol response to challenge (van der Pompe et al., 2001) when compared with age-matched control participants. There is also evidence that cancer-related stress is associated with lower natural killer cell activity in women with Stages 2 and 3 disease who are under active medical treatment (Andersen et al., 1998).

A major reason to explore these aspects of physiological adaptation follows from studies relating stress hormones to psychological changes and to potentially important immune system parameters. Psychosocial stressors relate to the activation of the hypothalamic–pituitary–adrenal axis concurrent with distress responses. These responses are characterized by the release of glucocorticoid hormones (i.e., cortisol) that have immunosuppressive effects (Munck & Guyre, 1986). Accordingly, we have conceptualized changes in cortisol and cellular immune functioning as indicators of physiological adaptation in breast cancer patients as they move through treatment. Stress- or distress-related changes in cortisol and cellular immune functions may contribute to infectious disease (Herbert & Cohen, 1993). Whether these physiological changes affect mortality and morbidity after treatment for breast cancer remains controversial (Antoni, 2003a; Antoni, Lutgendorf, et al., 2006). Thus, an important aspect to consider is whether teaching women with breast cancer to better manage stressors in the period surrounding surgery and adjuvant treatment would enhance both psychosocial and physiological adaptation, promoting optimal quality of life and physical health over time.

Developing a Model for Psychosocial Intervention

The findings about optimism, coping strategies, social support, anxiety reduction, and stress physiology pointed to specific foci that might be implemented in a psychosocial intervention to facilitate the adaptation process during the period after diagnosis and initial treatment for breast cancer. Cognitive coping responses and positive reframing represent one such focus. We hypothesized that interventions that teach people to use coping strategies (e.g., positive reframing) and to maintain a more optimistic outlook might be related to less distress and more benefit finding following diagnosis and surgery. Teaching women skills such as assertiveness could enable them to request support when it is needed, and make clear to family and friends which of their actions are helpful and which are not. We also reasoned that anger management skills would help manage negative emotions in interpersonal relationships, thereby mitigating the tendency for social support to erode over time. In addition, we hypothesized that a supportive group should foster resistance to withdrawal from other sources of support and other aspects of normal life activities. Finally, we thought that teaching anxiety reduction techniques such as relaxation, mental imagery and deep breathing could help offset anticipatory anxiety during the course of adjuvant therapy.

We used this information to help create a model to guide the ways in which to focus a multimodal intervention, cognitive–behavioral stress management (CBSM), for women undergoing treatment for breast cancer (see Figure 11.1). Largely on the basis of the results of our observational studies of patients with breast cancer and our use of CBSM with other medical populations faced with the challenges of diagnosis and treatment (e.g., HIV infection; Antoni, 2003b; Antoni et al., 1991), we reasoned that a CBSM intervention could be used to modify many of the factors that we had previously shown to be associated with better psychosocial adaptation (e.g., decreased distress, increased benefit finding). Recall that some of these factors included maintaining an optimistic attitude, greater use of coping strategies (e.g., acceptance, positive reframing, less use of avoidance and denial as coping strategies), and efficient use of social sup-

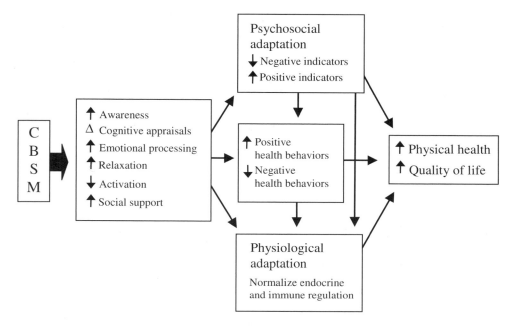

Figure 11.1. Theoretical model for cognitive–behavioral stress management (CBSM) intervention effects on psychosocial and physiological adaptation during treatment for breast cancer and putative effects on later quality of life and physical health. CBSM intervention targets are noted in the box on the far left side.

port networks. Hence, our CBSM intervention was designed to teach women techniques to (a) increase awareness of cognitive–affective processes; (b) change cognitive appraisals about stressors to be more rational and balanced; (c) increase time spent in emotional processing and cognitively restructuring their responses to stressors; (d) improve relaxation skills and other anxiety and tension reduction techniques, thereby decreasing physiological activation; and (e) increase the receipt of useful social support.

During the course of CBSM intervention, we also drew on observations of psychoneuroimmunological associations among person with HIV (for a review, see Antoni, 2003b). Those led us to hypothesize that, among women with breast cancer, improvements in psychosocial adaptation (e.g., decreased distress and anxiety, increased benefit finding) during CBSM might be accompanied by improvements in physiological adaptation, as indicated by endocrine and immunologic parameters. If altered cortisol and immunologic indicators—which, as noted, have been observed in breast cancer patients—are influenced by stress and anxiety, negative mood, coping, outlook, and social support, then a stress management intervention might help normalize cortisol and immune system regulation. It may do so by decreasing anxiety and negative affect (thereby possibly improving indicators of positive adaptation such as benefit finding) by teaching skills that enhance awareness, change appraisals, increase emotional processing, increase relaxation skill, and increase social support.

Finally, our model hypothesized that, along with improvements in health behaviors, improved psychosocial and physiological adaptation to breast cancer treatment could have positive implications for longer-term quality of life and physical health. As noted previously, we found that women who reported more benefit finding during initial treatment for breast cancer reported better quality of life up to 13 years later (Carver & Antoni, 2004). A fascinating question is whether similar processes might affect tumor growth processes that are possibly mediated by neuroendocrine and immunologic parameters (Antoni, Lutgendorf, et al., 2006).

Design and Results of the Intervention

Using the theoretical model outlined in Figure 11.1, we evaluated the effects of CBSM on indexes of negative and positive psychosocial adaptation among women who were recruited in the weeks after surgery for Stages 1 through 3 breast cancer. Early recruitment (i.e., prior to the start of adjuvant therapy) allowed us to minimize the influence of potential confounding variables and to evaluate the clinical utility of offering psychosocial intervention in the midst of the stressful period of medical treatment (Antoni, 2003c).

Our CBSM intervention uses closed, structured groups of 4 to 7 women with breast cancer and two female coleaders; groups meet weekly for ten 2-hour sessions (Antoni, 2003c). The CBSM techniques are taught with in-session experiential exercises and out-of-session assignments (e.g., practicing relaxation). Women receive recordings of one of their group leaders reciting relaxation exercises, which they are urged to use daily at work or at home. The intervention focuses on helping women to cope better with daily stressors and to optimize available social resources. We use group members and leaders as role models, encourage emotional expression, replace doubt appraisals with confidence about stress management skills (Beck & Emery, 1985), teach anxiety reduction skills using training in muscle relaxation and relaxing imagery (Bernstein & Borkovec, 1973), and provide conflict resolution skills through assertion training (Fensterheim & Baer, 1975) and anger management. Participants on average attend 7 or 8 sessions out of the 10 offered.

The intervention includes a therapist training manual and a participant workbook (Antoni, 2003c). For each of the trials we have conducted, interventionists were trained in the CBSM protocol over a 10-week period. All sessions were videotaped; treatment fidelity was ensured by two clinical psychologists who monitored the videotapes at multiple points during each cohort. Weekly group supervision meetings ensured that any deviations in intervention protocol were communicated to interventionists at the point at which they were detected.

First Trial of CBSM in Women Undergoing Treatment for Breast Cancer

We first tested a 10-week CBSM intervention that focused on women's needs during the postsurgery and adjuvant therapy period (Antoni et al., 2001). The initial assessment was 4 to 8 weeks after surgery, and the 10-week intervention began shortly after randomization to either this condition or a comparison condition that served as the control group. The comparison group received a 1-day stress management group seminar at roughly the time the 10-week intervention groups were ending. All participants were assessed prior to the intervention, at 3-months postintervention, and again at 6 and 12 months postsurgery.

PSYCHOLOGICAL OUTCOMES. Most of the women in the sample did not have clinically significant depression because of a stringent inclusion criterion that required them to have Hamilton Depression Inventory (Hamilton, 1959) scores of less than 15. However, CBSM decreased depressive symptoms in the subset of women who had elevated depression at study entry, based on Center for Epidemiologic Survey Depression (Radloff, 1977) scores of 16 or greater. Prevalence of moderate depressive symptoms was approximately 25% preintervention and decreased to 13% afterward. The intervention also enhanced reports of finding benefit in the cancer experience (Antoni et al., 2001). This elevation was maintained at the 6-month follow-up. We also found that the effects of CBSM on benefit finding were significantly larger in women who were lowest in optimism at study entry (Antoni et al., 2001). Reports of examining and expressing feelings were enhanced by the intervention and did not change in the control condition. However, these changes were not maintained in the long term. The intervention also caused a significant increase in optimism among those initially less optimistic compared with the control group. This variable had already proven to be a resilience factor for adjustment. Optimism is a stable personality trait (Scheier & Carver, 1992); this is the first time we are aware of in which a behavioral intervention improved optimism scores. It is important to note that benefit finding increases during the intervention were correlated most strongly with increases in emotional expression and examination. They were moderately associated with increases in optimism, and were independent of changes in depression (Antoni et al., 2001).

PHYSIOLOGICAL OUTCOMES. Using evening blood samples from a subset of participants in this study, we also examined associations among psychosocial, serum cortisol, and immune system variables. Immune measures were limited to those that were theorized to be relevant to the surveillance of breast cancer and possibly to the risk of recurrence or metastasis. These measures had been related in prior work to stress-related variables (e.g., stressors, distress, social support). Included were a set of measures that characterized cell-mediated immune functioning. One such measure was lymphocyte proliferation response (LPR) following stimulation of T-cell receptor with anti-CD3 antibody. At study entry, greater evening serum cortisol levels were related to lower LPR. It is of interest to note that greater LPR related to more total social support provisions, greater optimism, more use of positive reframing coping, and less use of behavioral disengagement coping. These results supported the notion that some of the psychosocial targets of our intervention (see Figure 11.1) are associated with individual differences in indicators of physiological adaptation.

We also found that CBSM participants had lower levels of serum cortisol after the intervention compared with control participants with equivalent baseline values (Cruess et al., 2000). Greater reductions in cortisol were also related to greater increases in benefit finding, but not to distress levels during the intervention. Path analyses suggested that the intervention's impact on cortisol change was mediated by change in benefit finding. This indicates that the intervention had an impact on an aspect of the body's stress response, and did so by creating a positive psychological change (i.e., increasing benefit finding). This is the first demonstration of such an effect in the context of CBSM intervention.

We also used blood samples from this subsample to investigate immunologic effects of the CBSM intervention by examining change from baseline to 3 months after intervention. We delayed the measurement of immune functioning to the 3-month follow-up because the women had by then completed rounds of chemotherapy or radiation therapy. This was done so that these treatments would be less able to distort immune assay results, although we acknowledge that their effects were likely still present to some unknown degree. Women who were assigned to the CBSM intervention showed greater LPR (McGregor et al., 2004). These findings held even after controlling for adjuvant therapy status at each time point. As in the case of CBSM-associated cortisol changes, women with the largest increases in benefit finding during the intervention showed the greatest lymphocyte responses 3 months later, an association that was not observed in control participants. This study provided preliminary support for our model specifying CBSM effects on both psychosocial and physiological adaptation after treatment for breast cancer (see Figure 11.1). Moreover, a normalization of physiological adaptation measures (i.e., decreased cortisol and increased LPR) was consistently associated with increases in benefit finding.

These analyses were limited by a small sample size, exclusion of women with clinically elevated levels of anxiety and depression, a limited number of indicators of positive adaptation, relatively short-term follow-up measures, and an inability to determine which aspect of this multimodal intervention was responsible for its effects.

Second Trial of Women Undergoing Treatment for Breast Cancer

Our second trial tested our model with a larger sample of women representing a wider range of distress who were followed over a longer period after the intervention with a larger array of psychosocial indicators of adaptation. We focus here on our observations of changes in benefit finding and some other indices reflecting positive adaptation. We also examined potential active ingredients of the intervention's psychological effects. To address this question, we created a set of items to assess participants' use of and comfort with the stress management skills in the intervention. The items, collectively called the Measure of Current Status (Carver, 2005), assess the ability to relax at will, recognize stressful situations, restructure maladaptive thoughts, be assertive in requesting support when needed, express anger effectively and appropriately, and choose appropriate coping responses. The items were framed to be appropriate to participants in both conditions.

This second intervention study collected baseline data on women 4 to 8 weeks postsurgery (Time 1) and followed them for 1 year, as did our first project.

Intervention effects from this study were tested by latent growth-curve model-ing (LGM; Muthén, 1997), a form of structural equation modeling. In LGM, a trajectory of change over repeated measurements is computed for each partici-pant (Llabre, Spitzer, Siegel, Saab, & Schneiderman, 2004). The properties of interest here are the intercept (i.e., the trajectory's starting value) and the slope of change over repeated measurements. The path from condition to slope reflects the extent to which change in the dependent variable over time relates to experimental condition.

PSYCHOSOCIAL OUTCOMES. Among the changes we observed in positive adap-tation indicators (Antoni, Kazi, et al., 2006), we found that women assigned to CBSM reported increases in benefit finding (Tomich & Helgeson, 2004), in perceived ability to attain positive states of mind (Horowitz, Adler, & Kegeles, 1988), in positive affect and emotional well-being on the Functional Assessment of Cancer Therapy (Cella et al., 1993), and in positive lifestyle changes. Decreases were found in interpersonal disruption as measured by the Sickness Impact Profile (Bergner, Bobbitt, Carter, & Gilson, 1981). Figure 11.2 shows a sample of CBSM effects on some of these indicators of positive psychosocial adaptation; these effects persisted through the final follow-up.

STRESS MANAGEMENT SKILLS. We next determined that CBSM participants compared with control participants had a greater increase in their confidence in being able to use relaxation skills to manage stress. This was the largest change that we observed among skill sets. We then tested mediation models, in which this difference between groups was examined as a mediator of the inter-vention's effects on benefit finding. Once the effect of relaxation confidence was taken into account, the effects of the intervention on benefit finding, as well as several other indicators of negative and positive adaptation, were no longer sig-nificant (Antoni, Kazi, et al., 2006). Subsequent analyses suggested that increases in emotional processing (i.e., emotional awareness and expression) during the intervention might also have acted to mediate the effects of CBSM on benefit finding (Antoni, Kazi, et al., 2006).

This pattern of results supports a model wherein CBSM-related increases in specific anxiety-reduction techniques such as relaxation, as well as increases in time spent processing emotions, may be the key active ingredients of CBSM's effects on benefit finding. We have yet to test whether other potentially impor-tant processes (e.g., changes in social support) could further explain the effects of CBSM on benefit finding in this population. We are also preparing to evalu-ate the effects of the intervention on indicators of physiological adaptation and to determine which processes explain such effects.

Lessons Learned

In our intervention work with patients with breast cancer, improvements in psychosocial adaptation, including increased reports of benefit finding, during CBSM appeared to depend in part on several factors. One is the acquisition of, or at least confidence about using, anxiety reduction skills, such as relaxation

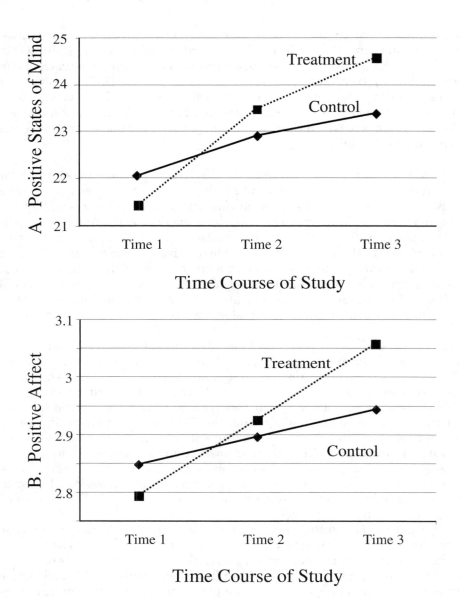

Figure 11.2. Comparison of slopes of change in indicators of positive adaptation among women undergoing medical treatment for breast cancer who were assigned to psychosocial treatment condition (i.e., cognitive–behavioral stress management) versus control condition. Time 1 = baseline measurement approximately 4 to 8 weeks postsurgery; Time 2 = 3 months postintervention; Time 3 = 9 months postintervention.

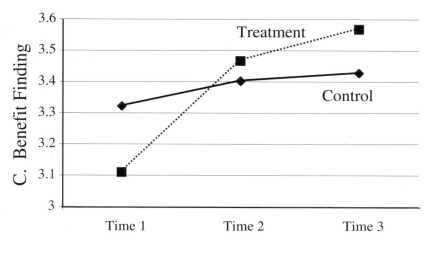

Time Course of Study

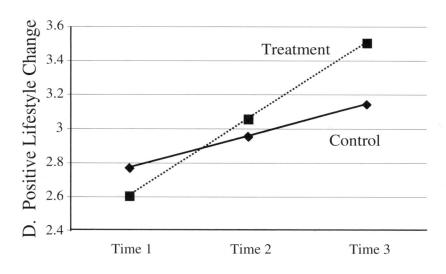

Time Course of Study

Figure 11.2.   (Continued)

and imagery. A second is increases in emotional processing. A third factor, yet to be tested, may be a receptive social network (i.e., the group setting). On the basis of these results, we offer three sets of processes that may be essential to psychosocial interventions seeking to improve indicators of adaptation in women with breast cancer (see Figure 11.3). These changes may occur in any order and may feed one another, contributing to their continued use and to the development of positive adaptation.

As has been described by others in other contexts (e.g., see Austenfeld & Stanton, 2004; see also chap. 10, this volume), individuals who remain open, aware, and expressive of their emotional experiences may be especially flexible about using coping strategies such as reframing and acceptance. Expressiveness may also make them more receptive to, and attractive to, sources of social support that can be used for emotional or instrumental purposes, provided that they are able to communicate clearly about their needs. Our prior work and that of others has suggested the importance of these cognitive and social processes during the breast cancer experience (e.g., see Alferi et al., 2001; Carver et al., 1993). Having adequate coping skills and social resources may help women process stressors more efficiently, resulting in less arousal and vigilance and a more positive attitude toward life (i.e., optimism) and their own abilities (i.e., self-efficacy). Bower, Epel, and Moskowitz (see chap. 9, this volume) noted that these processes were potentially important for facilitating benefit finding in cancer patients. These experiences may enhance a sense of increased benefit find-

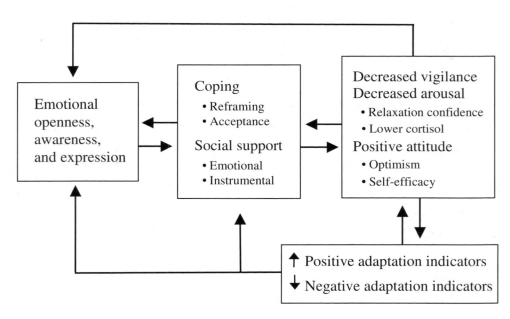

Figure 11.3. Model depicting how emotional expression, coping, social support, arousal, and attitudinal processes changing during psychosocial intervention may contribute to increases in positive adaptation indices (e.g., benefit finding) and decreases in negative adaptation indices (e.g., negative affect).

ing and other indicators of positive adaptation (e.g., positive states of mind, positive affect) and reduce negative adaptation (e.g., decreased negative affect). They may also increase the willingness to remain open to, aware of, and expressive of one's emotions, thereby strengthening the cyclical nature of these processes. The sense of having improved one's adaptation may itself feed back to any set of these processes depicted in Figure 11.3.

It may be that the most effective psychosocial interventions are those that are able to catalyze one or more of these processes singly or simultaneously. For example, emotional awareness and expression might be facilitated in a group setting in which stress appraisals are addressed in sessions, and homework focuses on identifying emotional reactions to daily challenges. This could set in motion a movement toward the facilitation of coping and social support changes. Alternatively, cognitive coping skills training might directly increase the use of positive reframing and acceptance and deter the use of avoidant strategies, whereas interpersonal skills training (i.e., anger management and assertiveness training) could improve communications to acquire resources from social networks. This training could teach women how to improve their coping economy, by learning to match emotional-focused strategies to uncontrollable elements of stressors, and problem-focused strategies to controllable elements (Folkman et al., 1991).

Interventions focused on anxiety reduction and arousal reduction skills, such as relaxation, imagery, deep breathing, and meditation, could provide individuals with a tangible stress reduction tool that they could use to decrease their vigilance in arousing situations. Use of such skills and their immediate effects on anxiety could have the secondary effect of enhancing the person's general (i.e., optimism) and self-specific (i.e., self-efficacy) outlook. These experiences could either feed back toward greater openness, awareness, and expression of emotions or feed forward to increases in positive adaptations such as benefit finding and positive affect.

This collection of skill sets learned in multimodal approaches such as CBSM might set the adaptation processes in motion indefinitely. More likely, however, these growth processes are self-limiting, and require either new challenging life events or psychosocial intervention booster sessions to reignite the growth process. The extent to which psychosocial intervention can catalyze physiological adaptation through a similar set of cascading processes is an empirical question, one that we are actively pursuing.

Future Directions

Our intervention trials provided evidence that group-based CBSM can produce substantial and durable improvements in diverse aspects of psychosocial adaptation, such as benefit finding in women undergoing treatment for early to midstage breast cancer. Effects emerged after 3 months and were sustained for 9 months after the intervention. Each effect appeared largely attributable to participants' confidence in having learned specific stress reduction techniques as well as their involvement in emotional processing. In contrast, there was no empirical support for the role of nonspecific factors arising from simply being in a supportive group with other women with breast cancer. Although it is impossible to totally rule out the role of group processes in this sort of design (i.e., in which both conditions were conducted in groups), these findings provide some support for the efficacy of an intervention that teaches specific stress management skills for use during and after the period of active medical treatment for breast cancer. In actuality, it is likely that group factors synergize with content-specific skills training to optimize the effects of the intervention.

The fact that we observed larger effects of this intervention in the second trial, which included more distressed women compared with the first, suggests the possibility that the intervention may have its greatest impact on women who are in greatest need. Future work should focus on the most distressed women, possibly sampling at a point in the breast cancer experience that is even more distressing (e.g., diagnosis, postadjuvant therapy during the reentry phase, recurrence). The fact that specific stress management skills and emotional processing may serve as the active ingredients of CBSM indicates that future research could dismantle the intervention and experimentally isolate and test these and other specific components to better understand causal pathways. Analyses of our CBSM effects in the second trial revealed that women who attended approximately half of the CBSM sessions seemed to fare nearly as well as those who attended all 10 sessions. Future work should therefore evaluate shorter versions of the interventions, possibly focusing on the development of those skills that were among its active ingredients. We are currently pursuing the answers to all of these questions to refine the ways one can intervene in the context of breast cancer to produce the greatest change in adaptation, over the longest period, using the shortest intervention format.

If the dismantling of intervention elements reveals the centrality of specific stress management techniques, this could suggest the importance of providing patients with a tangible, portable, and immediately applicable skill that they can use in a wide range of settings, including the physician's office, a social setting, or in the privacy of their home. It remains to be determined whether it is confidence in these skills, ability to perform them, or their actual use in daily life that is most important. Electronic daily diary studies that simultaneously measure use of stress management skills and objective measures of stress (e.g., salivary cortisol) would be informative. Another important next step is to follow each cohort of women over several years, to see whether intervention effects on psychosocial and physiological adaptation during active medical treatment predict longer-term quality of life effects and actual health benefits in breast cancer survivors. Recent work suggests that neuroendocrine substances such as cortisol may contribute to tumor growth processes directly or indirectly through changes in immune system parameters (Antoni, Lutgendorf, et al., 2006).

The studies in our program of research have yielded strong support for the efficacy of psychosocial intervention in effecting adaptation across many channels in women dealing with breast cancer. It would, however, be a mistake to assume that these effects can be generalized to all women confronted with this challenge. These samples were largely self-selected, middle class, educated, and Caucasian. It remains to be seen whether this form of intervention is equally effective in improving quality of life among minority women with breast cancer

(Wilmoth & Sanders, 2001). Determining whether this is so will require the use of culturally adapted versions of psychosocial intervention. This is a critical consideration for future work and one that should be implemented before moving these forms of intervention into clinical practice.

References

Alferi, S., Carver, C. S., Antoni, M. H., Weiss, S., & Duran, R. (2001). An exploratory study of social support, distress, and disruption among low income Hispanic women under treatment for early stage breast cancer. *Health Psychology, 20,* 33–41.

American Cancer Society. (2003). *Cancer statistics.* Available from http://www.cancer.org

Andersen, B. L., Farrar, W. B., Golden-Kreutz, D., Kutz, L. A., MacCallum, R., Courtney, M. E., & Glaser, R. (1998). Stress and immune responses after surgical treatment for regional breast cancer. *Journal of the National Cancer Institute, 90,* 30–36.

Antoni, M. H. (2003a). Psychoneuroendocrinology and psychoneuroimmunology of cancer: Plausible mechanisms worth pursuing? *Brain Behavior and Immunity, 17*(Suppl. 1), 84–91.

Antoni, M. H. (2003b). Stress management effects on psychological, endocrinological, and immune function in men with HIV: Empirical support for a psychoneuroimmunological model. *Stress, 6,* 173–188.

Antoni, M. H. (2003c). *Stress management intervention for women with breast cancer.* Washington, DC: American Psychological Association.

Antoni, M. H., Baggett, L., Ironson, G., August, S., LaPerriere, A., Klimas, N., et al. (1991). Cognitive–behavioral stress management intervention buffers distress responses and immunologic changes following notification of HIV-1 seropositivity. *Journal of Consulting and Clinical Psychology, 59,* 906–915.

Antoni, M. H., Kazi, A., Lechner, S., Wimberly, S., Gluck, S., & Carver, C. S. (2006). How stress management improves quality of life after treatment for breast cancer. *Journal of Consulting and Clinical Psychology, 74,* 1143–1152.

Antoni, M. H., Lehman, J., Kilbourn, K., Boyers, A., Yount, S., Culver, J., et al. (2001). Cognitive–behavioral stress management intervention decreases the prevalence of depression and enhances benefit finding among women under treatment for early-stage breast cancer. *Health Psychology, 20,* 20–32.

Antoni, M. H., Lutgendorf, S., Cole, S., Dhabhar, F., Sephton, S., McDonald, P., et al. (2006). The influence of biobehavioral factors on tumor biology, pathways, and mechanisms. *Nature Reviews Cancer, 6,* 240–248.

Austenfeld, J. L., & Stanton, A. L. (2004). Coping through emotional approach: A new look at emotion, coping, and health-related outcomes. *Journal of Personality, 72,* 1335–1363.

Beck, A. T., & Emery, G. (1985). *Anxiety disorders and phobias: A cognitive perspective.* New York: Basic Books.

Bergner, M., Bobbitt, R. A., Carter, W. B., & Gilson, B. S. (1981). The Sickness Impact Profile: Development and final revision of a health status measure. *Medical Care, 19,* 787–805.

Bernstein, B., & Borkovec, T. (1973). *Progressive muscle relaxation training: A manual for the helping professions.* Champaign, IL: Research Press.

Bolger, N., Foster, M., Vinokur, A., & Ng, R. (1996). Close relationships and adjustment to a life crisis: The case of breast cancer. *Journal of Personality and Social Psychology, 70,* 283–294.

Carver, C. S. (2005). *Measure of current status.* Unpublished instrument, University of Miami, Coral Gables, FL.

Carver, C. S., & Antoni, M. H. (2004). Finding benefit in breast cancer during the year after diagnosis predicts better adjustment 5 to 8 years after diagnosis. *Health Psychology, 26,* 595–598.

Carver, C. S., Pozo, C., Harris, S. D., Noriega, V., Scheier, M. F., Robinson, D. S., et al. (1993). How coping mediates the effect of optimism on distress: A study of women with early stage breast cancer. *Journal of Personality and Social Psychology, 65,* 375–390.

Carver, C. S., Smith, R. G., Antoni, M. H., Petronis, V. M., Weiss, S., & Derhagopian, R. P. (2005). Optimistic personality and psychosocial well-being during treatment predict psychosocial well-being among long-term survivors of breast cancer. *Health Psychology, 24,* 508–516.

Cella, D. F., Tulsky, D. S., Gray, G., Sarafian, E., Linn, A., Bonomi, M., et al. (1993). The Functional Assessment of Cancer Therapy scale: Development and validation of the general measure. *Journal of Clinical Oncology, 11,* 570–579.

Cruess, D. G., Antoni, M. H., McGregor, B. A., Boyers, A., Kumar, M., Kilbourn, K., & Carver, C. S. (2000). Cognitive–behavioral stress management reduces serum cortisol by enhancing benefit finding among women being treated for early stage breast cancer. *Psychosomatic Medicine, 62,* 304–308.

Fensterheim, H., & Baer, J. (1975). *Don't say yes when you want to say no.* New York: David McKay.

Folkman, S., Chesney, M., McKusick, L., Ironson, G., Johnson, D., & Coates, T. (1991). Translating coping theory into intervention. In J. Eckenrode (Ed.), *The social context of coping* (pp. 239–259). New York: Plenum Press.

Hamilton, M. (1959). The assessment of anxiety states by rating. *British Journal of Medical Psychology, 32,* 50–55.

Herbert, T. B., & Cohen, S. (1993). Stress and immunity in humans: A meta-analytic review. *Psychosomatic Medicine, 55,* 364–379.

Horowitz, M., Adler, N., & Kegeles, S. (1988). A scale for measuring the occurrence of positive states of mind: A preliminary report. *Psychosomatic Medicine, 50,* 477–483.

Llabre, M. M., Spitzer, S., Siegel, S., Saab, P. G., & Schneiderman, N. (2004). Applying latent growth curve modeling to the investigation of individual differences in cardiovascular recovery from stress. *Psychosomatic Medicine, 66,* 29–41.

Manne, S., Ostroff, J., Sherman, M., Heyman, R., Ross, S., & Fox, K. (2004). Couples' support-related communication, psychological distress, and relationship satisfaction among women with early stage breast cancer. *Journal of Consulting and Clinical Psychology, 72,* 660–670.

McGregor, B. A., Antoni, M. H., Boyers, A., Alferi, S. M., Blomberg, B. B., & Carver, C. S. (2004). Cognitive–behavioral stress management increases benefit finding and immune function among women with early-stage breast cancer. *Journal of Psychosomatic Research, 56,* 1–8.

Munck, A., & Guyre, P. M. (1986). Glucocorticoid physiology, pharmacology, and stress. *Advances in Experimental Medicine and Biology, 196,* 81–96.

Muthén, B. (1997). Latent variable modeling with longitudinal and multilevel data. In A. Raftery (Ed.), *Sociological methodology* (pp. 453–480). Boston: Blackwell.

Radloff, L. (1977). A self-report depression scale for research in the general population. *Applied Psychological Measurement, 1,* 385–401.

Scheier, M. F., & Carver, C. S. (1992). Effects of optimism on psychological and physical well-being: Theoretical overview and empirical update. *Cognitive Therapy and Research, 16,* 201–228.

Sephton, S., & Spiegel, D. (2003). Circadian disruption in cancer: A neuroendocrine-immune pathway from stress to disease? *Brain Behavior and Immunity, 17,* 321–328.

Spencer, S., Lehman, J., Wynings, C., Arena, P., Carver, C. S., Antoni, M. H., et al. (1999). Concerns about breast cancer and relations to psychological well-being in a multi-ethnic sample of early stage patients. *Health Psychology, 18,* 159–169.

Spiegel, D. (2002). Effects of psychotherapy on cancer survival. *Nature Reviews Cancer, 2,* 383–389.

Tomich, P. L., & Helgeson, V. S. (2004). Is finding something good in the bad always good? Benefit finding among women with breast cancer. *Health Psychology, 23,* 16–23.

Urcuyo, K. R., Boyers, A., Carver, C. S., & Antoni, M. H. (2005). Finding benefit in breast cancer: Relations with personality, coping, and concurrent well-being. *Psychology and Health, 20,* 175–192.

van der Pompe, G., Antoni, M. H., Duivenvoorden, H., De Graeff, R., Simonis, T., van der Vegt, F., & Heijnen, C. (2001). An exploratory study into the effect of group psychotherapy on cardiovascular and immunoreactivity to acute stress in breast cancer patients. *Psychotherapy and Psychosomatics, 70,* 307–318.

van der Pompe, G., Antoni, M. H., & Heijnen, C. (1996). Elevated basal cortisol levels and attenuated ACTH and cortisol responses to acute stress in women with metastatic breast cancer. *Psychoneuroendocrinology, 21,* 361–374.

Wilmoth, M. C., & Sanders, L. D. (2001). Accept me for myself: African American women's issues after breast cancer. *Oncology Nursing Forum, 28,* 875–879.

12

The Clinician as Expert Companion

Richard G. Tedeschi and Lawrence G. Calhoun

It is clear to us that positive changes can be experienced by some, perhaps many, of those who struggle to cope with traumatic events.[1] We believe we have also learned something about how to facilitate this process. This chapter is written primarily for clinicians who wish to put into practice the lessons about *posttraumatic growth* (PTG) that we have learned by conducting our own research and attending to the growing published work of others, and by listening carefully to the persons whom we have served in our clinical work, and who have participated in our research studies. We describe the clinician's role as that of an *expert companion* to focus attention on the kind of relationship that we think can be most helpful to persons dealing with highly challenging life circumstances (Tedeschi & Calhoun, 2004b, 2006).

What follows represents a general description of our ideas about PTG in clinical work, especially with patients in health care settings. First, we present our model of PTG and the clinician's role as expert companion. Next, we clarify commonly misunderstood concepts about PTG. Then, we describe specific strategies for being an expert companion. Finally, we provide an excerpt from a therapy session that exemplifies the expert companion role. We conclude with a note about the possibility for expert companions to experience vicarious PTG. A more extensive exposition of our views can be found in Calhoun and Tedeschi (1999). In this chapter, before considering how clinicians can facilitate PTG, we consider questions that some people have raised about this concept, so that clinicians who wish to attend to themes of growth in their applied work will have confidence that encouraging the process of PTG appears to be worthwhile for the patients with whom they work.

Our model of the clinician as expert companion has arisen from our clinical experience and the limited research available on this topic. We continue to develop a general framework for use by clinicians that is based on ideas developed in our own clinical work and on the initial phases of controlled research by

---

[1]A note of semantic clarification: As we have done elsewhere, we use the terms *trauma* and *traumatic events* in ways that are broader than the narrowly circumscribed criteria of the current *Diagnostic and Statistical Manual of Mental Disorders* (4th ed., text rev.; American Psychiatric Association, 2000). We interchange their use with expressions we regard as generally synonymous, including *major life stressors, crises, life crises,* and similar terms. Clearly, these terms would apply to persons facing major health problems and serious illness, including those who are diagnosed as terminally ill.

others (Cordova et al., 2007; Zöllner & Maercker, 2006). What we suggest is based on the best available information, but this information is limited.

A Model for Clinical Conceptualization

Our guide to clinical work is the model of PTG that we first proposed in the 1990s (Tedeschi & Calhoun, 1995). The evolving model we have proposed describes a process that unfolds over time (more extensive descriptions can be found in Calhoun & Tedeschi, 1998, 2004, 2006). Briefly, this model suggests that one of the clinician's most important tasks is to guide patients in moving from merely suffering, to suffering meaningfully. People may be more likely to seek psychological treatment when there is a loss of meaning, especially for religious or existential issues (Fontana & Rosenheck, 2005). Clinicians, if they are listening, will attend to much more than symptoms such as insomnia, anxiety, avoidance, and so forth; they will be adopting roles as practical philosophers who struggle alongside patients in the process of making sense of patients' illnesses and finding purpose in life following these medical events. Clinicians will be expert companions, who focus on uncovering strategies for moving beyond the stressful aspects of disease. It is important to keep in mind that recognition of PTG can allow people to be wiser, not just sadder, and to be more than mere survivors.

To the expert companion, one important consideration is the patient's premorbid personal characteristics. Even for patients who have suffered multiple stressors (Harvey, Barnett, & Rupe, 2006), it may be useful to develop some ideas of the kinds of people they were before the most recent event (e.g., symptoms and diagnosis of multiple sclerosis). Persons who tend toward positive affect (Stanton & Low, 2004), are open to experience, are extraverted, and take an active, problem-solving approach to difficulties are likely to report more PTG (Tedeschi & Calhoun, 1996). To the extent that patients have been prepared to respond constructively to their illness, the clinician can take a more active approach in addressing issues associated with being ill. Clinicians should also consider that those who are in the middle range of psychological adjustment might experience more PTG than people with great psychological vulnerabilities or those with extraordinary psychological strength (Tedeschi & Calhoun, 1995).

Another consideration is the nature of the life crisis or, as we have described it, the *seismic event* (Calhoun & Tedeschi, 1998). An event is seismic when it has an impact on the assumptive world (Janoff-Bulman, 2006), similar to that of an earthquake on physical structures, forcing the person to reconsider fundamental beliefs about the kind of person he or she is, the degree to which the world is benevolent, what the future may hold, why things happen in the world, the nature of human beings, the purpose of life, and other major existential issues (Cann, Calhoun, & Tedeschi, 2007; Janoff-Bulman, 1992, 2004, 2006; Koltko-Rivera, 2004). Clinicians must consider the specific details of the events in question because the challenges to the assumptive world and the philosophical questions that may be asked by the patient will differ on the basis of the characteristics of the diagnosis. Different conversations will ensue, some focused on blame, some on life paths and priorities, others on spiritual elements, and yet others on past choices about relationships. For example, a diagnosis of terminal cancer might prompt questions about justice, purpose in life, or thoughts about life priorities. In contrast, being diagnosed with HIV may generate questions about past sexual behavior and concerns about how to cope with a chronic life-threatening illness that requires decades of medical management to stay alive.

The interaction of the seismic, highly challenging event with the particular personality and coping styles of the person yields ways of responding in three important areas that the clinician should investigate: managing emotional distress, reconsidering beliefs and goals, and revising the course of the life narrative (Neimeyer, 2001, 2006).

Most approaches to assisting patients facing highly challenging health problems are designed to *manage emotional distress* or the kinds of symptoms associated with traumatic stress, such as arousal or intrusions. We will not review the well-known techniques that are used to deal with this aspect of traumatic response; rather, we refer readers to other sources that examine the general clinical approach to trauma treatment (e.g., see Cook, Schnurr, & Foa, 2004; Herman, 1992).

The recognition of PTG may, for some, produce a somewhat greater tolerance of the emotional distress regarding the event (Janoff-Bulman, 2006). Individuals may be able to tell themselves that the experience of illness is not in vain and that something worthwhile can emerge from it, thereby reducing some distress. Because PTG may take time to develop, perceptions of PTG may not be a part of the management of emotional distress early on. People who are coping with fear-provoking health scenarios may need to use basic anxiety management techniques such as appropriate dosing with fear-provoking scenarios and distraction, to allow themselves to move through the initial phases of self-management.

As the implications of the seismic event become apparent, patients often *reconsider their beliefs and goals,* or their assumptive world. In facing the challenges to the assumptive world, the clinician must use his or her expertise in helping the patient manage anxiety and other emotions that interfere with reflective rumination, which is the deliberate and constructive processing of trauma so that it is manageable, comprehensible, and finally, meaningful (Calhoun & Tedeschi, 1999; Tedeschi & Calhoun, 1995).

Although we are speaking here of rebuilding the assumptive world, it should be apparent that the new set of assumptions may be different from what has gone before. A hallmark of the assumptive world is that it typically is not closely examined. In contrast, the set of beliefs and guiding perspectives on living that is formed out of trauma and loss is often painstakingly built. Rather than a more gradually, and perhaps passively, developed assumptive world, the new set of beliefs based on the deliberate rumination that takes place after major stressors often includes pointed questions and challenges to the self: Should I believe this? Does that make sense? Can I live life believing this? What makes sense in light of what happened to me? Some goals may need to be reevaluated and perhaps abandoned.

There may be a sense of having one's life brought to a halt by illness, giving time for reflection on priorities and assumptions about living. This interruption of the normal course of living is in itself a *change in the life narrative,* and allows decisions to be made about what the patient will do after recovery, or in living with a chronic condition, or in facing a terminal illness. The life narrative often comes to be divided into the time before illness and the sometimes-strange new life that emerges (e.g., see Price, 1994).

The emotional distress, disrupted beliefs and life goals, and changed life narrative tend to produce rumination akin to symptoms of posttraumatic stress, such as reexperiencing the trauma and increased arousal. This "brooding" rumination (Nolen-Hoeksema & Davis, 2004) is a distressing experience that makes people doubt their ability to cope. It may also lead some to seek out others with whom to talk about what has happened. Some might start writing about their experiences, and others might pray. Clinicians may feel that they should help put an end to this pain as soon as possible. During the initial time of emotional distress and rumination, the focus for many patients and their clinicians is on minimizing and getting through the pain as quickly as possible. However, wholesale suppression of distress is not necessary for PTG and may in fact be counterproductive. Patients are usually engaged in managing distress and rebuilding their assumptive worlds in a process whereby gains in coping yield gains in PTG, which in turn yields a better ability to cope and less emotional distress. A certain degree of distress management is certainly necessary so that the distress does not overwhelm the patient's ability to think critically and constructively. It is important to keep in mind, however, that this cognitive activity is likely to become more constructive over time and may eventually be useful in producing PTG. The clinician's job is not necessarily to help suppress this rumination but to assist the patient in making the rumination more reflective in nature and less brooding (Nolen-Hoeksema & Davis, 2004).

As the ruminative process becomes more reflective, patients can focus on the more profound issues of meaning and purpose and their plan for the future. We have distinguished the latter from the former by sometimes referring to it as *cognitive engagement* because the term *rumination* has come to connote a depressogenic type of thinking process (Tedeschi & Calhoun, 2004b). The shift to the more productive thinking pattern of cognitive engagement is facilitated when the clinician is willing to listen carefully to the patient's specific concerns about the past, what they expect of the future, their wish that things could be undone so that the narrative could continue (i.e., *counterfactuals*), and the struggle to come to terms with the fact that a revised narrative is being written (Harpham, 1994). Attention to these concerns is necessary if we are interested in encouraging PTG.

An important element in making the transition from brooding rumination to more reflective cognitive engagement may be the presence of effective listeners and of people who are models for changed schemas that include elements of PTG (Calhoun & Tedeschi, 2006; see also chap. 8, this volume). Talking to others about the illness experience appears to be an important factor in PTG (Cordova, Cunningham, Carlson, & Andrykowski, 2001). Participation in support groups that comprise people enduring similar situations may assist the process of adaptation and perhaps PTG, provided that discussions about these experiences are valued by all concerned and that openness is encouraged. Of course, we must consider the patient's sociocultural context, including the primary reference groups of friends, family, neighbors, social circle, and larger societal macrosystems (Calhoun & Tedeschi, 2004, 2006). These groups will vary in the degree to which PTG is a concept that is familiar and encouraged, and how it is understood (e.g., as a spiritual experience, as a commonplace occurrence, as something to be valued, as something to be doubted).

To an extent, other people in the patient's social system can encourage or discourage disclosure about certain aspects of the illness and its aftermath, including PTG. Generally, clinicians find that almost regardless of cultural contexts, a major problem for most patients is the sense that others have finished considering the effects of their illness before they themselves have. Social support may be lacking. Some patients know few individuals who will allow them to express their feelings, fears, and concerns (see chap. 8, this volume); therapists are often the only ones who have the time and the patience to be fully present and listen as patients consider and reconsider, ruminate, and ultimately work through their feelings about the illness. Clinicians can expect a patient to consider his or her life before the illness, the stressors surrounding the illness itself, and the "new normal" that then must develop. This new reality initially can seem alien and not normal at all. Many of these concerns come up in therapy.

Themes of growth may not emerge until a few years after diagnosis (Cordova et al., 2001). If this is the case, developing from an event in the distant past seems much less likely. This sometimes may be due to a tendency to become preoccupied with fruitless ruminations. For example, a patient may search for meaning by focusing on why this happened to him or her (Collins, Taylor, & Skokan, 1990). It is the clinician's job to help patients identify ways to constructively ruminate so that they will not end up in these dead ends that tend to inhibit the possibility of growth. As Harvey et al. (2006) describe, the route to PTG may be torturous and include setbacks and additional stressors. Therefore, it is important for clinicians to focus on the particulars of the lives survivors have led. Growth might be interrupted or enhanced by additional traumas; as people respond to major stressors in their lives, it is often crucial to consider the kind of response they have received from the people around them. Clinicians become part of a patient's social support system and can have a crucial impact that facilitates growth.

Clarification of Commonly Misunderstood Concepts of Posttraumatic Growth

There may be some misunderstandings about the concept of PTG (Calhoun & Tedeschi, 1999, 2004). In this section, we repeat and clarify some of the positions we have taken on such issues, with a focus on the clinical context. These matters are important for practitioners to consider when working with persons facing serious medical issues.

It's Not the Illness, It's the Struggle

Clinicians would be wise to acknowledge that the positive changes patients may experience come not from the illness but from the confrontation and struggle to cope with it (Calhoun & Tedeschi, 1999; McQuellon & Cowan, 2007). In this struggle, most, but not all, people are focused on "making it through," rather than on any aspect of PTG. In the struggle to survive and adapt, cognitive engagement with the fundamental issues of life—existential issues of meaning, responsibility, impermanence, and death—may produce a deepening of character. The aftermath of illness can be a laboratory in which life lessons can be explored and understood.

Posttraumatic Growth Does Not Necessarily Relieve Distress

A general assumption among some PTG researchers is that PTG should lead to, or at least be accompanied by, a reduction in distress. In fact, however, it is more likely that PTG and distress coexist, at least in the relatively short-term following a diagnosis and unpleasant treatments. Although the literature has not expanded to examine enough prospective investigations into the long-term trajectories of PTG, cross-sectional studies suggest that distress is present for years in survivors of many traumas who also report PTG (Lev-Wiesel & Amir, 2003). Our model of PTG is explicit: A certain threshold of distress is initially necessary to define a medical event as traumatic and to start the process that may lead to PTG. We have suggested that enduring distress may be necessary to maintain the edge, the sharpness of pain that produces a continued involvement in existential issues and a continuing sense that perspectives have changed (Calhoun & Tedeschi, 1998). Substantial distress is necessary at the start for events to be worthy of the label *traumatic,* and continuing distress may be necessary for people to have a sense that they remain in a condition in which they are able to recognize PTG.

Patients May Reject Posttraumatic Growth at One Point and Embrace It at Another

Because the development of PTG appears to be a long-term process in many persons, there are likely to be times when the possibility of PTG is unrecognized and even unwelcome. Psychological pain and physical distress may be initially overwhelming, preventing a patient from appreciating anything relating to the notion of PTG. In some situations, acknowledgment of PTG may seem to be a sort of betrayal. For example, it can be seen as a betrayal of a loved one who has died or of others who still struggle with similar illnesses (Tedeschi & Calhoun, 2007a).

When the possibility of PTG is unwelcome, the clinician must carefully evaluate whether to attempt to foster PTG. No amount of empirical data can determine whether pursuing PTG is beneficial for each individual patient, so clinicians must make their own ethical decisions about their patients' best interests. We can say confidently that most people with whom we have worked, although this is clearly not a random sample, have gradually come to appreciate their growth in the aftermath of trauma. For some patients, PTG can come as a surprise. Clinicians should take a long-term perspective on the development of PTG in patients and recognize that these developments may come to fruition only after direct clinical contact has ended.

Posttraumatic Growth May Be Most Common in the Middle Range

We have suggested that people in the broad middle range of psychological fitness will be more likely to experience PTG than people who are very high or very low in resilience and other adaptive resources (Tedeschi & Calhoun, 1995). Unlike people who lack resilience and have low psychological fitness, people with average coping skills are likely to have enough resources to successfully manage the initial distress and rumination that accompanies trauma, setting the stage for PTG. People in this middle range also have some lessons to learn or strengthening to experience. People at the highest levels of psychological fitness may not have any additional room to grow.

Similarly, people in the broad middle range of physical fitness may be more likely to experience PTG than those who are very healthy or very ill. Chronic, debilitating illnesses may be too stressful for some patients to experience PTG because their coping resources are being constantly overwhelmed. However, those who are challenged by their medical situations but have the ability to cope fairly well, may report a good deal of PTG (see chap. 1, this volume). In an early study with people who had been paralyzed, we found this to be true for people with physical disabilities. Even seriously and permanently disabled persons reported PTG (Tedeschi & Calhoun, 1988).

Reports of Posttraumatic Growth May Be Real or Illusory

Some of our colleagues (e.g., see Bonanno, 2005; McFarland & Alvaro, 2000) tend to be skeptical about PTG, regarding such reports as essentially illusory or, at the least, consisting primarily of either automatic or deliberate attempts on the part of the person to make things better by seeing them in a somewhat unjustifiably positive light. Most psychologists trained in doctoral programs that have emphasized an exclusively scientific, experimental tradition, or those trained in the scientist–practitioner (a description we apply to ourselves) model, have been socialized to be skeptical about phenomena such as PTG. This is not necessarily a bad thing because it stimulates discourse and clinical research.

We have long acknowledged that PTG may partly be "a function of a general cognitive bias to retroactively see one's life as always improving" (Tedeschi & Calhoun, 1995, p. 120) and that people exposed to great stress may report PTG "because they are comparing their current state with a past state of great psychological distress" (Tedeschi & Calhoun, 1995, p. 120). Certainly, it is possible that some people reporting PTG are functioning under some illusions.

But what should be the clinician's stance when dealing directly with a patient facing difficult life circumstances who talks about how life is now somehow better than before the illness? What should be the clinical response to Hamilton Jordan, survivor of several different kinds of cancer, who talks about how things have changed for the better for him, with life taking on some new, joyful meaning (Jordan, 2000)? For clinical purposes, it is probably useful to discern whether patients seem to be whitewashing the severity of the health problem and its aftermath or are failing to acknowledge the difficulty of their struggle.

With rare exceptions, when the individual's psychological state is unambiguously delusional, we think it is desirable to work within the patient's framework and to accept reports of PTG as valid. We take this stance for several reasons.

First, the experience of growth may indeed be empirically valid (Dohrenwend et al., 2004; Park, Cohen, & Murch, 1996). If some distortions do occur, they appear to be rare (Dohrenwend et al., 2004), and reports of growth tend to be corroborated by others (Park et al., 1996).

Second, for many persons, PTG is an experience in which the way they think, view the world, and see their place in it has been changed, sometimes radically so. Scientific attempts to legitimatize such experiences by giving them the imprimatur of empirical veracity may seem not only inappropriate but also arrogant. Clinicians have long realized that an empathic therapeutic relationship is fundamental to any possibility of change. The clinician's most appropriate approach is to first assume that the patient's perceptions have validity and are worth understanding, rather than to meet the patient with skepticism. That is not to say that a good clinician is gullible and will believe anything a patient says. Quite to the contrary, the eclectic, cognitive constructivist–narrative stance that we take is based on the understanding that all of a patient's experience is in some way constructed and subjective. Joining the patients in his or her subjective experience (Taylor & Brown, 1988) can allow the patient to more fully express the understandings and perspectives that are forming in the aftermath of trauma, enhancing the appreciation for those perspectives by the clinician and, consequently, by the patient as well.

Third, the majority of seriously ill persons seen by clinical health psychologists will be involved in personal struggle and be experiencing great physical discomfort. They will have little doubt that any lessons they learn will be hard won and real. They are real because they are not learned intellectually, but with a strong affective component (Calhoun & Tedeschi, 1998). If this affect endures, the associated lessons may remain accessible. In the midst of pain and fear that have been managed to an extent that can allow reflective rumination, persons may retain the edge in their thinking that comes from being in the crisis rather than reflecting back on it from a distance. We have heard people who have survived cancer for some time without setbacks say that they are concerned that without the fear, they may take things for granted or return to previous ways of living life. It appears that negative affect, especially in the lives of people who have a good capacity for positive affect, may fuel the process of maintaining and enhancing PTG. This implies that the clinician's role is not to suppress negative affect too readily or too completely.

Various Routes to Growth

Certainly, people who experience PTG are not the only ones who learn and put into action important lessons about living life well. There are routes to this maturity and wisdom other than through major life crises (see chap. 5, this volume). Life experiences that have a substantial impact on schemas may produce effects similar to those that we see in PTG. We emphasize here, however, that the lessons associated with major stressors are particularly powerful because of the affective component that is involved. To the extent that affect is involved in other pathways, such as vicarious PTG (Arnold, Calhoun, Tedeschi, & Cann, 2005), extraordinary positive events (Ihle, Ritsher, & Kanas, 2006), more commonplace or normative developmental events, or the impressive teachings of a mentor, growth may occur in domains similar to those seen in PTG.

To Just Keep on Going Is Good Enough

PTG is not necessarily the primary desirable outcome from the loss of one's physical health. Another desirable outcome, perhaps for most patients, is to "just keep on going" (Harvey et al., 2006). Certainly, we do not judge people who manage in this way as having failed to achieve a real resolution of trauma. Furthermore, when people experience a cluster of many losses (Harvey, Barnett, & Overstreet, 2004), PTG may be difficult to achieve. Distress may become so overwhelming that people remain focused on emotional management rather than proceeding to the more constructive cognitive engagement of reflective rumination, mentioned earlier. Harvey et al. (2004) see the task of survivors who encounter these aggregations of trauma as being stimulated to do new work that can lead to PTG when the latest major trauma occurs, but that in many instances the goals should be more modest. Still, people who have experienced some of the harshest traumas do report some PTG (e.g., Holocaust survivors; Lev-Wiesel & Amir, 2003). Clinicians should never underestimate the potential for growth in people who have faced even the most severe health crises.

Specific Strategies for Expert Companionship

Adopt the General Attitude of an Expert Companion

The clinician companion is an expert at being a companion, in that he or she is curious about what has happened and what may happen to the patient, allowing for different possibilities, accepting of the worst but also of the best. The expert companion is not someone who attempts or encourages a whitewashing of the worst of the situation, or who offers platitudes or easy solutions. There is a constant recognition, and sometimes overt statements, about how terrible the situation appears to be to the patient, and how the problems faced may be extremely difficult, and perhaps impossible, to solve. Even when growth is being discussed, it is made clear that this is a hard way to learn, change, and develop.

Show Humility and Empathy

Much can be accomplished by establishing a companionate relationship with patients, in which the psychologist is more a learner than an expert. In this approach, the clinician practices with sincere humility in the presence of patients, conveying the message that "this may be hard to get through and it may take the both of us." There are a number of thoughts, perspectives, and statements that clinicians can keep in mind, and sometimes say, to remain expert companions. For example, some situations are so horrible that it is helpful for clinicians to have the normal human response of "I'm not sure I could have handled that" or "No wonder you are seeking support." This is helpful for patients who fear for their sanity (Tedeschi & Calhoun, 2007a). They can feel relieved to hear their "expert" proclaim that anyone would need help with something so extraordinary or so tragic.

In operating this way, the expert companion relates to the patient primarily as someone from whom much can be learned, rather than as a person who needs to be changed or treated. It is important for the clinician to listen to the patient in a way that allows the clinician to be emotionally affected and to be changed by the encounter. This way of being with patients allows clinicians to be more effective in the moment with their patients, and with other patients in the future.

The humble and empathic stance of expert companionship is also helpful because it relieves clinicians of the impossible responsibility for solving the problems associated with major life difficulties. Working with persons who are very sick, perhaps dying, can be hard on the soul, and it is useful to recognize the limitations of one's expertise (McQuellon & Cowan, 2007). In a world where empirically supported treatments, the promotion of new therapies, and a fascination with techniques that purport to speed the process of trauma recovery, such as eye movement desensitization and reprocessing, are the norm, we are admittedly recommending something that may appear to be little more than supportive therapy. However, we have tried to provide clinical examples that reveal the subtle ways in which the clinician accompanies the survivor through the process we describe in our model of PTG (see Calhoun & Tedeschi, 1998, 1999, 2004, 2006, and Tedeschi & Calhoun, 2004b, for more extensive descriptions and examples).

Appreciate the Paradoxes of Intervention

PTG requires an appreciation of paradox on the part of the clinician and the patient. The basic paradox is that loss can produce gain, or at least coexist with it. We have described other paradoxes that appear to be involved with PTG (Calhoun & Tedeschi, 1999): a combination of action and acceptance, a recognition that helpful others are important but that surviving trauma is inherently lonely, and the notion that in vulnerability there can be strength. For the clinician, an appreciation of paradox is important because, in our view, good practice with seriously ill persons is paradoxical. The concept of expert companionship (Tedeschi & Calhoun, 2004a) is inherently paradoxical. The best route to success for clinicians is to downplay expertise and overt attempts to solve the problems of the trauma survivor and instead facilitate PTG by being an expert companion to the patient. The expert companion operates on the following principles:

1. Acknowledge the difficulty of the situation.
2. To the extent possible, be there through the difficulties.
3. Be willing to listen to the hard parts of the story.
4. Relate to the patient through his or her worldview.
5. Accept apparent "illusions" as useful to the patient.
6. Help the patient manage anxiety and other emotions.

7. Help the patient move from brooding rumination to more constructive reflection.
8. Notice and remark about the strengths and changes that come from the struggle.
9. Do not offer platitudes.
10. Listen in a way that allows you to be changed.

Avoid Direct Interventions on Posttraumatic Growth

We begin here with the premise that for most patients, most of the time, it may be desirable for the clinician to listen for themes of PTG. Under some circumstances, it may be desirable to encourage it. However, we are skeptical at this point about the wisdom of trying to engage in interventions designed directly to help individuals to experience PTG. A potential unintended consequence of such an approach may well be one of the dangers against which Wortman (2004) has so wisely warned us: By giving the message that PTG is somehow normative, and that it is to be expected, clinicians may actually increase the burden of persons whose suffering is already great. Direct attempts to teach patients to grow may inadvertently add to a general "tyranny of positive thinking" (Holland & Lewis, 2000, p. 13) that will not be helpful and may indeed make patients feel greater distress. In addition, we think that in clinical work, PTG is best viewed in the context of a wide array of possible strategies designed to assist persons to cope with difficult life challenges, and not as a posttraumatic intervention per se.

Pass on What Has Been Learned by Others

Since we began to document PTG in the 1980s, we have considered a large extent of our work in the area to be a retelling of the stories of the people in our clinical sessions and research studies (e.g., see Calhoun, Tedeschi, & Uhrich, 1986; Tedeschi & Calhoun, 1988; Tedeschi, Calhoun, Morrell, & Johnson, 1984). As clinicians, we find it useful to be able to retell these stories in clinically appropriate ways at appropriate times. We can maintain our humility by saying, "Some other people have told me that it helps them to. . . . That may be something you could consider." Indeed, by listening carefully, there are many ideas and strategies that can be gleaned from people who are attempting to manage difficult medical conditions.

Be in It for the Long Run

There are few, if any, easy solutions to the impact of devastating illnesses, and the process of meaning making often seems to be alien to people struggling to survive their losses, griefs, and fears (Tedeschi & Calhoun, 2007b). The expert companion accepts that adaptation may be a lengthy process, perhaps a lifelong one, and demonstrates that he or she will accompany the patient long after other supportive people in the patient's proximate culture may have become frustrated, frightened, or simply uncomfortable. Often, only professionals are able to continue to listen for months or years to horrific stories told by those whose beliefs and hopes may have been shattered.

Helping Patients in the Three Ways They Cope With Seismic Events

As discussed previously, people typically cope with seismic (i.e., highly challenging) events in three basic ways: by managing emotional distress, by reconsidering beliefs and goals, and by revising the life narrative. The following sections discuss ways to help patients with these three areas. However, the expert companion must first consider the particular personality and coping styles of patients prior to their health problems, and how they may have dealt with previous life challenges.

Encouraging discussion of the pre-crisis character of a person can reveal things that can be useful in considering the possibilities for PTG. For example, extraversion is modestly associated with PTG (Tedeschi & Calhoun, 1996). This can be used by encouraging the individual to stand up to the challenge of his or her traumatic event. The story of the symptoms, medical tests, diagnosis attempts, and treatment will typically be part of the first phases of clinical contact and may include reference to the challenged or shattered belief system and to the feelings of panic and hopelessness often found in the early stages of a serious medical problem (McQuellon & Cowan, 2007). After considering the personality and coping skills of the individual, the expert companion can assist the patient in the three areas of coping in the following ways.

Helping the Patient Manage Emotional Distress

Assistance can be given in managing anxiety and unproductive, brooding rumination. For example, the technique of scheduling time to ruminate, and doing it actively with a pen and paper, drawing materials, or computer helps many ruminators gain a sense of some control over themselves. This technique acknowledges a paradox of trauma: Feelings associated with trauma need to be expressed but patients also need time to avoid thoughts of illness and distraction. Patients can be made aware that letting the trauma have its way or expressing feelings is good to a point. However, as we have mentioned before, a wholesale suppression of distress is not necessary for PTG, and may be counterproductive. Patients are usually engaged in managing distress and rebuilding their assumptive worlds in a process whereby gains in coping yield gain in PTG, which in turn yields a better ability to cope and less emotional distress. A certain degree of distress management is certainly necessary so that the distress does not overwhelm the patient's ability to think critically and constructively.

Helping the Patient Reconsider Beliefs and Goals

Key to the process of developing PTG is work on the shattered assumptive world. Patients will begin in different places with regard to this. Some will find themselves adrift in a world that no longer makes any sense, whereas others will actively reconstruct their ideas about relationships, God, life priorities, and other domains of PTG. It can be disconcerting for the clinician as well as the patient when the assumptive world has failed. Clinicians who are expert companions might find themselves wondering along with the patient what it makes sense to believe. Indeed, one of the benefits of being a clinician who works with people involved in traumatic events is that one is more attuned to these aspects in one's own life. We find it useful to truly be companions in the patient's struggle, asking some of the questions ourselves, and leaving the responses open and ambiguous rather than jumping in with easy answers. In fact, the best expert companions in clinical health psychology may be those who are a little uncertain of the answers themselves. These clinicians will be more likely to join the suffering patient rather than to be detached because of their sense that they have already thoroughly learned these lessons.

In helping the patient reconsider previous beliefs and goals, the expert companion's role is to join in the patient's practical philosophizing (Baltes, Staudinger, Maercker, & Smith, 1995). There may not be a clear resolution during the time of treatment, and in fact, it may be useful for patients to continue with this sort of thinking, that the assumptive world is never quite finalized but is continually in revision. Still, there must be enough of a basis for moving forward with life that the patient has a sense that certain actions are more important than others. In the patient's search for new beliefs and goals, the clinician can also assist by helping the patient find others who have gone through similar health events. This aspect of social support provides models of coping and PTG and allows patients to make the often surprising discovery that they can be of help to others as well (Calhoun & Tedeschi, 1999). This can become an essential element of their new assumptive world.

Helping the Patient Revise the Life Narrative

The expert companion can also think of him- or herself as a ghostwriter who helps the patient develop a meaningful account of the life events that have changed the narrative trajectory. By the end of treatment, patients may be able to accept their current state and develop ideas of how to progress. Many go further than this, declaring that their previous life choices were not up to the revised standards for meaning that they have developed, and so reject their old ways. Recovery from addiction often reflects this kind of thinking, as does the aftermath of life-threatening diseases and accidents.

Encouraging the Patient to Face the Worst Things Directly

While helping the patient manage emotional distress, reconsider beliefs and goals, and revise the life narrative, the expert companion usually encourages the patient to face the worst things directly. An honest focus on the negative and distressing aspects of illness runs counter to the assumption by some that PTG work is encouraging illusion or denial. In fact, when we are working with persons in health crises and with other trauma survivors, we try always to acknowledge that something terrible has happened to them.

Facing Ambiguity

Serious health problems often leave people with a sense of ambiguity about what to believe and how to live (i.e., a shattered assumptive world). The clinician must remain close to the patient who is unsure about how to proceed with his or her life, and not give in to the temptation to foreclose on the struggle prematurely. In a way, people may find themselves in an identity crisis. However, as Erikson (1964) described, some role confusion can be a good thing. The ambiguity plays an important role in the cognitive processing of serious illness.

Facing Mortality

Health challenges that are highly stressful seem to have an element of mortality. People are faced with loss, ending, and a recognition that they have only a limited amount of time left. Of course, some situations, such as terminal disease, are obvious mortality threats. The clinician who is an expert companion in these circumstances must be able to discuss life and death, and not steer away from the possibility of death, the ugliness of it, or the relief that may come with it. Other medical patients may not face mortality per se, but are disfigured or may have lost the use of various body functions. These patients are also dealing with issues related to major loss, albeit not loss of life.

Struggling With Counterfactuals

Most serious health problems seem to put people in the position, at least early on, to wish that things were not the way they are, and yearn to undo them. This appears to be the basis for imagining how the outcome could have been different, and the degree to which one's own actions might have affected it. These counterfactuals (Davis & Lehman, 1995) can form the basis for much rumination, which is generally unproductive. However, expert companions can support patients as they engage in this rumination, because simple reassurances or encouragement have minimal lasting effects. Most people have heard these things from others already. In our experience, what seems to be most effective is to deal straight away with the patient's counterfactual thinking, going over the exact details of what they wish they had done and the likely outcomes, even though the clinician may not have a clear sense of where this might lead. There is relief for most patients in having permission to think through the counterfactuals explicitly. Sometimes this kind of exercise produces a continuing ambiguity about what the outcome might have been if other paths had been taken. Even this can be tolerated well if the patient feels that the counterfactuals have been thoroughly explored. Sometimes this results in the dissipation of the counterfactual rumination.

Using Metaphors

We have described elsewhere (Calhoun & Tedeschi, 1999) how seismic events can often lead people to try to describe their experience using metaphors. We have also illustrated how we use metaphors to demonstrate positive changes that patients may have difficulty seeing. Staying within the experience of the patient is extremely important. For example, a photographer whose son died was able to understand the gradual emergence of personal change when the clinician used a metaphor of photos emerging in developing fluid (Calhoun & Tedeschi, 1999). A man who was frustrated that listening to his bereaved wife did not seem to quickly help her, was able to grasp the benefits of patience when the clinician referred to all the preparations he made prior to going out to chop wood (Tedeschi & Calhoun, 2004a).

Encouraging Reflection Instead of Brooding

Although some initial rumination that is automatic and nonproductive may be an expected part of the PTG process, this cognitive hand-wringing should be directed to evolve into more useful reflection. The best way to encourage this evolution is by directly joining it. After awhile, most patients want us to help them move to a new way of adapting to their changed life circumstances. After saying repeatedly that they cannot believe that it happened, or how angry or afraid they are about it, patients often begin to say things about planning, responding, deciding, and so forth. Another approach is illustrated in Tedeschi and Calhoun (2004a). In this case, a mother was worried about her dead daughter being cold in her grave. By directly exploring her thinking and taking it seriously, showing her how it was an extension of her maternal impulses, the mother was able to let go of her concern that she was "being crazy" and start to consider other ways of continuing to love and care for her daughter. It is not desirable to be formulaic about the best clinical approach in such situations, but in all cases, we have found direct, respectful, and patient communication to be key. Coupled with an understanding of the patient's progress toward PTG and using the model of PTG as a guide, suggesting the next moves can encourage patients in their struggle toward growth.

Noticing the Evolving Domains of Growth

Some authors in the benefit-finding literature refer to "meaning making" as an important part of the process. As clinicians, we have tended to eschew this kind of talk with patients. Most patients find the terminology obscure, and the discussion of making meaning out of their situation seems to leave most people unsure of what to do. Instead, we discuss the more concrete and specific changes outlined in the Posttraumatic Growth Inventory (PTGI; Tedeschi & Calhoun, 1996). It is fairly easy for most patients to talk about how their relationships have changed, how their appreciation for life has changed, how they may feel stronger, how their life paths and priorities are different, and how they have grown spiritually. Indeed, because the items on the PTGI were derived from a review of the literature on major life stressors and suffering, and from qualitative analyses of interviews with persons facing difficult circumstances, it is easy to see how trauma survivors can relate to such discussions. We encourage expert companionship in the direct and common language used in therapy.

An Example of Expert Companionship

The following excerpt from therapy shows expert companionship with a focus on PTG. The therapist is working with a 25-year-old woman (patient) who has suffered a stroke that has left her with some muscle weakness and some cognitive impairment. She had been a champion swimmer in high school and had just started law school when the stroke occurred. Excerpts from interviews approximately 9 months into her rehabilitation follow.

Patient: I am not sure I can handle school like this.
Therapist: The time it takes to write would make it tough.
Patient: Not just the physical part, but getting my thoughts together. I can do it pretty well when speaking, but writing doesn't come so easily anymore.
Therapist: You have certainly been working on it.
Patient: I wonder how much more improvement I will make. I have to get a follow-up on the neuropsych tests again soon. I'm not sure they'll look too good.
Therapist: I know it was discouraging last time.
Patient: Yes, especially the recommendation I should apply for disability. How do they know I'm all washed up?
Therapist: You do have a determination that they may not have taken into account.
Patient: They don't know me.
Therapist: You've been going at this like you did your swimming. You have made progress.
Patient: I'm not sure it will be enough, but I'm not giving up now.
Therapist: You can still be determined, even in this new reality.
Patient: I know I've lost a lot. I just want to make sure I don't lose any more.
Therapist: You are recognizing these losses almost every moment, even when you are determined to push on.
Patient: Well, just when I am doing certain things.
Therapist: Sometimes they are more obvious.
Patient: [starting to cry] Yes, some things are.
Therapist: And you grieve these losses.
Patient: Grief—that's it.
Therapist: Like there have been some deaths.
Patient: Yes, but that's not all. I see the gains, too.
Therapist: What gains do you notice?
Patient: Oh, I have more understanding for people.
Therapist: Understanding?
Patient: Like that people are all dealing with something, and you can't assume things about people. Everyone has something they are dealing with that is affecting them. People assume things about me that aren't fair, accurate. I've learned not to do this with others.
Therapist: You can't know what is going on with people that might figure into how they seem to be.
Patient: I knew this last summer. I could think it, even when I couldn't really talk yet. You learn this, hanging around with stroke vic-

	tims all summer. It's like I know things old people know, but I'm only 25.
Therapist:	You have a different feel for people.
Patient:	I'm more compassionate.
Therapist:	Are there other ways you see yourself differently?
Patient:	I'm still figuring that out; trying to figure out what I have, and what may come back. I know I've lost stuff. I'm not sure what I can do.
Therapist:	Still figuring that out, and it is a moving target, isn't it. You are still getting changes.
Patient:	And that's a good thing. I'm still improving.
Therapist:	Yes, it just makes it hard to plan what you will be able to do.
Patient:	I'm pushing as hard as I can, and I know John wants me to, to take advantage of this window for recovery. But sometimes I just need to take a break for a day, and just be what I am right now, and not really do anything.
Therapist:	Is that OK by you?
Patient:	Well, I think John can get upset, so I don't tell him. I think he wants me to give 100%. He's had to put up with a lot, more than I remember, because I don't remember much of anything about the beginning, and I was in the coma. So I want to do all I can.
Therapist:	But a break for a day seems to be a normal thing for everyone from time to time.
Patient:	Not me. I might have given myself a half a day, if I worked hard the first half. That's how I've been.
Therapist:	You've changed a little on this?
Patient:	Yes, sometimes I just have to let it all be.
Therapist:	You are figuring out how to do this your way.
Patient:	I'm not sure what I am doing.
Therapist:	You are making it up as you go, a new life.
Patient:	I really don't know what it is, or will be. But I know that to some extent I need to let myself be who I am, or who I am becoming.
Therapist:	I'm thinking that you've spent your whole life prior to the stroke learning about who you are, your capabilities, tendencies, mental and physical abilities, personality, and such. You've been observing yourself and evaluating yourself for a lifetime. Now you are different, and you have had only a few months to assess, and like I said before, you have been changing all along.
Patient:	That's true.
Therapist:	So it's hard to know yourself like you used to, and hard to know who you will become.
Patient:	Hard to figure out what to do with myself.
Therapist:	How could you know that now?
Patient:	It would be easier if I did, and easier on John, too. I think he wants those questions answered.
Therapist:	That clarity would be easier to adjust to.
Patient:	Everyone seems to want me to have this sorted out. I guess I disappoint them like this. My sister wants me to find God, and she keeps talking to me about it. But you know, I'm not ready for that.

Therapist:	She has her own notions about that.
Patient:	Yes, but I don't want to be talking about spirituality and such right now. I don't think about why this happened to me. I just figure it did, why not? And statistically if it happened to me it doesn't happen to someone else, like you.
Therapist:	But it doesn't work exactly that way.
Patient:	Well, I mean statistically. And I think, it happened to me, and I saved someone else from this kind of thing.
Therapist:	But there are questions your sister wants you to consider.
Patient:	Yes, well, it's just not something I'm interested in discussing with her, because I can tell she wants me to think a certain way.
Therapist:	Maybe it will be okay sometime to discuss it with someone who doesn't have a certain agenda about it.
Patient:	Yeah, but everybody seems to.
Therapist:	How about me?
Patient:	No, that's why I come here. This is the place I figure things out on my own. Well, I mean you help, but here I can just be free to think on my own. I need that. Because there are lots of changes, bad ones, sure, but some good ones that I am trying to do, too.

In this excerpt, it is evident that this patient can recognize both gains and losses, and be realistic about them. The clinician shows interest in these points and helps her expand on them, but it is clear that she wants to do it her way, so it is important not to push the idea of growth, or imply any expectations. One possible illusion emerges when she talks about taking this stroke on so someone else will not have to. This is gently challenged, but it is clear she needs to think about this aspect of her situation. This is her contribution to others, and the expert companion allows for this. It is not harmful to her or anyone else. It may be part of her newfound compassion for others. It is also clear that she is not only in the initial stages of rehabilitation but also in the initial phases of PTG, and her view of herself physically, cognitively, socially, and emotionally is changing. One area she clearly states she is not willing to discuss is spirituality, but this may be more a reaction to her sister's demands, and it may be possible that she will address this with the therapist at some point. She says at the end that the therapist allows her to find her own way, yet is helpful. This is a good sign that the proper balance of expert companionship has been established.

Final Note: Posttraumatic Growth for the Clinician?

As a clinical health psychologist treating persons who are survivors of highly stressful events, you will come face to face with mortality, pain, fear, and the ambiguities of how to live life meaningfully in situations characterized by your patients' agonies. If you practice expert companionship, you will be touched more deeply by the life situations of your patients; you will likely be more hurt and struggle to protect yourself from the hurt you experience. You may even experience compassion fatigue (Figley, 1995). Thus, you should practice good self-care (see Calhoun & Tedeschi, 1999, for some suggestions). However, you may also experience a form of growth akin to that of trauma survivors, a vicarious version of PTG (Arnold et al., 2005).

Just as we ask patients to be open to the psychological impact of serious challenges to their health, we encourage clinicians to remain open emotionally to allow the greatest possibilities for vicarious growth: closer relationships, more clearly developed priorities and appreciation for life, a deeper spiritual life, and a sense of personal strength. We emphasize that the expert companions in this work should listen to their patients in a way that allows themselves to be changed, rather than focusing exclusively on trying to change the patient (Tedeschi & Calhoun, 2006). Many psychologists who are researching PTG or who are working with patients facing difficult health problems may find themselves returning to this work because of the fascinating and encouraging stories of people who have done so well in desperate circumstances. Many of us may hope that we would do as well as our patients when tragedy befalls us. Perhaps we can learn some lessons from our patients that can be applied to our own lives, both now and in the future.

References

American Psychiatric Association. (2000). *Diagnostic and statistical manual of mental disorders* (4th ed., text rev.). Washington, DC: Author.

Arnold, D., Calhoun, L. G., Tedeschi, R. G., & Cann, A. (2005). Vicarious posttraumatic growth in psychotherapy. *Journal of Humanistic Psychology, 45,* 239–263.

Baltes, P. B., Staudinger, U. M., Maercker, A., & Smith, J. (1995). People nominated as wise: A comparative study of wisdom-related knowledge. *Psychology and Aging, 10,* 155–166.

Bonanno, G. (2005). Clarifying and extending the concept of adult resilience. *American Psychologist, 60,* 265–267.

Calhoun, L. G., & Tedeschi, R. G. (1998). Posttraumatic growth: Future directions. In R. G. Tedeschi, C. L. Park, & L. G. Calhoun (Eds.), *Posttraumatic growth: Positive change in the aftermath of crisis* (pp. 215–238). Mahwah, NJ: Erlbaum.

Calhoun, L. G., & Tedeschi, R. G. (1999). *Facilitating posttraumatic growth: A clinician's guide.* Mahwah, NJ: Erlbaum.

Calhoun, L. G., & Tedeschi, R. G. (2004). The foundations of posttraumatic growth: New considerations. *Psychological Inquiry, 15,* 93–102.

Calhoun, L. G., & Tedeschi, R. G. (2006). The foundations of posttraumatic growth: An expanded framework. In L. G. Calhoun & R. G. Tedeschi (Eds.), *Handbook of posttraumatic growth: Research and practice* (pp. 1–23). Mahwah, NJ: Erlbaum.

Calhoun, L. G., Tedeschi, R. G., & Uhrich, J. (1986, March). *Positive aspects of critical life problems: Recollections of grief.* Paper presented at the annual meeting of the Southeastern Psychological Association, Kissimmee, FL.

Cann, A., Calhoun, L. G., & Tedeschi, R. G. (2007, August). *Core Beliefs Inventory: A brief measure of the assumptive world.* Poster session presented at the annual meeting of the American Psychological Association, San Francisco, CA.

Collins, R. L., Taylor, S. E., & Skokan, L. A. (1990). A better world or a shattered vision? Changes in life perspectives following victimization. *Social Cognition, 8,* 263–285.

Cook, J. M., Schnurr, P. P., & Foa, E. B. (2004). Bridging the gap between posttraumatic stress disorder research and clinical practice: The example of exposure therapy. *Psychotherapy: Theory, Research, Practice, Training, 41,* 374–387.

Cordova, M. J., Cunningham, L. L. C., Carlson, C. R., & Andrykowski, M. A. (2001). Posttraumatic growth following breast cancer: A controlled comparison study. *Health Psychology, 20,* 176–185.

Cordova, M. J., Giese-Davis, J., Golant, M., Kronenwater, C., Chang, V., & Spiegel, D. (2007). Breast cancer as trauma: Posttraumatic stress and posttraumatic growth. *Journal of Clinical Psychology in Medical Settings, 14,* 308–319.

Davis, C. G., & Lehman, D. R. (1995). Counterfactual thinking and coping with traumatic life events. In N. J. Roese & J. M. Olson (Eds.), *What might have been: The social psychology of counterfactual thinking* (pp. 353–374). Hillsdale, NJ: Erlbaum.

Dohrenwend, B. P., Neria, Y., Turner, J. B., Turse, N., Marshall, R., Lewis-Fernandez, R., & Koenen, K. C. (2004). Positive tertiary appraisals and posttraumatic stress disorder in U.S. male veterans of the war in Vietnam: The roles of positive affirmation, positive reformulation, and defensive denial. *Journal of Consulting and Clinical Psychology, 72,* 417–433.

Erikson, E. (1964). *Childhood and society* (2nd ed.). Oxford: Norton.

Figley, C. (1995). *Compassion fatigue: Coping with secondary traumatic stress disorder in those who treat the traumatized.* Philadelphia: Brunner/Mazel.

Fontana, A., & Rosenheck, R. (2005). The role of loss of meaning in the pursuit of treatment for posttraumatic stress disorder. *Journal of Traumatic Stress, 18,* 133–136.

Harpham, W. S. (1994). *After cancer: A guide to your new life.* New York: Norton.

Harvey, J. H., Barnett, K., & Overstreet, A. (2004). Trauma growth and other outcomes attendant to loss. *Psychological Inquiry, 15,* 26–29.

Harvey, J. H., Barnett, K., & Rupe, S. (2006). Posttraumatic growth and other outcomes of major loss in the context of complex family lives. In L. G. Calhoun & R. G. Tedeschi (Eds.), *Handbook of posttraumatic growth: Research and practice* (pp. 100–117). Mahwah, NJ: Erlbaum.

Herman, J. (1992). *Trauma and recovery.* New York: Basic Books.

Holland, J. C., & Lewis, S. (2000). *The human side of cancer: Living with hope, coping with uncertainty.* New York: HarperCollins.

Ihle, E. C., Ritsher, J. B., & Kanas, N. (2006). Positive psychological outcomes of spaceflight: An empirical study. *Aviation, Space, and Environmental Medicine, 77,* 93–101.

Janoff-Bulman, R. (1992). *Shattered assumptions.* New York: Free Press.

Janoff-Bulman, R. (2004). Posttraumatic growth: Three explanatory models. *Psychological Inquiry, 15,* 31–35.

Janoff-Bulman, R. (2006). Schema-change perspectives on posttraumatic growth. In L. G. Calhoun & R. G. Tedeschi (Eds.), *Handbook of posttraumatic growth: Research and practice* (pp. 81–99). Mahwah, NJ: Erlbaum.

Jordan, H. (2000). *No such thing as a bad day.* Atlanta, GA: Longstreet Press.

Koltko-Rivera, M. E. (2004). The psychology of worldviews. *Review of General Psychology, 8,* 3–58.

Lev-Wiesel, R., & Amir, M. (2003). Posttraumatic growth among Holocaust child survivors. *Journal of Loss and Trauma, 8,* 229–237.

McFarland, C., & Alvaro, C. (2000). The impact of motivation on temporal comparisons: Coping with traumatic events by perceiving personal growth. *Journal of Personality and Social Psychology, 79,* 327–343.

McQuellon, R. P., & Cowan, M. A. (2007). *Living in mortal time: Conversations for those who have never died.* Winston-Salem, NC: Author.

Neimeyer, R. A. (2001). *Meaning reconstruction & the experience of loss.* Washington, DC: American Psychological Association.

Neimeyer, R. A. (Ed.). (2006). Re-storying loss: Fostering growth in the posttraumatic narrative. In L. G. Calhoun & R. G. Tedeschi (Eds.), *Handbook of posttraumatic growth: Research and practice* (pp. 68–80). Mahwah, NJ: Erlbaum.

Nolen-Hoeksema, S., & Davis, C. G. (2004). Theoretical and methodological issues in the assessment and interpretation of posttraumatic growth. *Psychological Inquiry, 15,* 60–64.

Park, C. L., Cohen, L., & Murch, R. (1996). Assessment and prediction of stress-related growth. *Journal of Personality, 64,* 645–658.

Price, R. (1994). *A whole new life: An illness and a healing.* New York: Atheneum.

Stanton, A. L., & Low, C. A. (2004). Toward understanding posttraumatic growth: Commentary on Tedeschi and Calhoun, *Psychological Inquiry, 15,* 76–80.

Taylor, S. E., & Brown, J. D. (1988). Illusion and well-being: A social psychological perspective on mental health. *Psychological Bulletin, 103,* 193–210.

Tedeschi, R. G., & Calhoun, L. G. (1988, August). *Perceived benefits in coping with physical handicaps.* Paper presented at the annual meeting of the American Psychological Association, Atlanta, GA.

Tedeschi, R. G., & Calhoun, L. G. (1995). *Trauma and transformation: Growing in the aftermath of suffering.* Thousand Oaks, CA: Sage.

Tedeschi, R. G., & Calhoun, L. G. (1996). The Posttraumatic Growth Inventory: Measuring the positive legacy of trauma. *Journal of Traumatic Stress, 9,* 455–471.

Tedeschi, R. G., & Calhoun, L. G. (2004a). *Helping bereaved parents: A clinicians' guide*. New York: Brunner-Routledge.

Tedeschi, R. G., & Calhoun, L. G. (2004b). Posttraumatic growth: Conceptual foundations and empirical evidence. *Psychological Inquiry, 15*, 1–18.

Tedeschi, R. G., & Calhoun, L. G. (2006). Expert companions: Posttraumatic growth in clinical practice. In L. G. Calhoun & R. G. Tedeschi (Eds.), *Handbook of posttraumatic growth: Research and practice* (pp. 291–310). Mahwah, NJ: Erlbaum.

Tedeschi, R. G., & Calhoun, L. G. (2007a). Grief as a transformative struggle. In K. J. Doka (Ed.), *Living with grief: Before and after the death* (pp. 107–122). Washington, DC: Hospice Foundation of America.

Tedeschi, R. G., & Calhoun, L. G. (2007b, April). *Strange blessings: Grief and posttraumatic growth*. Invited keynote address presented at the Association of Death Education and Counseling, Indianapolis, IN.

Tedeschi, R. G., Calhoun, L. G., Morrell, R. W., & Johnson, K. A. (1984, August). *Bereavement: From grief to psychological development*. Paper presented at the annual meeting of the American Psychological Association, Toronto, Ontario, Canada.

Wortman, C. B. (2004). Posttraumatic growth: Progress and problems. *Psychological Inquiry, 15*, 81–90.

Zöllner, T., & Maercker, A. (2006). Posttraumatic growth and psychotherapy. In L. G. Calhoun & R. G. Tedeschi (Eds.), *Handbook of posttraumatic growth: Research and practice* (pp. 334–354). Mahwah, NJ: Erlbaum.

Afterword

The authors in this volume have presented a thorough overview of what is currently known about positive life change in the context of medical illness. The subtitle of our book—*Can Crisis Lead to Personal Transformation?*—poses a provocative question, one that we hope our readers feel more equipped to answer after reading this volume. Still, we conclude this book with the unsettling feeling that although much is known about positive life change, far more remains to be learned. We close with a brief integration of a knowledge base that seems to be fairly solidly established and our ideas about what we have left to learn.

Positive Life Change Following Illness Captures Attention

The proliferation of research on this topic over the past 15 years makes it clear that somehow the notion of overcoming adversity, and transforming oneself as a result, resonates with the need to derive meaning from life's seemingly uncontrollable events (Joseph & Linley, 2005). This concept of positive psychological growth may be concomitant with physical recovery from illness, but it is something that is also qualitatively distinct, given that those living with medical conditions that are chronic, progressive, and even terminal also frequently report that they have experienced positive life changes. To date, findings on growth suggest that encounters with the personal and existential challenges that accompany illness may prompt positive personal change rather than simply a return to a pre-illness baseline.

Reports of Positive Life Change Are Common in Those Experiencing Medical Conditions

The wealth of recent research leads us to the conclusion that many persons with serious medical conditions have grown from the experience. Although we initially theorized that the extent and types of growth people might experience would be partially determined by the context of their illness, there are now data to suggest that specific aspects of various medical conditions may determine growth. For example, as discussed in chapter 3, a moderate level of threat is related to more perceived growth than higher or lower levels of threat. In chapter 6, the authors compared and contrasted the experiences of individuals with cancer and HIV in terms of their perceptions of benefits. The authors of chapter 7 presented qualitative and quantitative findings regarding similarities and differences in growth across different medical conditions. However, much remains to be learned about how levels or types of growth or perceived benefits may vary by specific illness characteristics, such as pain, disability, and chronicity.

Perceptions of Positive Life Change May or May Not Be Reflected in External Markers of Change

Although much of the research on growth assumes that self-reports are accurate reflections of positive life change, there are reasons to doubt the validity of these reports (see chap. 2). Many researchers and clinicians remain keenly interested in the phenomenon of growth as a reflection of important changes in the life of the person struggling with highly stressful situations such as illness. Others, however, maintain that the perception of change is the factor that actually matters, postulating that an individual's perception of benefits is all that can ever be assessed and that these perceptions are sufficient. The chapters in this volume capture the ongoing struggle with these fundamental issues.

Positive Life Change May or May Not Arise Through the Shattering of Global Meaning Systems

Reports of growth appear to arise in the midst of struggle; many people report benefits while still actively engaged in coping with their illness. Such growth may be part of the process of reconstructing one's global beliefs and goals, a notion consistent with the findings regarding the need for significant threat to experience growth (see chaps. 1, 3, and 8). However, although a variety of rich theories of growth have been proposed, little research has actually tested these theories, and we know little about how growth and perceived benefits arise.

Positive Life Change Following Illness May or May Not Be Related to Well-Being

As a number of chapters in this volume have demonstrated, reports of growth are inconsistently related to various aspects of well-being, including biological correlates (see chap. 9) and physical and emotional factors (see chaps. 10 and 11). These inconsistencies may be due to design and measurement issues, but they suggest that the links between perceptions of growth and well-being are not straightforward.

Developmental Context of Illness Appears to Matter in Positive Life Change

Several chapters in this volume suggest that life course and life span issues may affect the experience of growth in children (see chap. 4) and adults (see chap. 5). However, little research to date has examined these developmental issues, and many questions remain. For example, illnesses that occur at nonnormative times may create more distress and, subsequently, more growth; however, it is also plausible that they may leave a person less able to resolve their feelings of loss, leading to less growth as a result of illness. Research on developmental issues, as well as clinical interventions for changing the trajectories of those at higher risk for distress and lack of growth, remains an agenda for the future.

Positive Life Change May Have Important Clinical Applications

Clinicians have been interested in the therapeutic role of positive life changes and in ways to implement therapeutic techniques to facilitate growth (see chaps. 11 and 12). Much remains to be learned about whether growth should in fact be facilitated clinically and the type of training therapists should have prior to attempting such interventions. Applying what we have learned to clinical practice remains a challenge, although this is one of the primary objectives of research in this area. On the basis of the content of the chapters in this book, we suggest that clinicians may need to remain well-informed about new developments in this area to apply this material in therapeutic settings.

It is our hope that the evaluation of the existing research base and the perspectives of the authors in this volume encourage serious consideration of these issues, ranging from the philosophical to the practical, and that researchers, clinicians, educators, administrators, and policymakers take on the challenge of furthering our understanding of whether and how medical illness can lead to positive life change.

Reference

Joseph, S., & Linley, A. P. (2005). Positive adjustment to threatening events: An organismic valuing theory of growth through adversity. *Review of General Psychology, 9,* 262–280.

Author Index

Numbers in italics refer to listings in the references.

Subject Index

About the Editors

Crystal L. Park, PhD, is associate professor of psychology at the University of Connecticut. She studies coping with highly stressful events, including the roles of religious beliefs and religious coping, the phenomenon of stress-related growth, and the making of meaning from those stressful life events. She has recently been examining these issues in the context of cancer and congestive heart failure. She is currently examining mediators of the effects of spirituality on well-being in congestive heart failure patients and testing a meaning-making writing intervention for posttraumatic stress disorder. She is associate editor of *Psychology of Religion and Spirituality, Psychology and Health,* and *The International Journal for the Psychology of Religion.*

Suzanne C. Lechner, PhD, is a member of the University of Miami (UM) Sylvester Cancer Center within the Biobehavioral Oncology and Cancer Control Program. She holds the title of scientist within the Braman Family Breast Cancer Institute of UM Sylvester. She is a licensed clinical health psychologist and research assistant professor of psychiatry and psychology at the UM Miller School of Medicine. Dr. Lechner's clinical research program focuses on benefit finding and growth as well as on other indexes of positive adaptation to cancer. She is heavily involved in trials to test the efficacy of psychosocial interventions for persons living with breast cancer to ultimately attenuate the psychological burden of disease.

Michael H. Antoni, PhD, is professor of psychology and psychiatry and behavioral sciences at the University of Miami (UM) Miller School of Medicine. He leads the Biobehavioral Oncology and Cancer Epidemiology Program at the UM Sylvester Cancer Center and is a licensed psychologist in Florida. His research examines stress and stress management effects on quality of life, health, and biobehavioral mechanisms in persons diagnosed with viral infections and different cancers. Dr. Antoni is a fellow of the Society of Behavioral Medicine and is associate editor of the *International Journal of Behavioral Medicine* and *Psychology and Health.*

Annette L. Stanton, PhD, is professor of psychology and psychiatry/biobehavioral sciences at the University of California, Los Angeles (UCLA). She is a senior research scientist at the UCLA Cousins Center for Psychoneuroimmunology and a member of the Division of Cancer Prevention and Control Research in the UCLA Jonsson Comprehensive Cancer Center. Her research centers on specifying factors that promote psychological and physical health in individuals who confront health-related adversity, with a particular focus on coping with cancer. Dr. Stanton has been honored with the Senior Investigator Award from Division 38 (Health Psychology) of the American Psychological Association.

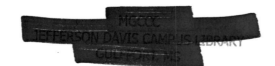